The Mixed Methods Research Workbook

This book is dedicated to (1) my family—Sayoko, Kori, Tomoyuki, Kazuhisa, and Takashi—for relinquishing time for me to write; (2) John W. Creswell, my friend and colleague, who encouraged me to write this book; (3) the participants in my mixed methods workshops; (4) my host Professor Yali Cong and my students, who took my mixed methods course at Peking University Health Science Center in Fall Semester 2016 in the People's Republic of China and where I served as Fulbright Distinguished Chair in the Social Sciences; (5) my colleagues in the University of Michigan Mixed Methods Program who have worked with me to further develop and refine many activities in this workbook through our workshops; (6) to my colleagues Timothy C. Guetterman, Melissa DeJonckheere, Justine Wu, Jane Forman, Ellen Rubinstein, and Sergi Fàbregues, who generously reviewed draft versions of various chapters; and (7) Rania Ajilat and Lilly Pritula, who provided invaluable technical support.

Sara Miller McCune founded SAGE Publishing in 1965 to support the dissemination of usable knowledge and educate a global community. SAGE publishes more than 1000 journals and over 600 new books each year, spanning a wide range of subject areas. Our growing selection of library products includes archives, data, case studies and video. SAGE remains majority owned by our founder and after her lifetime will become owned by a charitable trust that secures the company's continued independence.

Los Angeles | London | New Delhi | Singapore | Washington DC | Melbourne

The Mixed Methods Research Workbook

Activities for Designing, Implementing, and Publishing Projects

Michael D. Fetters

Mixed Methods Program and Department of Family Medicine, University of Michigan

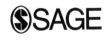

Los Angeles | London | New Delhi
Singapore | Washington DC | Melbourne

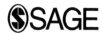

FOR INFORMATION:

SAGE Publications, Inc.
2455 Teller Road
Thousand Oaks, California 91320
E-mail: order@sagepub.com

SAGE Publications Ltd.
1 Oliver's Yard
55 City Road
London EC1Y 1SP
United Kingdom

SAGE Publications India Pvt. Ltd.
B 1/I 1 Mohan Cooperative Industrial Area
Mathura Road, New Delhi 110 044
India

SAGE Publications Asia-Pacific Pte. Ltd.
18 Cross Street #10-10/11/12
China Square Central
Singapore 048423

ISBN: 978-1-5063-9359-9

Acquisitions Editor: Leah Fargotstein
Editorial Assistant: Claire Laminen
Production Editor: Astha Jaiswal
Copy Editor: Lana Todorovic-Arndt
Typesetter: C&M Digitals (P) Ltd.
Proofreader: Lawrence W. Baker
Indexer: Wendy Allex
Cover Designer: Dally Verghese
Marketing Manager: Shari Countryman

19 20 21 22 23 10 9 8 7 6 5 4 3 2 1

BRIEF CONTENTS

DETAILED CONTENTS

SERIES EDITORS' INTRODUCTION

Applying research methods to address real-world situations has never been an easy task. It may be more difficult when you plan to use mixed methods research to meaningfully integrate quantitative and qualitative approaches within a study. The complexity of the mixed methods research process arises because it is shaped by multiple personal, interpersonal, and social contexts and related methodological considerations (Plano Clark & Ivankova, 2016a). This complexity presents a significant challenge to researchers who are new to mixed methods research and who are faced with methodological decisions about how to integrate different methods. By working through guided exercises and application activities informed by the mixed methods literature, researchers new to mixed methods research can both learn about mixed methods research and apply this knowledge to design, implement, evaluate, and publish a mixed methods project.

The Mixed Methods Research Workbook: Activities for Designing, Implementing, and Publishing Projects by Michael D. Fetters is a practical resource on how to apply a mixed methods approach building on existing knowledge about mixed methods research. The book has a workbook format so that readers can actually work through their project ideas using the activities provided in the book. This strategy combines the pedagogical benefits of project-based learning with real-world examples of mixed methods studies from different disciplines. Drawing on his extensive experience of leading mixed methods workshops, Fetters engages readers in step-by-step activities useful for conceptualizing, designing, implementing, and publishing a mixed methods study. One of the unique features of the book is its collaborative focus, because many activities can be performed in pairs where workbook users interact with each other about the study design and implementation components.

As editors of the Mixed Methods Research Series, we are excited to endorse *The Mixed Methods Research Workbook: Activities for Designing, Implementing, and Publishing Projects* as the seventh volume in the series. Although its workbook format differs from other books in the series, *The Mixed Methods Research Workbook* clearly fits the series' purpose to provide researchers, reviewers, and consumers of mixed methods with a how-to perspective on the essential aspects of conducting mixed methods research in the social, health, and behavioral sciences. *The Mixed Methods Research Workbook* is an innovative and creative contribution to the series that offers a practical approach to learning how to apply mixed methods research through examples, exercises, and activities. We believe the book will be of interest to students, instructors, and researchers due to its unique applied focus and effective pedagogical features. So, we wish the book readers an enjoyable process as they get to work on creating their mixed methods research projects.

Nataliya V. Ivankova and Vicki L. Plano Clark
Editors, Mixed Methods Research Series

PREFACE

If you are working on a mixed methods research or evaluation project, I developed this workbook to support you in your project using applied activities. If you are teaching graduate students how to plan, implement, or publish a mixed methods research or evaluation project, I developed these activities to support them in their projects. The workbook could be especially useful in a graduate dissertation course. Each chapter includes activities that can be used in a course, workshop, or research group or lab. Researchers already engaged in mixed methods projects will find the workbook chapters stand alone for supporting specific mixed methods integration activities. This workbook differs from other published mixed methods books, given that its primary focus on activities will help you apply essential and cutting edge mixed methods concepts to your mixed methods projects.

The workbook features a particular focus on essential concepts and activities for integration. This emphasis reflects, and benefits from, my service as a co-chief editor of the *Journal of Mixed Methods Research*. When becoming one of the co-chief editors of *JMMR* in 2015, I helped set a new explicit focus on integration in mixed methods scholarship. The integration challenge, conceptually stated in the formula of 1 + 1 = 3, emphasizes an integrated approach pushing researchers to achieve a whole greater than the sum of the individual parts. The integration trilogy conceptualizes how integration can occur in fifteen dimensions of mixed methods research and evaluation projects. This explicit emphasis distinguishes modern mixed methods from a past tendency of casually using qualitative and quantitative research at the same time, but not fully leveraging integration to reap fully the rewards of mixed methods projects.

I wrote the workbook to be useful for three groups of mixed methods researchers. First, for someone just getting started in mixed methods, the chapters are written in a logical order for developing, conducting, and publishing a mixed methods project, such that each chapter builds on the previous chapter. In this way, the workbook can be used as a companion to most graduate-level mixed methods research coursebooks. Second, the workbook can be used as a primary source for mixed methods research workshops, given the focus on essential mixed methods content and work activities. Third, for more experienced researchers already engaged in research and evaluation projects, the chapters were designed to be independent and accessible for specific integration activities, e.g., creating a data sources table, identifying integration during data collection and analysis, developing a joint display, publishing mixed methods papers. Hence, the workbook chapters and activities can be used selectively according to specific research project needs.

Each chapter follows a similar structure and begins with a list of learning objectives. After briefly presenting essential material about the chapter topic, I provide Workboxes: first a completed example as a Workbox illustration, and then a Workbox with the same structure to be filled out according to your specific project. Some chapters contain figures to provide a conceptual understanding of more abstract concepts, and or tables to organize complex material. Many chapters contain "Stories From the Field," anecdotes about real experiences that illustrate in more detail the ideas from the chapters. Each chapter features Application Activities appropriate for use in classrooms or workshops or in lab or work groups. These are followed by a checklist for reflection and a self-assessment of progress in achieving chapter objectives. Each chapter ends with a select list of Key Resources.

The mixed methods research workbook represents the culmination of many experiences in conducting, teaching, consulting, and mentoring about mixed methods research. I personally have been conducting mixed methods research projects in the social and health sciences and medical education since 1992, and have previous experience as the principal investigator, or the mixed methods lead investigator, from 14 funded mixed methods projects in many complex multicultural and multilinguistic settings. The workbook activities evolved over the course of teaching mixed methods research through many one to five-day workshops in eleven countries. I expanded workshop activities into a full course at Peking University of Health Science in where I taught the first known graduate-level course on mixed methods research in the People's Republic of China. My experiences led to serving as an expert consultant on both the 2013 National Institutes of Health Best Practices for Mixed Methods Research from the Office of Behavioral and Social Science Research and the 2019 PCORI Qualitative and Mixed Methods Research Guidelines. As mentor to multiple junior colleagues on their mixed methods investigations and as a consultant to senior colleagues less familiar with mixed methods, I continue to find the applied activities presented here useful.

Chapters 1 to 5 support your completion of the upfront work needed for successfully executing a mixed methods research and evaluation project. Chapter 1 will help you identify a topic appropriate for a mixed methods project, review essentials of mixed methods research and the rationale, and consider potential feasibility issues. Chapter 2 supports identifying and beginning to refine a topic for mixed methods research. Chapter 3 will help you choose among different types of literature reviews and support your choice of a search strategy. Chapter 4 helps facilitate your incorporation of your personal background, theory, and worldview into your project. Chapter 5 provides a concise structure for articulating relevant background, research objectives, and questions for your project.

Chapters 6 to 12 provide the essential knowledge and activities required for collecting your mixed methods data. Chapter 6 provides an approach for explicitly identifying your qualitative and quantitative data sources. In Chapter 7 you will choose among one or more core mixed methods designs and begin the process of developing a procedural diagram. In Chapter 8 you will learn about scaffolded (also known as complex, intersected, or advanced) designs and how you can integrate multiple core designs together, or bring theory or other types of designs into a mixed methods study. In Chapter 9, you will choose among different strategies for sampling in your project, while in Chapter 10 you will learn about and choose among different integration strategies by the intent of the data collection and analysis. In Chapter 11, you will learn about three uses of an implementation matrix and create one appropriate for the stage of your project. In Chapter 12, you will systematically consider the ethical conduct of mixed methods research and evaluation projects.

Chapters 13 to 16 provide prerequisite information for conducting mixed data analysis and activities that will ensure you can maximize the potential of your mixed methods project. Chapter 13 introduces to you seven essential steps of mixed methods data analysis and will assist in your identification of the strategies for use in your own project. In Chapter 14, you will learn about joint display planning, joint display analysis, and joint display presentation. In Chapter 15, you will learn about other advanced procedures for mixed methods analysis and choose an approach for your project. In Chapter 16, you will consider systematic issues relevant to the research integrity of your project and choose a framework for assessing threats in your project.

Too many mixed methods research and evaluation projects never fully achieve their potential for publication. Chapters 17 and 18 will support two crucial aspects of publishing: preparing for submission and then using the hourglass design model to write empirical mixed methods papers.

I am indebted to a number of individuals who have influenced the writing of the workbook. Pierre Pluye from McGill and I first developed several of the core activities and refined them further in a series of workshops we convened at North American Primary Care Research Group meetings, the first in 2009. Rikke Jorgensen persisted in her invitation for me to conduct my first full-week mixed methods workshop at the excellent research methods course in Aalborg Psychiatric Hospital, Aarhus University Hospital, Aalborg, Denmark, in 2011. The Michigan-Aalborg connection continues through ongoing teaching and exchange of a series of erudite Danish mixed methods researchers. I am highly grateful for the opportunity provided by Fulbright Program, which supported my sabbatical of teaching and conducting mixed methods at Peking University Health Science Center. Professor Yali Cong provided the infrastructure and support necessary for my leading the first known graduate-level course on mixed methods research taught in China, and my students pushed me to expand and refine the mixed methods activities. University of Michigan Family Medicine Departmental support has proven critical for sustaining our program of teaching, developing, and expanding mixed methods activities. As noted in the book's dedication, many of my colleagues at the University of Michigan Mixed Methods Program have shaped my thinking about mixed methods research and provided feedback on early chapter drafts. I am highly grateful to the Mixed Methods Research Series Editors, Nataliya Ivankova and Vicki Plano Clark, and Leah Fargotstein, Editor for Research Methods, Statistics, and Evaluation, SAGE Publishing, for their patience, support, and guidance.

I am grateful to the reviewers of various chapters of the mixed methods workbook.

Mehmet Ali Dikerdem, Institute for Work Based Learning, Middlesex University

Clare Bennett, University of Worcester, England

Joke Bradt, Department of Creative Arts Therapies, College of Nursing and Health Professions, Drexel University

Janine Chitty, University of Arkansas Fort Smith

Xiaofen D. Keating, The University of Texas at Austin

Charles A. Kramer, University of La Verne

Betsy McEneaney, UMass-Amherst

Arturo Olivarez Jr., The University of Texas at El Paso

David Preece, Centre for Education and Research, University of Northampton, UK

Douglas Sturgeon, University of Rio Grande

Karthigeyan Subramaniam, University of North Texas

Eric D. Teman, University of Wyoming

Kristen Hawley Turner, Drew University

Karen L. Webber, The University of Georgia

Finally, and most important, the encouragement for me to write this book came from my colleague and mentor John W. Creswell, a leading international author on qualitative and mixed methods research. When we co-founded the Mixed Methods Program at the University of Michigan in 2015, we set as one of our program goals providing mixed methods research workshops three times per year. Eager for the workshops to have a focus on *work*, our group chose to use many of these activities as the primary framework for our two- to three-day workshops. These workshops, with highly motivated and inquisitive scholars, have provided a highly fertile soil for nurturing and growing new ideas and activities. By the time the Workbook went to press, we had conducted 12 mixed methods workshops, each attended by 23 to 40 interdisciplinary participants with backgrounds in education, social science, and health sciences fields who have utilized many of the activities now available to you in this workbook. Participants in our workshops, thus far numbering 349, have hailed from across the United States including Puerto Rico and far reaches of the globe including: Australia, Brazil, Canada, China, Colombia, Denmark, Guyana, India, Ireland, Jamaica, Japan, Korea, Lithuania, Nigeria, Philippines, Puerto Rico, Singapore, South Africa, Thailand, Trinidad and Tobago, and the UK. The summer mixed methods dissertation workshop has been among the most popular of our workshops, and we have been especially fortunate to engage international graduate students based on the generous support of the Sara Miller McCune Foundation. My greatest reward in writing this book will be your finding it useful in your mixed methods research and evaluation projects. I hope you will drop me a note if you do and please include any suggestions for improvements.

IDENTIFYING A TOPIC, RATIONALE, AND POTENTIAL FEASIBILITY ISSUES FOR CONDUCTING A MIXED METHODS RESEARCH OR EVALUATION PROJECT

Around the world, researchers are turning to mixed methods research (MMR) to take on the most complicated and challenging research questions in the health sciences, education, business, and the broader social sciences. While eager to begin, you may feel like an artist staring at a blank canvas, excited about all the potential yet overwhelmed with how to start putting concepts onto that white space. This chapter and its activities will help you clarify your topic, articulate a rationale for conducting a mixed methods study, and support a candid assessment of feasibility issues. As a key outcome, you will articulate a rationale for using a mixed methods approach for your topic.

LEARNING OBJECTIVES

The ideas presented here will help you to

- Consider the overarching context for conducting your MMR and evaluation studies
- Develop a preliminary topic for your MMR or evaluation project
- Identify the advantages of using qualitative and quantitative approaches, and develop the rationale for your MMR project or evaluation study
- Explore potential feasibility issues of conducting MMR or a mixed methods evaluation about your topic of interest

MIXED METHODS RESEARCH IN CONTEXT

If you came into my office asking how to get started on an MMR or evaluation project, I would want to make sure you first knew fundamental features and rationales for using qualitative, quantitative, and mixed methods procedures. For the purposes of this MMR workbook, **mixed methods research** refers to the integrated use of qualitative and quantitative approaches in a sustained program of inquiry with due consideration of the philosophical, methodological, and approaches in practice.

Conceptually, MMR is straightforward. It means bringing together the strengths of qualitative research procedures and the strength of quantitative research procedures to achieve something more, or a new whole greater than if you had used either approach alone. The equation 1 + 1 = 3 represents this idea and resonates with many seeking a conceptual understanding (Fetters, 2018; Fetters & Freshwater, 2015a). The goal of this workbook is to engage you in activities that will help you plan a project that will achieve a whole greater than the sum of the individual parts. The content and activities emphasize how to achieve integration in the key aspects of a mixed methods study. **Integration** refers to "the linking of qualitative and quantitative approaches and dimensions together to create a new whole or a more holistic understanding than achieved by either alone" (Fetters & Molina-Azorin, 2017b).

Many activities you will complete in this workbook can be used as drafts for inclusion in dissertation proposals, grant proposals, oral and poster presentations, and publications. But rather than restricting how you will develop, conduct, and present your project, they are meant as a starting point, and you should feel free to adapt them to your needs. As illustrated in the Story From the Field 1.1, rules were made for novices.

STORY FROM THE FIELD 1.1
To Be Structured or Unstructured, That Is the Question

The activities in this workbook provide structure for developing elements of an MMR study. The field of MMR remains very young, and directions in which the field will go remain unclear. Indeed, many mixed methods methodologists feel scholars should resist the inertia to fall into the existing academic lines and boundaries. After publishing an editorial on writing a mixed methods article for publication (Fetters and Freshwater, 2015b), I received an email from a highly respected, but alarmed, MMR colleague. He wrote, "I liked your editorial, and plan to share with my students, but don't you think that you have gone too far in prescribing the structure for writing mixed methods?" This illustrates a tension in MMR relative to writing creatively but also incorporating structure for consistency as many authors do follow a particular structure. To my esteemed colleague, I pointed out a disclaimer we wrote in the editorial: "Rules are for novices" (Fetters and Freshwater, 2015b). In other words, someone new to MMR often desires to complete work in the "correct" or "accepted" way, and for such an audience, the structures and templates provided here will prove to be helpful. But as aspiring mixed methodologists became more experienced, they find opportunities and needs for stretching the boundaries and adapting the templates to their own needs.

Designing and conducting mixed methods studies challenge researchers who need not only the knowledge and skills to conduct both qualitative and quantitative methodologies but also the knowledge and skills to integrate these methodologies as an MMR project. Abbas Tashakkori, a pioneer in the field of MMR, advises considering whether a **monomethod research** (i.e., qualitative or quantitative project alone) will suffice for answering your research question before embarking on a mixed methods project (Fetters & Molina-Azorin, 2017c).

The chapter activities will help you consider common rationales for using qualitative, quantitative, and MMR, and confirm your justification for a mixed method or monomethod research project. Both qualitative and quantitative traditions are well established, and to some extent, staying within one of these traditions feels more secure. But if you have a perplexing issue that cannot be addressed using one methodology alone, many exciting developments in the field of MMR can facilitate a rigorous investigation. Compared to the late 1980s and early 1990s when there was just a handful of books and resources, now there are many dozens of mixed methods books, and many are written with examples and applications in specific fields such as education, business, the health sciences, and social work, evaluation among others. The Mixed Methods Research Workbook uniquely focuses on applied activities to support your mixed method research and evaluation projects.

GETTING TO WORK

Every research project needs to start somewhere, and I advise starting with a topic. The remainder of Chapter 1 is designed to help you identify a preliminary topic and then determine if a mixed methods approach will help you address your topic.

Identifying a Preliminary Topic

A **preliminary topic** refers to the content, subject matter, or point of concern for your MMR or evaluation project. While many research experts urge starting with the research question, in reality, many people begin by experimenting with topics. As you progress, you may refine your topic, and then start developing research questions that derive from your topic. You will have more time to work on clarifying and committing to a topic in Chapter 2. For considering the potential of qualitative, quantitative, and mixed methods procedures, having a topic in mind will help you.

Activity: Identifying a Preliminary Topic

Using Workbox Illustration 1.1.1 as a reference, in Workbox 1.1.2, write a *preliminary topic* for your MMR project. By putting your topic into writing, you will commit more concretely to developing your idea further and consider how a mixed methods project could be applied. In Workbox Illustration 1.1.1, examples from completed studies are extrapolated back to their days of question formulation.

Workbox Illustration 1.1.1: Preliminary Research Topics of Featured Studies

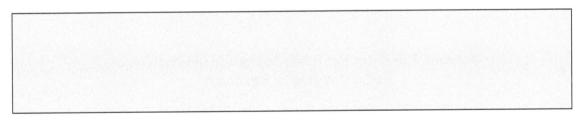

Business: Corporate environmental strategy and organizational capability
Education: School culture and academic achievement
Health Sciences: Teaching communication skills with virtual humans

Business – see Appendix A (Sharma & Vredenburg,1998); Education – see Appendix B (Harper, 2016); Health Sciences – see Appendix C (Kron et al., 2017)

Workbox 1.1.2: Preliminary Research Topic

How This Workbook Will Help Plan and Conduct Mixed Methods Research

There are many resources about conducting qualitative, quantitative, and MMR projects. Even a general overview of qualitative and quantitative procedures would extend well beyond the confines of this workbook. Thus, the MMR workbook will prove most useful if you have at least basic knowledge about both qualitative and quantitative data collection procedures. Or, you can use it in parallel to an introductory textbook. Alternatively, if you are working on a team, ideally you should have membership of someone with more than a superficial knowledge of each type of research. The workbox activities in this chapter will have you start by identifying a topic, and considering advantages and limitations of qualitative, quantitative, and MMR.

BRIEF REVIEW OF KEY ELEMENTS OF QUALITATIVE RESEARCH

Overview of Qualitative Research

Qualitative research is particularly useful for examining *how* and/or *why* a phenomenon of interest occurs, or to examine in depth the experiences of a population relative to a central phenomenon of interest. Qualitative researchers generally are informed by a worldview based on the notion that reality is constructed from human experiences and their interactions with others (see Chapter 4). Qualitative researchers openly acknowledge that their own experiences provide lenses for how they view and interpret the world, including their interpretations of data that emerge during the research process. They seek to use preconceptions in their work to inform and explore questions they have about a phenomenon, but also to make conscious inquiry for counter interpretations of data. To explore a central phenomenon or idea, they typically work with a smaller number of participants. They ask open-ended, general, or broad questions. Additionally, if they want to understand behaviors, qualitative researchers will invest time in observing participants. Qualitative researchers collect information by using the participants' words, images, or observed actions.

Identifying the Rationale for Using Qualitative Research

For advancing your mixed methods project, a critical consideration is why you want to conduct qualitative research. Creswell and Plano Clark (2018) in their book *Designing and Conducting Mixed Methods Research* provide a succinct summary of advantages of using qualitative research. These can include obtaining detailed perspectives of a small sample of people, capturing the voices of participants, seeking an understanding of participants' experiences in context, obtaining the views of participants, and appealing to people's enjoyment of stories, to name a few.

There also are a number of perceived limitations by quantitative researchers about qualitative research. Elucidated textual data is sometimes construed as soft data by researchers who favor the so-called hard or objective data of quantitative research. They may consider as limitations the relatively few people in studies, the research being subjective, and the hazards of relying on others to "produce" or "generate" the data through interviews or observations. Largely, these concerns are based on misunderstood intents of qualitative researchers who have different purposes.

Activity: Identifying Advantages and Limitations of Using Qualitative Research

These advantages and perceived limitations have been incorporated into Workbox 1.2, where you should consider the potential application to your own project. Check off the potential advantages and limitations you perceive of using qualitative research procedures for the preliminary topic you identified in Workbox 1.2. If you have other advantages or limitations, add these to the lists. Thereafter, indicate *why* you believe data collected in the ways you have checked will be useful or perceived as a limitation in *your* research.

Workbox 1.2: Potential Advantages and Limitations of Using Qualitative Research

Advantages of Using Qualitative Research
☐ Provides detailed perspectives of a few people
☐ Captures the voices of participants
☐ Allows participants' experiences to be understood in context
☐ Is based on views of participants, not of the researcher
☐ Appeals to people's enjoyment of stories
☐ Other _____
Why?
Limitations of Using Qualitative Research
☐ Has limited generalizability
☐ Provides soft data (not hard data such as numbers)
☐ Studies few people
☐ Creates subjective data
☐ Researcher relinquishes control of the data produced
☐ Other _____
Why?

BRIEF REVIEW OF KEY ELEMENTS OF QUANTITATIVE RESEARCH

Overview of Quantitative Research

Quantitative research almost invariably involves multiple measurements of a phenomenon and the examination of associations. A researcher may be measuring how much, how many, how often, or the magnitude of a phenomenon of interest. Quantitative research is often used to examine associations between variables, to look at causality, or for assessing if one approach is more effective than another approach. Quantitative researchers commonly view reality as being objective and reproducible (see Chapter 4). Quantitative researchers typically focus on narrowly defined research questions or hypotheses. Quantitative researchers utilize highly structured close-ended questions or items as they seek to measure a phenomenon of interest. These may take form of scales for ratings, or selection among a series of items or statements. Quantitative researchers take steps to eliminate or reduce bias, as the purpose is to identify objective findings, rather than "subjective" interpretations provided by qualitative researchers.

Identifying the Rationale for Using Quantitative Research

For advancing your project, another critical early decision requires consideration of why to conduct quantitative research as part of your mixed methods project. Creswell and Plano Clark (2018) provide a succinct summary of advantages of using quantitative research that has been incorporated into Workbox 1.3, where you should consider the potential application to your own project. Advantages of using quantitative procedures can include drawing conclusions from a large sample, analyzing data efficiently, examining relationships in data, examining probable causes and effects, controlling for bias, appealing to some researchers' preference for numbers, among other things. But there are potential limitations of quantitative research as well, such as being distanced, impersonal, and dry, neglecting the voices of participants, providing limited understanding of context of the participants, and being driven by the researcher's agenda or goals rather than concerns of participants.

Activity: Identifying Advantages and Limitations Using Quantitative Research

These potential advantages and disadvantages have been listed in Workbox 1.3. Check off the potential advantages and limitations you perceive of using quantitative research procedures in your MMR project. If you have another reason or rationale as an advantage or disadvantage, add it to the respective list. Thereafter, indicate *why* you believe data collected in the ways you have checked will be useful or perceived as a limitation in *your* research.

Workbox 1.3: Potential Advantages and Limitations of Using Quantitative Research

Advantages of Using Quantitative Research
☐ Draws conclusions for large numbers of people
☐ Analyzes data efficiently
☐ Integrates relationships within data
☐ Examines probable causes and effects
☐ Controls bias
☐ Appeals to people's preferences for numbers
☐ Other _____
Why?
Limitations of Using Quantitative Research
☐ Is impersonal and dry
☐ Does not record the words of participants
☐ Provides limited understanding of the context of participants
☐ Is largely researcher driven
☐ Other _____
Why?

BRIEF REVIEW OF KEY ELEMENTS OF MIXED METHODS RESEARCH

Overview of Mixed Methods Research

A growing number of leaders in the field consider integration to be important in all dimensions of a program of MMR or evaluation (Fetters & Molina-Azorin, 2017c). For example, Teddlie and Tashakkori (2009) introduced the idea of a fully integrated approach to mixed methods procedures, though their discussion focused primarily on the methods. Elizabeth Creamer (2018) expands this notion in her book titled *An Introduction to Fully Integrated Mixed Methods Research*. She advocates for researchers to intentionally mix or integrate qualitative and quantitative strands of the study through all phases. Fetters and Molina-Azorin (2017b) envision mixed methods researchers integrating qualitative and quantitative elements through all dimensions of the mixed methods enterprise.

Identifying the Rationale for Using Mixed Methods Research

Mixed methods researchers seek to incorporate specific advantages of both qualitative and quantitative procedures. After conducting an intervention in a classroom to improve test scores on an achievement test, educational researchers may want to explore why they obtained certain results. When examining increases in productivity in manufacturing, business researchers may want to know how it occurred. In addition to examining the nature of a group's experience with a phenomenon qualitatively, the mixed methods researcher may also want to estimate quantitatively how commonly the identified experiences occur among all users.

Mixed methods researchers accept that qualitative and quantitative traditions often have differing world views (though recent scholars have proposed single world views), that some issues are highly informed by personal experiences, while other phenomena can be reasonably and meaningfully measured, and accept both as valid (see Chapter 4). Mixed methods researchers may be interested in both a specific phenomenon, as well as generalizability. Mixed methods researchers accept using preconceptions in the qualitative component of a mixed methods project while also controlling for bias in quantitative data collection. Mixed methods researchers will utilize procedures that produce both qualitative and quantitative data based on rigorous procedures, as defined within the tradition of data collection, that is, either qualitatively or quantitatively. Mixed methods researchers will be comfortable with text data from interviews, observations, and other sources, as well as numerical data elicited through a variety of closed-ended data collection procedures.

Activity: Identifying Potential Advantages and Limitations of Using Mixed Methods Research

When embarking on an MMR project, all investigators should pause to consider the advantages and limitations of using a mixed methods approach rather than a monomethod approach, that is, exclusively qualitative or exclusively quantitative approach. In Workbox 1.4, check off the potential advantages and limitations of using MMR procedures you perceive in your project. Thereafter, indicate *why* you believe that to be the case.

Workbox 1.4: Potential Advantages and Limitations of Using Mixed Methods Research

Advantages of Using Mixed Methods Research (MMR)
☐ Uses the strengths of qualitative and quantitative research to offset respective weaknesses
☐ Enhances the breadth and depth of the research
☐ Compares data from both types of research to examine different, similar, or seemingly discordant findings about a phenomenon
☐ Uses results of one type of data for collection to build procedures for the collection of the other type of data
☐ Develops a model qualitatively and tests it quantitatively
☐ Constructs a theoretical model quantitatively and validates it qualitatively
☐ Other _____

Why?
Limitations of Using MMR
☐ Perceived incompatibility of qualitative and quantitative paradigms
☐ May not need the complexity of MMR to answer the research question
☐ Difficult to have the skills to conduct both qualitative and quantitative together
☐ Requires more resources
☐ Extends beyond the scope of usual procedures, or not widely recognized in one's field
☐ May require the expertise of multiple team members
☐ Challenge of publishing MMR
☐ Other _____
Why?

Identifying the Advantages of Using Qualitative and Quantitative Procedures to Develop an Integrated Mixed Methods Research Approach

Having considered the various advantages and limitations for using qualitative, quantitative, and mixed methods procedures in your project, it is prudent to articulate these in writing for your own research. Workbox Illustration 1.5.1 provides examples from business, education, and the health sciences.

Workbox Illustration 1.5.1: Advantages for Specific Mixed Methods Research Projects: Examples of Three Fields

Field	Qualitative Research	Quantitative Research	Mixed Methods Research
Business (Sharma & Vredenburg, 1998)	• To obtain detailed perspectives of a few people, e.g., interviews in seven firms in the Canadian oil and gas industry to ground the resource-based view of the firm within the domain of corporate environmental responsiveness • To allow participants' experiences to be understood in context, e.g., the researchers explored potential linkages between environmental strategies and the development of capabilities and understand the nature of any emergent capabilities and their competitive outcomes	• To examine relationships between variables, e.g., the extent proactive environmental strategies are associated with the emergence of competitively valuable organizational capabilities	• Findings from the phenomenon explored in qualitative study were supplemented by the literature from corporate performance, environmental strategies, organizational learning, and the resource-based view of the firm and were used to build a survey that was used to examine the association proactive environmental responsiveness strategies and the emergence of organizational capabilities
Education (Harper, 2016)	• To understand the context of middle school principal's responses to survey questions about academic optimism • To explore wide variations in scoring	• To understand the influence of academic optimism on school achievement • To assess for differences between math and reading achievement	• Results of the surveys were analyzed and *used to create questions* for the second strand to explore how principals influenced academic optimism

(Continued)

(Continued)

Field	Qualitative Research	Quantitative Research	Mixed Methods Research
Health sciences (Kron et al., 2017)	• To understand the experiences of medical students when exposed to the intervention and the control • To understand the findings based on the perspectives of the participating medical students	• To draw conclusions based on a large number of participants across three medical schools • To examine whether exposure to the intervention predicted better performance than exposure to the control in actual performance in a real-life scenario	• Qualitative results were used to *illustrate why students* who were exposed to the intervention performed better than students exposed to the control, based on students' perceptions of their experiences

Activity: Identifying Advantages of Using Qualitative, Quantitative, and Mixed Methods Research Procedures

In Workbox 1.5.2, write the *advantages* of conducting your mixed methods project from the perspective of the qualitative, quantitative, and mixed methods perspectives, as illustrated in Workbox Illustration 1.5.1. This workbox will be most useful if you use specific statements as related to the topic you raised in Workbox 1.1.2.

Workbox 1.5.2: Advantages of Using Qualitative, Quantitative, and Mixed Methods Research Procedures

Qualitative Research	Quantitative Research	Mixed Methods Research

FEASIBILITY ISSUES AND MIXED METHODS RESEARCH

Numerous researchers have devised eloquent research plans that turned out to be impractical to execute. Because MMR involves complex procedures, feasibility issues can undercut even the best designed proposals. In Workbox 1.6, your task is to begin thinking about feasibility issues that could affect your MMR project.

Feasibility issues may include lack of resources, lack of skills, lack of funds to finance the study including payment of participants, limited timing to collect data due to time restrictions for when a phenomenon of interest occurs (e.g., the solar eclipse of 2017 came and went), access to the population of interest, or any other concerns. Identifying potential concerns about feasibility issues early will inform your decision making about the process and potentially allow you to address them proactively.

Activity: Identifying Potential Feasibility Issues for Conducting Qualitative and Quantitative Data Collection

Using Workbox 1.6, write down at least five considerations regarding *feasibility* for collecting both qualitative and quantitative data for your identified preliminary topic.

Workbox 1.6: Potential Feasibility Issues
for Conducting Qualitative and Quantitative Data Collection

1.

2.

3.

4.

5.

6.

7.

8.

Application Activities

The Mixed Methods Workbook and Peer Mentoring

Based on numerous courses and workshops, I have discovered that a great source of feedback about your MMR or evaluation project is a **peer mentor**. A peer mentor is someone who you consider to be a colleague, namely, someone with roughly equal qualifications or ability, who will also help mentor, that is, advise or provide consultation to you. If you are in a course, on a team, or in a lab, you may find a peer mentor who can be your partner, that is, someone with whom you discuss your workbook activities, and someone who you will listen to and provide peer mentoring support. When you are presenting your Mixed Methods Workbook ideas, you are honing the valuable skill of articulating your ideas. As you listen to your partner and provide feedback, you are learning and honing the valuable skills of critiquing. Good luck to you and your partner(s) in peer mentoring!

1. **Peer Feedback**. If you are working on your project as part of a class or in a workshop, pair up with a peer mentor, and one of you spend about 5 minutes talking about your chosen topic. Take turns talking about your

topic and giving feedback. Your goal is to help your partner refine the project topic.

2. **Peer Feedback Guidance**. You might want to reflect on why this topic is important to the partner. Does the project topic and the rationale match? Do you feel your partner has a personal investment in the topic? Does the topic have face validity as something that has importance not just at a personal level but also at a broader level? Has your partner understood enough about the essentials of qualitative, quantitative, and MMR? Has your partner identified the potential advantages and limitations of using only qualitative research or only quantitative research? Has your partner identified a justification for using both qualitative and quantitative procedures as a mixed methods project?

3. **Group Debrief**. If you are in a classroom, large group, or lab setting, volunteers can present their preliminary topic, as well as the potential advantages for using both qualitative and quantitative methods. Individually, reflect on how these same issues may play out in your own project.

Concluding Thoughts

Use this checklist to assess your progress in achieving the Chapter 1 objectives:

☐ I considered the overarching, general context of conducting MMR and evaluation studies.

☐ I developed a preliminary topic for my mixed methods project.

☐ I identified advantages of using qualitative and quantitative approaches and how they contribute

to developing the rationale for my MMR project or evaluation study.

☐ I explored potential feasibility issues of conducting MMR about my topic of interest.

☐ I reviewed Chapter 1 outputs with a peer or colleague to refine my project focus.

As you build on these completed objectives, Chapter 2 will help you develop a topic for your research or evaluation project.

Key Resources

1. **FURTHER READING ON QUALITATIVE RESEARCH**

- Creswell, J. W. (2016). *30 essential skills for the qualitative researcher*. Thousand Oaks, CA: Sage.
- Creswell, J. W., & Poth, C. N. (2018). *Qualitative inquiry and design: Choosing among five traditions* (4th ed.). Thousand Oaks, CA: Sage.
- Denzin N. K., & Lincoln, Y. S. (2018). *The SAGE handbook of qualitative research* (5th ed.). Thousand Oaks, CA: Sage.

2. **FURTHER READING ON QUANTITATIVE RESEARCH**

- Martin, W. E., & Bridgmon, K. D. (2012). *Quantitative and statistical research methods: From hypothesis to results*. San Francisco, CA: Jossey-Bass.
- Salkind, N. J. (2017). *Statistics for people who (think they) hate statistics* (6th ed.). Thousand Oaks, CA: Sage.
- Tokunaga, H. T. (2016). *Fundamental statistics for the social and behavioral sciences*. Thousand Oaks, CA: Sage.
- Vogt, W. P. (2006). *Quantitative research methods for professionals in education and other fields*. New York, NY: Pearson.

3. **FURTHER GENERAL READING ON MIXED METHODS RESEARCH**

- Bergman, M. M. (2008). *Advances in mixed methods research*. Thousand Oaks, CA: Sage.
- Creamer, E. G. (2018). *An introduction to fully integrated mixed methods research*. Thousand Oaks, CA: Sage.
- Creswell, J. W., & Plano Clark, V. L. (2018). *Designing and conducting mixed methods research* (3rd ed.). Thousand Oaks, CA: Sage.
- Curry, L., & Nunez-Smith, M. (2015). *Mixed methods in health sciences research: A practical primer*. Thousand Oaks, CA: Sage.
- Johnson, R. B., & Christensen L. (2017). *Educational research: Qualitative, quantitative and mixed approaches*. Thousand Oaks, CA: Sage.
- Mertens, D. M. (2015). *Research and evaluation in education and psychology: Integrating diversity with quantitative, qualitative, and mixed methods*. Thousand Oaks, CA: Sage.
- Plano Clark, V. L., & Ivankova, N. (2016). *Mixed methods research: A guide to the field*. Thousand Oaks, CA: Sage.
- Teddlie, C., & Tashakkori, A. (2009). *Foundations of mixed methods research*. Thousand Oaks, CA: Sage.

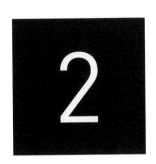

GETTING STARTED: IDENTIFYING A RESEARCH TOPIC FOR A MIXED METHODS PROJECT

The work researchers invest in narrowing the focus of a topic for a mixed methods research (MMR) or evaluation project can easily be underestimated. In the struggle to refine and revise your research topic, you may find it help-ful to connect with a narrative that led you to the topic. This chapter and its activities will help you discover how to develop your project topic, learn how the development of the project topic, purpose, and title is a cycle, recognize how meaningful project topics come from real-life problems and stories, propose a project idea, and identify how the project derives from a personally meaningful experience. As a key outcome, you will use logical procedures and activities to help you develop the topic for your project.

LEARNING OBJECTIVES

This chapter aims to

- Explore one or more ideas for your project to see if it intrinsically motivates you, and to articulate the experience, story, or rationale for why pursuing this project has merit
- Learn how the development of the project topic, purpose, and title is a cycle
- Recognize how good project topics come from real-life problems and stories
- Propose an idea for your project
- Identify the story/rationale underlying why the topic has a personal meaning to you

IDENTIFYING YOUR RESEARCH TOPIC

There are many pathways to identifying a **research topic** (Walsh & Wigens, 2003). Relative to the problem of identifying a research topic, John Creswell has noted that research fundamentally seeks to solve problems (Creswell, 2015). He has observed the tendency for novice researchers to emphasize what is already known rather than identifying what problem needs to be fixed. A good place to start is by asking yourself, "What is the problem I am trying to solve?" Johnson and Christensen suggested four sources where you might find these problems: (1) everyday life, (2) practical issues you encounter through your work, (3) past research, and (4) theory (Johnson & Christensen, 2014).

Based on experience mentoring many others, I believe the best topic for your research project is something that you are passionate about. So, you want to start out by asking yourself, "What is a topic that I am really interested in pursuing?" When I began my research career, my well-meaning mentors would ask, "What is your research question?" What I am proposing is you must first think about what is a research topic that interests you or puts "fire in your belly" (Ewigman, 1996). Once you have identified your topic, you can begin the process of honing it into a research question. As illustrated by Figure 2.1, going from a topic to research problem to a working purpose leads to a cycle of iteratively developing the researchable question, assessing feasibility, developing a plan to address the question, and reassessing the purpose. This cycle ultimately achieves a clear purpose and a project title.

FIGURE 2.1 ■ Cycle for Moving Between the Topic, Purpose, and Title

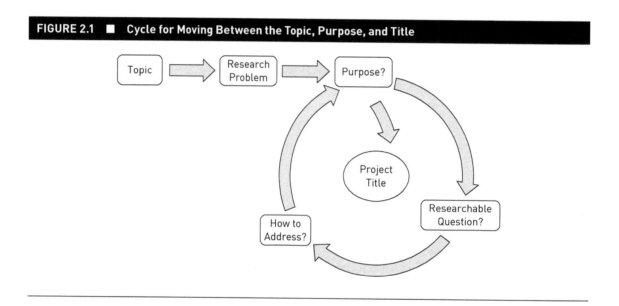

Why does your passion matter? From my observations as both a researcher and a mentor, projects that often face the most difficulty for completion occur when someone is assigned a topic, just to gain experience. If you are assigned or have negotiated a topic that you can take a lead and have specific tasks to work on, this can be a great way to get started. However, if you are trying to develop your own project, ideally you should feel curiosity and interest.

What is the difference between feeling passionate and not feeling passionate about a topic? As a physician in training, you often spend nights covering the hospital service, and this is called "on call." To balance the many competing demands of life, I often worked in the evenings on my research. I fondly called this "research call." What amazed me was that I would work on projects late into the evening, and then go to bed. The next day, I wouldn't actually remember how late I worked on the project. Why? Because I was so engulfed in my work that the time I spent didn't matter.

So why does this matter to you? If you are looking at your watch every time you are working on your project, it may mean that you don't have passion for the project and that you might be better off looking into something else (see Story From the Field 2.1). Use caution in comparing lack of passion with mind block, which is when you are not sure what you want to do next. This workbook can help you feel the excitement of taking a project from concept to completion. But you need to find your own passion, and it often takes time.

STORY FROM THE FIELD 2.1
WHY FINDING AN INTERNALLY MOTIVATED PROJECT IDEA MATTERS

During my research training, my colleague, a brilliant person, stumbled repeatedly relative to identifying a topic and finally took one that was assigned. He struggled with the research as he was not internally motivated to do the project. While he went through the steps of the project, and ultimately completed it, barriers kept "popping up" that slowed the work. In the end, he met the requirements for the program but never wrote up the results of the project. The source of the problem was not a lack of intelligence but a lack of internal motivation.

TRANSLATING YOUR "IDEA" TO "INK"

One of the best ways to get started is by writing down a topic of interest. For all the magnificent ideas you carry around in your head, if they are not in ink, they remain too abstract and not concrete. On many occasions, I was convinced I had the project plans worked out in my head, but then it wasn't so clear when I tried to put the plans on the page. In this way, writing is thinking!

GOOD RESEARCH IDEAS COME FROM STORIES

Regardless of your discipline, one of the best sources of good ideas will be your own experiences. In your field, life, work, and readings, you'll inevitably stumble upon problems and issues. These experiences are "stories" rooted in real issues that spawn ideas for research (Miller & Crabtree, 1990). These can be considered as "eyebrow-raising," something that made you "stop and think," something you observe(d) in your daily work that "didn't make sense." Perhaps, you have read something and then thought "that doesn't make any sense!" or you'll ponder the many choices about how you could do something, but there is "no clear best choice." An inspiration for your work might be an article you have read about an injustice that occurred in your community, or perhaps there was a national event. What are the stories that have driven you to thinking about the topic you raise? (See Story From the Field 2.2.)

STORY FROM THE FIELD 2.2
A MEDICAL STUDENT'S MOTHER'S PAIN INSPIRED HER WORK TO UNDERSTAND DOCTORS' PERSPECTIVES ON PAIN

In an article by Miller, Yanoshik, Crabtree, and Reymond (1994), published in the journal *Family Medicine*, the authors conducted a qualitative research project about doctors' and patients' views on pain. The impetus for the study came from a team member shocked by how poorly her mother's chronic pain was treated by her doctors. She worked with her mentors to channel her passion into a research project to explore doctors' and patients' views about pain. The experience and story helped to identify a compelling clinical question that led to their research study on how doctors handle pain.

Activity: Identifying a Topic

Using Workbox Illustration 2.1.1 as an example, write down in Workbox 2.1.2 a research topic that interests you. If you like, you can write two or three. I advise writing out your topic(s) using a full sentence or several sentences.

Workbox Illustration 2.1.1: Project Idea—Example From the MPathic-VR Mixed Methods Medical Education Study

My idea is to bring advances in gaming technology to the classroom to teach medical students, medical residents, and other learners about verbal and nonverbal communication skills.

Source: Fetters, M.D. and Kron, F.W. (2012–15). *Modeling Professional Attitudes and Teaching Humanistic Communication in Virtual Reality (MPathic-VRII).* National Center for Advancing Translational Science/NIH 9R44TR000360-04.

Workbox 2.1.2: Project Idea—The Problem I Want to Solve

Activity: Identifying the Story Behind Your Topic

Using Workbox Illustration 2.2.1 as an example, in Workbox 2.2.2, write down why you are interested in the topic. If you are a graduate student, the odds are that you have chosen your field for a compelling personal reason, consciously or unconsciously. Ideally, the rationale you identify will be helpful to discern your level of passion. For example, if you have an interest in improving your city's air quality, perhaps you have a family member with asthma. As an instructor, you may have witnessed certain students struggle, who you know to be very intelligent. In a business internship, you may have observed waste in company procedures that you felt could be improved. By articulating your fundamental interest, you can hone your idea into a research question.

Workbox Illustration 2.2.1: The Story Behind the Topic—Example From the MPathic-VR Mixed Methods Medical Education Study

As a family doctor, I have realized how important communication skills are to the doctor-patient relationship. But it took me many years working as a clinician to hone my own skills. As I saw advances in gaming technology based on my own sons' strong interest in gaming, I was struck by the ability of gaming to sustain their attention. This triggered an interest in utilizing serious gaming technology to teach communication skills.

Source: Fetters, M.D. and Kron, F.W. (2012–15). *Modeling Professional Attitudes and Teaching Humanistic Communication in Virtual Reality (MPathic-VRII).* National Center for Advancing Translational Science/NIH 9R44TR000360-04.

Workbox 2.2.2: The Story Behind the Topic

Application Activities

1. **Peer Feedback.** If working on your project as part of a class or in a workshop, pair up with a peer mentor. First, one of you spend 5 minutes talking about your topic. Take turns talking about your projects and giving feedback. Tell the story that prompted your idea. As you discuss your topic, make a candid assessment about your motivation and interest. Is what you have observed or read about this topic been of just passing interest or did it really strike a note? If you feel passionate, that is a great sign. If you are uncertain, that could be okay. The uncertainty may be due to a lack of confidence or lack of passion about the topic you are considering. Seeds of good topics may take weeks, months, or even years to germinate.

2. **Peer Feedback Guidance.** As you listen and give feedback to your partner, you are learning and honing the valuable skills of critiquing. Help your partner refine the project idea. Help reflect on why this topic is important to the partner. Does the project idea and the rationale match? Can you feel this person has a personal investment in the topic? Does the topic have face validity of importance, not just at a personal level, but at a broader level?

3. **Group Debrief.** If in a classroom or large-group setting, volunteers can present their ideas and stories. Listen for their passion. Reflect as to whether the project idea is interesting but lacks utility or applicability.

Concluding Thoughts

Use this checklist to assess your progress in achieving the Chapter 2 objectives:

☐ I explored the underlying motivation for the project idea and considered how personal experience, story, or rationale helps explain the topic's merit.

☐ I learned how the development of the project topic, purpose, and title is a cycle.

☐ I discovered how good project topics come from real-life problems and stories.

☐ I proposed an idea for my project.

☐ I identified the story/rationale underlying why my project is personally meaningful.

☐ I improved my idea by presenting it to a peer mentor and incorporating feedback.

☐ I sharpened my knowledge of the material by critiquing a peer mentor's idea and providing feedback.

Now that you have completed these objectives, Chapter 3 will help you refine your topic.

Key Resources

FURTHER READING ON IDENTIFYING A TOPIC

- Creswell, J. W. (2015). Steps in designing a mixed methods study. In J. W. Creswell, *A concise introduction to mixed methods research.* Thousand Oaks, CA: Sage. ISBN: 978-1483359045.

- Johnson, R. B., & Christensen, L. (2014). How to review the literature and develop research questions.

In R. B. Johnson & L. Christensen, *Educational research: Quantitative, qualitative and mixed approaches.* Thousand Oaks, CA: Sage. ISBN: 978-1412978286.

- Walsh M., & Wiggins L. (2003). Introduction to research. *Foundations in nursing and health care.* Cheltenham, UK: Nelson Thornes. ISBN: 978-0748771189.

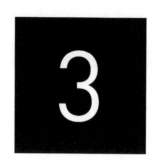

REVIEWING THE LITERATURE FOR A MIXED METHODS PROJECT

As in any research or evaluation project, mixed methods projects require examination of the literature supporting the project. While you may have heard of the benefits or requirements for a literature review for your mixed methods project, you may feel uncertain about how to choose among different types of literature reviews. This chapter and its activities will support your distinguishing between different types of literature reviews, choosing search terms to identify existing literature, conducting a literature search on the project topic, and examining the breadth and depth of previous research to frame your mixed methods project. As a key outcome, you will identify key qualitative, quantitative, and mixed methods empirical studies that will inform your mixed methods project.

LEARNING OBJECTIVES

This chapter aims to introduce you to the different types of literature searches so you will be able to

- Distinguish among the different types of literature reviews you can conduct
- Identify search terms that will help you find relevant literature
- Conduct a search that will inform your own mixed methods project
- Examine the breadth and depth of previously completed research, and identify limitations in the published literature to frame your own project

PURPOSE OF YOUR MIXED METHODS RESEARCH LITERATURE REVIEW

The purpose of your literature search is very simple. You need to answer the basic question, "What do we know about my topic already?" *We* here signifies the academic community as written in the existing literature. When your topic is too broad, it means *we* already "know" a lot about it, as illustrated by voluminous literature. This chapter will help you narrow the scope of your project. You can engage a peer mentor to help you clarify your own topic, and you can help clarify your partner's topic as well.

Literature Review as a Quintessential Step for Designing Your Mixed Methods Research and Evaluation Projects

All research, mixed methods or not, should start out with a literature review. Any research project submitted for funding will review the literature in the background or introduction section of the proposal. A well-kept secret is that you will probably want to do your literature search at least twice, once when you are starting your project to justify your research, and a second time when you have completed your data collection and analysis and are ready to write up your dissertation or paper(s) for publication. Some services automatically will send you interval updates on newly published papers based on key words you provide. There are different foci of the two searches. In the first, you need to justify your project, while in the second, you need to identify literature relevant to your primary research findings. When writing for publication (see Chapter 18), some researchers recommend writing the methods and results first, and the introduction/background section last, in parallel with the discussion (Fetters & Freshwater, 2015b). Hence, the need for an ongoing, or a full-blown second literature search. But before getting too far ahead, you need to understand the different literature review types.

UNDERSTANDING DIFFERENT TYPES OF LITERATURE REVIEWS

For the purposes of your project, literature reviews fall into three categories: (1) a focused narrative literature review that will be less intense but adequately informs your mixed methods project; (2) a more advanced scoping review; and (3) a highly advanced systematic review, a full undertaking as a research endeavor.

Narrative Review

A narrative review involves an intensive search of the literature and then summarization of key topics using a narrative format. A focused narrative review can suffice for a dissertation proposal and the background of a specific paper. If conducted in an exhaustive way, a narrative review can be published as a scholarly work and provide informative background about a current topic. In previous work, I have conducted such exhaustive narrative reviews with students, for example, about the translation of instruments for use into other languages (Garcia-Castillo & Fetters, 2007) and the role of free clinics in the health care system (Schiller, Thurston, Khan, & Fetters, 2013). A narrative review may be less involved than the complex procedures involved in a scoping or systematic review. As narrative reviews are less complex, they are also less resource intensive, both in terms of the costs of procuring a narrower range of articles but also for the time costs involved.

Scoping Review

A scoping review is a more advanced review of the literature than a narrative review, and it addresses a broader topic than a systematic review as the latter focuses on stricter criteria. In a scoping review, the researcher examines the extant, range, and nature of research activity relative to a single phenomenon or topic of interest (Arksey & O'Malley, 2002). A scoping review uses a protocol with the following major steps: (1) identifying the research question; (2) identifying relevant studies; (3) selecting studies for inclusion; (4) charting the data; and (5) collating, summarizing, and reporting the results. A scoping review may be of particular interest to mixed methods researchers because a broader range of study types are included (e.g., not just qualitative studies as in a meta-synthesis, or just randomized controlled trials as may be the case in a meta-analysis). A scoping review also differs from other systematic reviews as the latter involves a formal assessment of study quality, which is not necessarily a feature of a scoping review. If conducted rigorously, the scoping review qualifies as a systematic review and can be highly informative. Campbell et al. (2017) conducted a scoping review to comprehensively describe characteristics of mixed methods studies on coronary artery disease and major risk factors such as diabetes and hypertension.

Systematic Reviews

Many doctoral students are required to conduct an advanced literature search, often a systematic review. Systematic reviews are research projects unto themselves. For your mixed methods project, you should understand what the different types of systematic reviews involve and choose accordingly for your own project.

There are four types of systematic reviews: a meta-analysis, a meta-synthesis, systematic mixed studies review, and meta-integration. A meta-analysis involves rigorous quantitative procedures and uses statistical procedures as part of the systematic review (Higgins & Green, 2011). A meta-synthesis involves the use of qualitative procedures for rigorously conducting a systematic review of qualitative studies (Sandelowski, Docherty, & Emden, 1997). A mixed methods research (MMR) synthesis, also called a mixed studies research synthesis, involves rigorous procedures for examining mixed studies, that is, quantitative, qualitative, and mixed methods studies (Heyvaert, Hammes, & Onghena, 2017). A meta-integration involves systematically identifying diverse QUAL, QUAN, and mixed methods studies, and using advanced mixed methods procedures such as fractionating, data transformation, and integration (Frantzen & Fetters, 2015). See Story From the Field 3.1 for the work involved in a systematic review.

STORY FROM THE FIELD 3.1
CASE STUDY OF AN ADVANCED LITERATURE SEARCH USING A MIXED METHODS STUDIES REVIEW

Kirsten Frantzen invited me to collaborate on her dissertation project about parental self-perception in autism spectrum disorder (ASD). To conduct her systematic mixed studies review of the literature, she used a search strategy that consisted of three separate blocks (Frantzen et al., 2015). The first consisted of ASD-specific keywords. The second block contained keywords related to the three psychological constructs central to her systematic review (*competence*, *self-efficacy*, and *locus of control*), as well as *stress* and *coping* to ensure that key-related literature was detected. The third block consisted of parent-related keywords such as *values*, *beliefs*, *culture*, *involvement*, *burden*, *attitude*, and *quality of life*. Using three different databases, Pubmed, PsycINFO, and Embase, her initial search and two subsequent searches yielded a total of 911 potentially applicable articles. After reducing the total number by reading the abstract, there were 389 articles. After applying two additional levels of exclusion criteria, she identified 53 articles for inclusion in her systematic review. As this case illustrates, pursuit of systematic review should not be taken by the weary at heart as much work is involved, but it can be highly rewarding when done!

Determining the Type of Literature Review Appropriate to Your Topic

Now that you understand the major types of literature review, you should now commit to a specific type of review. Using Workbox Illustration 3.1.1, complete Workbox 3.1.2. Record the type of literature review appropriate for your topic and project, and write why you've chosen this approach. For example, you may choose a narrative approach citing the rationale of (1) you have a specific paper you are working on already, and (2) it is not feasible given the resource issues, e.g., time, money, etc. Alternatively, you might record that you will conduct a systematic search that is (1) required as part of your dissertation, (2) will allow you to write a manuscript based on the chapter for publication, and (3) you want to refine your project based on a comprehensive review.

Workbox Illustration 3.1.1: Example of Choosing a Basic Literature Review Based on the MPathic-VR Project Mixed Methods Medical Education Study

Literature Review Type
☑ Narrative literature review
☐ Scoping review
☐ Systematic review and type proposed:
Rationale:
The project only requires a sufficient review of the background literature, and in the context of working on grant writing, the focus was on the details of the justification for the grant rather than examining systematically the literature about use of virtual human technology in education.

Source: Fetters, M.D. and Kron, F.W. (2012–15). *Modeling Professional Attitudes and Teaching Humanistic Communication in Virtual Reality (MPathic-VRII).* National Center for Advancing Translational Science/NIH 9R44TR000360-04.

Workbox 3.1.2: Choosing a Literature Review Appropriate to Your Project

Literature Review Type
☐ Narrative literature review
☐ Scoping review
☐ Systematic review and type proposed:
Rationale:

CONDUCTING A FOCUSED
LITERATURE REVIEW OF YOUR TOPIC

As you can see, you could pursue various degrees of depth in your literature searches prior to conducting your mixed methods project. In the interest of not getting slowed down by an advanced systematic review, for the purposes of the workbook, you will need to focus your literature review to inform and justify your project. Of course, if you have the time or requirements to do a systematic review, I highly encourage you to do so as these are very informative, and other researchers cite them frequently. It will not preclude your ongoing use of the workbook, either.

Keeping the Background Literature Manageable

The amount of literature on general topics can be overwhelming (see Story From the Field 3.1 for example of a systematic review). For example, a search with the term *diabetes* might yield tens of thousands of articles. But when the term is narrowed down to "new onset Type 1 diabetes during pregnancy," you could imagine that there would be a much smaller amount of literature. There are key strategies you can employ to efficiently identify relevant research.

Activity: Keeping the Project Topic in Focus

To keep your literature search for your mixed methods project in focus, write your current research topic/question into Workbox 3.2. As discussed previously, it usually takes time for your research idea to evolve into a research question. Try and be as specific as possible.

Workbox 3.2: Working/Revised/
Updated Idea or Title of Your Project

Getting Peer Feedback

Pair up with a peer mentor to discuss your working title. Explain how your topic has evolved since you started and why. As you review a peer's topic, think critically about the changes made and the impact. Is this a more searchable topic and adequately focused title now? See if you can help improve your partner's suggested idea/title! If possible, review your **revised title** with your class professor or a colleague.

RIGHTSIZING THE LITERATURE REVIEW

You can now work with your title to identify relevant readings. A good place to start is to identify several conveniently available articles. Ask a professor or colleague if they have read any good articles on the topic. Perhaps you have stumbled upon one or two in a class or professional meeting that triggered your interest in the topic. If you already have a few articles such as these, skim the literature cited by the authors in the back. You can also look to see who has cited that particular article by doing a forward search. A forward search looks to see what authors have cited an article published in the past.

Activity: Identify Search Terms for Your Literature Review

To do a search, you will want to identify **search terms** relevant to your topic. If you found any articles close to your own topic, then look at the search terms in the article. Start by writing these down in Workbox 3.3. You should write out at least 5 to 7 key search terms for your project to avoid a "mountain of literature." The search terms should identify literature about the content area of your research. Another strategy is to include terms that will help identify methodologically relevant terms. Think about how you will identify qualitative and MMR titles.

**Workbox 3.3: Write Out
5 to 7 Key Search Terms for Your Project**

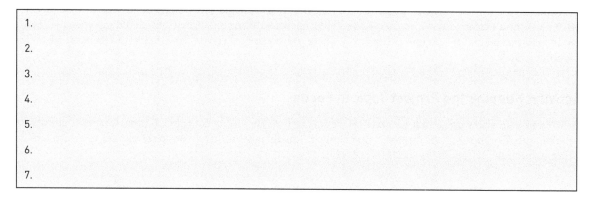

1.

2.

3.

4.

5.

6.

7.

Peer Review of Your Search

Pair up with a peer mentor to discuss your key search terms. As you review a peer's topic, think critically about the choices made and the impact. In most cases, the search terms identified do not provide a sufficiently narrow scope. See if you can help narrow your partner's scope! If possible, review your revised list with your class professor or a colleague.

What Should I Do? I Have a Mountain-High Level of Potential Article Hits!

Don't get discouraged by the initial breadth and depth of previous research. While there may be related literature, there will always be some aspects that were problematic or limited. Perhaps the previous research hasn't covered certain aspects of the project, or the research needs to be replicated because it was done in a different population, or the research has become dated. There are many other reasons. Many of the articles will not be relevant. Many can be eliminated by reviewing the title or quickly reading of the abstract. You will often find this information in the limitations section of the papers you read. So, if feeling overwhelmed by the sheer volume of papers, expedite the process by focusing on the limitations section.

Refine and Update Your Search Terms

Now that you have a better sense for the terms relevant to your project, update Workbox 3.3. While this may seem a menial task, you would be surprised how easily you can forget the search terms that you used when it comes to writing the background for your dissertation or research paper. If you are meticulous and methodical now, you will be able to retrieve these search terms easily. This information is needed for dissertations and published papers alike. Better to include them up front than to wait for an unnecessary criticism during the peer-review process. If you are still getting a very large number of articles back in your search, you may need to further refine your terms.

Working With an Information Science Specialist—Bring in Professional Talent!

You can learn a lot by first attempting the search yourself and then consulting with an information science specialist. As you will find, one of the most coveted articles for many researchers is a narrative, scoping, or systematic review about their topic. Perhaps you want to rethink doing an advanced search! If at all possible, enroll the assistance of an information science specialist (i.e., librarian). Information scientists are so smart! They have an extensive grasp of potentially relevant databases and can help identify search terms and strategies that will narrow your search. In your graduate library/media center, perhaps an information science specialist can help you identify terms and search JSTOR (short for Journal Storage), an online digital library. Alternatively, a health sciences information specialist can help you identify official Medical Subject Headings, i.e., MESH terms, that is, a hierarchically organized terminology for indexing and cataloging biomedical information.

Scan the Article Titles, Reduce Further

Once you have identified some 20 to 50 titles relevant to your project, you will most likely want to reduce this even further. In Frantzen's paper (Story From the Field 3.1), just reading the abstracts helped to reduce the number of articles by over 50%. There is no magic number about the number of articles. Conducting a literature search involves iteratively trying the search, looking at the results, and then going back to the literature. Saturation, a criteria used in qualitative research to guide when you can stop data collection, reflects the point when you are no longer learning new information. If you are conducting a systematic review, you will not be able to stop at saturation as a systematic review requires your inclusion of all studies identified based on your search criteria. In a focused review, you may not need to read in detail all the articles you have identified. But it is good practice to at least read through the abstracts (remember this value of the abstract later when you work on writing an effective mixed methods abstract in Chapter 18).

Retrieve and Read the Most Promising Articles

You will now want to retrieve and read the articles. Some prefer using hard copies, some reading electronic copies. When reading a hard copy, researchers can write in the margins notes, concepts, or questions. Others prefer electronic copies because it does not require paper, and this can conserve resources as well as avoiding a heavy, back-breaking backpack. While still a bit awkward, taking notes on electronic copies is an option also. The potential downside of using an electronic version is organizing thoughts or ideas that come as you read them. While reading through these articles, look not only at the content and the results of the study about that content but also the methods used and how the methods were applied. Be sure to read the limitations section as you can often find areas ripe for research. Some highly efficient researchers use qualitative data analysis software to organize and retrieve articles. This can be very helpful if you want to group articles according to subtopics irrespective of the methodology used.

IDENTIFYING QUALITATIVE, QUANTITATIVE, AND MIXED METHODS STUDIES

As you develop your mixed methods topic, separate out the qualitative, quantitative, and mixed methods studies. By separating these studies, you will be able to think like an MMR methodologist. This can help you understand not only what findings there have been but also methodologically what has been tried and worked or not worked well, as well as what has not been tried. Equally important, this will help you understand the most relevant limitations from qualitative, quantitative, and mixed methods perspectives. This language—qualitative, quantitative, and mixed methods—is used by MMR methodologists and increasingly by researchers as a way to think about the procedures and challenges of doing MMR, commonalities, and potential differences. If you are uncertain if the study was qualitative or quantitative, consider asking yourself if the authors used closed-ended questions (classify as quantitative), open-ended questions (classify as qualitative), or used a combination of both qualitative and quantitative questions (mixed methods). Also be mindful that the language authors use to describe their studies occasionally is not accurate, so remember there is more to the article than the title.

Activity: Identifying Relevant Qualitative Research

Researchers who publish their qualitative studies sometimes do, and sometimes don't, use the word *qualitative* in their papers. So, this is a good term to use, but you may also want to try language specific to qualitative research. There are many possible classifications. John Creswell uses *narrative, phenomenology, grounded theory, ethnography,* and *case study* to distinguish between 5 types of qualitative research (Creswell, 2013), and you may want to use these terms. You may also find the terms reflecting the data collection approach, for example, *interviews, focus group,* or *observations,* as useful search terms for identifying qualitative studies. Keep your eyes open for a meta-synthesis, a systematic review of qualitative studies. Using Workbox 3.4, add 3 to 5 articles (or more) of the most important studies related to your research that used *qualitative* research.

Workbox 3.4: Articles About
Your Topic Using Qualitative Methodology

1.

2.

3.

4.

5.

Activity: Identifying Relevant Quantitative Research

Researchers who publish results of surveys, randomized controlled trials, secondary dataset analyses, etc., generally do not use the word *quantitative* to describe their work. However, this language is used by MMR methodologists as a way to think about the challenges of doing MMR, to identify commonalities and potential differences across various quantitatively focused data collection procedures, and for teaching students. Keep your eyes open for a meta-analysis, a systematic review of quantitative studies. Using Workbox 3.5, add 3 to 5 articles (or more) of the most important studies related to your research that used *quantitative* research.

Workbox 3.5: Articles About Your
Topic Using Quantitative Methodology

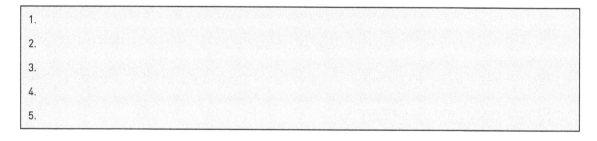

1.

2.

3.

4.

5.

Activity: Identifying Relevant Mixed Methods Research

Recent authors of MMR may use the term *MMR*, or even one of the common design terms, for example, *exploratory sequential, explanatory sequential, convergent*, etc. However, older studies may have used language such as *mixed studies, mixed method, multi-method, integrated, combined, multi-methodology, mixed-method*, or *qualitative and quantitative method*. A caveat is that some authors may even call their studies MMR even though the study may not meet criteria as a mixed methods study. Keep your eyes open for a mixed methods synthesis or meta integration, a systematic review of qualitative, quantitative, or mixed methods studies. Using Workbox 3.6, add 3 to 5 articles (or more) of the most important studies related to your research that used MMR.

Workbox 3.6: Articles About Your Topic Using
Mixed Methods, Multi-method, or Qualitative and Quantitative Methodology

1.

2.

3.

4.

5.

Activity: Review an Empirical Mixed Methods Journal Article

Select one of the mixed methods empirical articles you found. You should choose an article where the authors conducted original research by collecting and analyzing both qualitative and quantitative data. In your review, succinctly present the content of the research, summarize the mixed methods components in the article, and critique the strengths and weaknesses of the article. Your review should be 2 to 3 double-spaced pages in length. Submit your review and an attached copy of the article to your instructor. Alternatively, you can exchange reviews with a peer mentor and provide feedback. Workbox 3.7 offers criteria when assessing the quality of a mixed methods empirical article.

Workbox 3.7: Criteria for Assessing a Mixed Methods Empirical Article

1. Did the authors justify in the background literature the rationale for collecting and integrating both qualitative and quantitative data?

2. Did the authors cite mixed methods literature, and to what extent was it general or focused on the specific methodological approach used by the authors?

3. Did the authors present a MMR question?

4. Did the authors collect both qualitative (open-ended) and quantitative (closed-ended) forms of data, and if so, what type?

5. How did the authors integrate both forms of data in the design, and do they give the design a name?

6. What sampling relationship did the authors use?

7. How did the authors link the two types of data collection?

8. What was the rigor and depth of the quantitative data collection?

9. What was the rigor and depth of the qualitative data collection?

10. What is the rigor and depth of the quantitative data analysis?

11. What is the rigor and depth of the qualitative data analysis?

12. How did the authors conduct an integrated analysis? Did they merge the data, and if so, how?

13. Did the authors use any philosophical or conceptual framework, and if so how?

14. Does the study seem to convey significant findings that extend the literature or fill a gap in existing literature in the content area?

15. Did the authors speak to how the study adds to the mixed methods literature?

16. Do the authors use terms associated with MMR, such as *quantitative and qualitative*, *mixed methods*, *multi-method*, *integrated methods*, and so forth to search databases for mixed methods articles?

Application Activities

1. **Peer Feedback.** Share with your partner or peer mentor the results of your search. Explain how you have chosen these particular articles. Were there any articles that you found difficult to classify? Which are the most informative for your topic? How have you rethought the title of your project?

2. **Peer Feedback Guidance.** As you critique your partner's lists of titles, assess the relevance. Do the articles seem to inform the topic? Does the presenter understand the articles that were identified? Give candid feedback as to how you think the search could be improved.

3. **Group Debrief.** If in a classroom or large group setting, have volunteers present their literature search stories. What type of literature review is proposed? Was the search strategy successful? How much variation occurs by topic amongst different presenters for identifying mixed methods studies? Listen for the presenters passion. Has reviewing the literature helped to pique interest in the topic?

Concluding Thoughts

Use this checklist to assess your progress in achieving the Chapter 3 objectives:

☐ I learned about different literature review types and identified one appropriate to my topic.

☐ I identified key search terms for my project.

☐ I conducted qualitative, quantitative, and mixed methods literature searches for my project.

☐ I examined the breadth and depth of previously completed research and identified limitations in the published literature to help frame my project.

☐ I reviewed my Chapter 3 outputs with a peer or colleague to refine my literature review approach.

Now that you have completed these objectives, Chapter 4 will help you incorporate your personal contexts into your research or evaluation project.

Key Resources

1. **FURTHER READING ON A COMPREHENSIVE LITERATURE REVIEW**

   - Onwuegbuzie, A. J., & Frels, R. K. (2016). *Seven steps to a comprehensive literature review: A multimodal and cultural approach.* London, UK: Sage.

2. **FURTHER READING ON MIXED METHODS RESEARCH SYNTHESIS**

   - Heyvaert, M., Hannes, K., Onghena, P. (2016). *Using mixed methods research synthesis for literature reviews.* Thousand Oaks, CA: Sage.

3. **FURTHER READING ON META-INTEGRATION**

   - Frantzen, K. K., & Fetters, M. D. (2016). Meta-integration for synthesizing data in a systematic mixed studies review: Insights from research on autism spectrum disorder. *Quality & Quantity, 50*(5), 2251–2277. doi.org/10.1007/s11135-015-0261-6

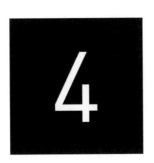

INCORPORATING PERSONAL BACKGROUND, THEORY, AND WORLDVIEWS INTO MIXED METHODS RESEARCH

"Personal contexts in mixed methods research" represents language used by Plano Clark and Ivankova (2016) to describe the role of the researcher's background knowledge, theoretical models, and philosophical assumptions, and how this personal context influences mixed methods research (MMR) projects. Like many, you may never have considered how your own background, theory, and worldviews can influence mixed methods studies. This chapter and its activities will help you identify your personal context; reflect on how personal experiences, values, and training can contribute to the research; explore the value of theoretical models; and delineate how the philosophical assumptions undergird mixed methods projects and apply them. As a key outcome, you will consider how your personal contexts can be used in the design and implementation of mixed methods projects.

LEARNING OBJECTIVES

This chapter aims to help you identify your "personal context" as articulated by Plano Clark and Ivankova (2016), namely, your own background experiences, theory, and worldview so you will be able to

- Reflect on how your personal context comprised of your personal background, theoretical models, and philosophical assumptions can influence your MMR proposal

- Identify how your own personal experiences, values, and training cumulatively inform your personal background and to clarify and use these experiences in your research

- Explore the value of a theoretical model, follow a general process for identifying one appropriate to your mixed methods project, and consider how to apply it

- Delineate how philosophical assumptions undergird MMR projects and how to apply them

INTRODUCTION TO THE "PERSONAL CONTEXTS" CONCEPT

While many people feel paralyzed when they hear the words *theory* and *philosophy*, these concepts are not to be feared, but embraced. They will strengthen your MMR. Conceptually, the **personal contexts** notion is easy. It simply asks you to consider very carefully how your own background experiences and readings of literature influence you as a researcher. Of course, there is a great deal of depth and scholarship around this topic, but keeping focused on this simple idea will make your work with theory and philosophy rewarding.

Developed by Plano Clark and Ivankova (2016), the personal context concept refers to "the philosophical assumptions, theoretical models, and background knowledge that shape mixed methods practice" (p. 193). This includes the philosophical assumptions about the kinds of knowledge that can be obtained through research and the role of the researcher in knowledge generation. Moreover, it includes theoretical models about the nature of the topic and related facts. Finally, it includes your personal expertise and experience related to the topic of your research. Essentially, the concept of personal context encourages researchers to think about how they each have their own "lens" as a product of their personal experiences, research background, theory, and philosophical assumptions. As there are publications devoted to these concepts, the workbook concepts and activities will challenge you to consider your own "lens" and continuously reflect about the impact on your own mixed methods project.

In Plano Clark and Ivankova's (2016) model, they organize their discussion from the most abstract to the least abstract: philosophical assumptions, theoretical models, and personal and research background (here referred to as just personal background). But for our purposes, the order will be flipped. You will start with the most concrete and personally obvious, namely, your personal background, and then build on consideration of theoretical models, and finally extend to the most abstract, the philosophical. While reflecting about what personal factors have been influential in your own life, scaffold on specific theory and philosophical views that resonate, and use this for defending your choices made relative to theory and philosophical assumptions.

PERSONAL AND PROFESSIONAL EXPERIENCE

While often not explicit, our personal and professional experiences strongly influence thinking about certain topics. In fact, researchers are often drawn to a particular topic precisely because of their own experiences. Cumulatively, our experiences create unique lenses, dispositions, and preferences that forge our views and interpretations.

Reflexivity in Qualitative and Mixed Methods Research

Reflexivity is a concept from the field of qualitative research that refers to how a researcher engages in honest, explicit, self-aware analysis of their own role in the research process (Finlay, 2002). Qualitative researchers use the process of reflecting to increase trustworthiness (language often used to indicate research integrity (see Chapter 16) of qualitative research. The expectation for researchers to be reflexive stems from the understanding that subjective elements influence data collection and analysis. Incorporating reflexivity is very important for maintaining the research integrity of all mixed methods projects, but particularly so for qualitatively driven mixed methods projects.

Activity: Identifying Your Personal and Professional Influences

While engaging in reflexive analysis is difficult and subjective, you need to start somewhere. Many people find the easiest approach is to begin with the first time in memory that you encountered this topic or phenomenon and consider the various influences that encounter had on your own thinking. In Workbox Illustration 4.1.1, I provide reflections about experiences that have influenced my interest in research on the topic of cancer. This is a truncated version as I have had additional experiences as a family doctor and as a health and social science researcher that have further influenced my thinking. If I were to write this out fully, it would be (and has been on various projects) many more pages long. This truncated, bulleted form provides an example of what a personal inventory can look like. A potential next step on the personal inventory format is to further divide this summary into two columns with the first column reflecting your knowledge and professional influences and a second column to include an *interpretation* about the potential impact on your work.

Workbox Illustration 4.1.1: Personal Background Influences on Cancer Research

- When in high school, an upperclassman had cancer (in retrospect a childhood lymphoma I presume) and missed school for a month or more. When he returned, he was bald and his hair grew back slowly. This experience influenced me to believe that cancer was something traumatic and terrible but survivable.

- When in high school and into college, both my grandmother and aunt developed breast cancer and both ultimately required surgery. This more personal experience led me to think of cancer as curable but that treatment had a cost of disfiguring surgery.

- Not many years after I started medical school, my aunt developed a recurrence and developed metastases. I was angered because I learned she had never been in a recurrence surveillance program. As her cancer was incurable, I also witnessed explorations of my extended family into alternative medical treatments (now called integrative medicine) in their desperation to save her. She tragically died many decades before she should have.

- When I lived in Japan in my undergraduate years during a study abroad program, I learned that patients were typically not told they had cancer.

- In medical school, I attended lectures and studied intensively about pathophysiology, pharmacology, genetics, and other basic science aspects about cancer that influenced my thinking about the science behind understanding and treating cancer.

- When in medical school during my third year, I started on the clinical wards for an oncology rotation. It was the first time that a patient who was assigned to me died. I witnessed intensive cardiopulmonary resuscitation that was ultimately futile and felt that end-of-life care was rather brutal.

- In my U.S. medical school, I learned that disclosing cancer to patients was routine, that U.S. physicians had historically withheld cancer from patients, and that some bioethicists framed disclosing cancer as "truth telling."

- As a medical resident eager to espouse the ethical principles of my profession, I strongly advocated for patient participation in decision making. However, I experienced an elderly male patient with terminal, metastatic cancer who also was mildly demented. Physicians are taught to help orient patients each day, and I would daily remind the patient where he was at, and that he was in the hospital for treatment of cancer. Every day he seemed to forget discussions from the previous day. His granddaughter, who was very involved in his care, one day took me aside and asked me to stop emphasizing cancer to her grandfather every day as she felt it unnecessary and emotionally difficult for him. This greatly tempered my view about the mantra of compelling patients to face cancer.

- Cognizant of differences between Japan and the United States, and eager to do research in Japan, I received funding to examine cancer communication in Japan in the 1990s. I soon realized that it was very awkward for me to discuss with doctors about their experiences diagnosing and treating patients using the language of "truth telling" as it implicated those who did not reveal cancer to be "liars," language not conducive to investigating the topic in Japan. I switched my language to that used in Japan, gan kokuchi, namely, "cancer disclosure."

- During my research, I encountered a Japanese breast surgeon who had trained in the United States. When discussing my project with him, he said that after he returned to Japan after his U.S. training, he felt strongly about the importance of the Western approach to full disclosure and informed consent. But after he disclosed the diagnosis of breast cancer to a patient who had a very early, completely curable tumor, he learned that shortly later she later committed suicide by self-immolation. His story chilled my naive belief about the unequivocal appropriateness of a Western approach to cancer disclosure in Japan.

- My experiences strongly influenced a research interest in prevention and early detection of cancer, as well as optimizing palliative care at the end of life.

- As a clinically active family physician, I have seen a number of patients who have both benefited from advances in cancer treatment and those who have succumbed and experienced palliative care. But the process has often been complicated both for cases that were cured and cases that received palliative care and succumbed to cancer, including my father.

- All these experiences have left me with strong clinical, teaching, and research interests in cancer prevention and early detection, cancer communication, and palliative care.

Why Does Conducting a Personal Inventory Matter?

In the Workbox Illustration 4.1.1 example, you can see why I personally would have an interest in the spectrum of prevention and early detection, cross-cultural approaches to communication, and enhancing transitions to palliative care for cancer patients. These have been dominant themes in my teaching and research career. As illustrated in Story From the Field 4.1, conducting a review of my own personal reflections led to epiphany on the value for the research process of understanding personal bias. I was collaborating with a colleague from Japan on a cross-cultural project on the topic of approaches to cancer disclosure in the United States and Japan. The process of independent self-reflection, and then candid discussion, helped us to understand that we were thinking about our cross-cultural work from very different perspectives. Ultimately, this enabled us to use our biases to more thoroughly look at the findings. For more examples of authors who have been self-reflective, and discovered those influences, see Crabtree and Miller's (1999) book, *Doing Qualitative Research*.

STORY FROM THE FIELD 4.1
EPIPHANY OF THE VALUE OF A PERSONAL BACKGROUND INVENTORY IN CROSS-CULTURAL CANCER RESEARCH

Shortly after I took my first faculty position after training as a researcher, I engaged in a cross-cultural research project with a similarly junior colleague from Japan. As we were preparing for the project, we underwent a personal inventory review as illustrated in Workbox Illustration 4.1.1. (Of course, I do not have the same perspectives now as then as my life has continued to change.) After we both independently completed our respective personal inventories, we reflected together about what we had learned. As we sought to frame our thoughts relative to the topic at hand, approaches to cancer communication, I told my colleague rather bluntly, "My review leads me to wanting to know why doctors in Japan do not tell patients they have cancer." He responded almost equally bluntly, "I am interested in why and how doctors in America tell patients they have cancer." While I had read about the importance of a personal inventory, and how we all have personal lenses about the work we do, I credit this as my first epiphany about (1) how much my own experiences were influencing my interests in the topic, and (2) how we could use our mutual biases (his perspective about how and why doctors disclose cancer to patients in the United States, and my bias to understand why doctors in Japan do not disclose cancer) to conduct more balanced and comprehensive cross-cultural comparative research.

Activity: Identifying Your Personal Background Influences

Workbox 4.1.2 is designed to engage you in thinking about your own background knowledge. Record what background knowledge—for example, personal experiences, professional learning, and occupational experiences—that you can foresee as *potentially* having an impact on your work. As an activity, jot down some notes of key experiences or events, and then expand them into a longer document using a word-processing program. Recall personal experiences, family experiences, or other experiences of close family, friends, or acquaintances that were memorable, inspirational, or traumatic, or some combination thereof. List courses you have taken, films you have seen, books you have read, and documentaries that you have watched. If you are an experienced researcher, cite previous research or articles you have read or perhaps written yourself. While not an exhaustive list, all of these previous experiences contribute to your background influences.

There is no one "correct" way to do a personal inventory, but it does require honest, personal reflection to probe below the surface and reflect about what you bring to the project. You can compose this using a bullet format or using a narrative format. The only constraining factor is your ability to recognize experiences that have influenced your worldview. Some scholars characterize a personal inventory as leading to an understanding, when you are conducting your project of "What is you in the data, and what are the data?" In other words, are you just confirming your own ideas and preconceptions, or are you truly letting the data "speak" such that a story can emerge? The process needs to occur among team members. The process can begin by one team member discussing reflections from the review with others asking questions framed by the potential impact on the research. Done well, the process takes time. There is no substitute.

Workbox 4.1.2: Identifying Your Personal Background Influences

THEORETICAL AND CONCEPTUAL MODELS

Generally, theoretical and conceptual models are assumptions about the characteristics of a topic or phenomenon. Simply stated, these provide ideas about how something works. Theoretical and conceptual models are distinguishable, but how they differ depends in part on conventions and "standards," explicit or implicit, in your own field (Nilsen, 2015). One interpretation of the defining features of theory is that it "is (a) 'a set of interrelated propositions, concepts, and definitions that present a systematic point of view'; (b) specifies relationships between / among concepts; and (c) explains and / or makes predictions about the occurrence of events, based on the specified relationships" (Imenda, 2014). In contrast, characteristics of a conceptual model are that it is (a) an organized presentation of theoretical terms and ideological conflicts, (b) an image or symbolic representation of a phenomenon that is frequently context specific, and (c) a complex mental formulation that conveys abstract ideas. Conceptual models are often associated with qualitative inquiry, while theoretical models are often, but not exclusively, associated with quantitative theory (Imenda, 2014).

The Office of Behavioral and Social Sciences Research (OBSSR) at the National Institutes of Health (NIH) in the United States is charged with enhancing, coordinating, and communicating health-related behavioral and social sciences research. The OBSSR released in 2011 "Best Practices for Mixed Methods Research in the Health Sciences" with the purpose of guiding the rigorous development and evaluation of MMR applications. This was updated with a second edition in 2018 when the OBSSR reported that the guideline was its most accessed link (NIH Office of Behavioral and Social Sciences, 2018). In the guideline, theory is defined to be ". . . a set of interrelated concepts, definitions, and propositions that explain or predict events or situations by specifying relations among variables" (NIH Office of Behavioral and Social Sciences, 2018). Rather than being construed as universal laws of science, theories are expected to be applied and work in a rather limited range of settings. Given the blurry line between the use of theoretical and conceptual, for the remainder of this chapter, I will use the language of theoretical model to refer to both theoretical and conceptual models.

Theory: The Specific and the General

Theoretical models may fall under broad frameworks (larger overviews or outlines with general ideas at the societal) or serve as middle-range theories (more specific in focus on particular phenomenon). Some examples of broad theoretical frameworks are feminist theory, critical theory, complexity theory, a theory of justice, or ecological theory. H. Russell Bernard, in the field of cultural anthropology, describes a spectrum of middle-range theories from idiographic or elemental theories that account for a single "case," meaning a single study, to nomothetic theories that account for multiple cases. Figure 4.1 represents a conceptual presentation of this continuum. Idiographic refers to theory that has been based on a specific population or cultural sharing group. Nomothetic accounts for facts in many cases. Bernard (1995) suggests that the more cases a theory accounts for, the more nomothetic it will be. Hence, it may be helpful to conceptualize theory along a continuum with the most applied, being idiographic, and as there are more cases that the theory applies to, the more nomothetic. For example, Bernard illustrates how multiple idiographic theories about paying a dowry that were group specific evolved to become nomothetic over time as they came together to form a more generally applicable theory.

FIGURE 4.1   ■   The Spectrum of Theory From More Specific to More Generalizable

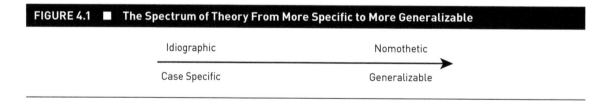

As in the Bernard example, theory is often field specific and context specific. For example, the Health Belief Model grew from problems the Public Health Service in the United States encountered from 1950 to 1960 with people being reluctant to accept preventive services for problems such as tuberculosis, cervical cancer, dental disease, rheumatic fever, polio, and influenza (Rosenstock, 1974). The Health Belief Model is one of several theories, such as the transtheoretical model, social cognitive theory, and the ecological model, that are frequently used in public health and health-promotion interventions (Glanz & Bishop, 2010). The stress process model has been used by Israel and colleagues in community-based participatory research (Israel et al., 2006). A number of theories, models, and frameworks have come to be used in the field of implementation science (Nilsen, 2015). The American Educational Research Association has numerous special interest groups, each centered on a specific theory (Johnson & Christensen, 2014). For example, social development theory (Bandura, 1971; Vygotsky,

1978) and unified learning theory (Shell et al., 2010) are two examples of theory used in educational research. Organizational theory is an example of theory used in business research (Jones, 2012). For examples of reviews of use of theory in business, the interested reader may refer to Armenakis and Bedeian (1999) regarding organizational change, or Yuki (1989) for a review of managerial leadership. There are numerous other theories, and many yet to be conceived—perhaps even yours!

Examples of Theory Use in Empirical Mixed Methods Research Studies

In your mixed methods project, you may engage in constructing and testing or justifying a theory (Johnson & Christensen, 2017). Another relatively common procedure is to use MMR research to adapt an existing model into a new sociocultural context and sometimes new languages. A theoretical framework can be used as an overarching stance for conducting MMR. Mixed methods researchers my use an inductive approach to develop theory qualitatively and then test it quantitatively, or take a qualitatively developed theory and deductively test the theory quantitatively (see Chapter 10).

Theory can be used as the rationale for conducting and/or implementing, or framing the analysis and presenting the research. Workbox Illustration 4.2.1 provides three examples of how theory has been used in mixed methods studies. In a business example, Sharma & Vredenburg (1998) used an interpretation of competitive theory to examine linkages between environmental responsiveness strategies and the emergence of competitively valuable organizational capabilities. As an educational research example, in his project, "Exploring the role of the principal in creating a culture of academic optimism: a sequential QUAN to QUAL mixed methods study," Harper predicated his research on a model of academic optimism that was formulated based on the three constructs of faculty trust, collective efficacy, and academic emphasis (Hoy, Tarter, & Hoy, 2006). Harper further used multiple theories to justify, organize, and execute the research process. For example, he used theory of organizational culture, theory of social capital, theory of efficacy, theory of organizational effectiveness, theory of transformational leadership, as well as academic optimism (Harper, 2016). In a health sciences example, Kron et al. (2017) utilized multimedia learning and interactive instructional theory (Domagk, Schwartz, & Plass, 2010; Sorden, 2012) to inform their approach to the design of an interactive virtual human system.

Workbox Illustrations 4.2.1: Theory Use in the Three Exemplar Projects

Field	Example of Role Theory Played in Selected Mixed Methods Research Studies	Discussion of Theory Tenets
Business (Sharma & Vredenburg, 1998)	Examined the validity of theory hypothesizing linkages between environmental responsiveness strategies and the emergence of competitively valuable organizational capabilities.	The resource-based view of the firm is an interpretation of competitive theory of the firm (Barney & Zajac, 1994) and argues that a firm's competitive strategies and performance depend significantly upon firm-specific organizational resources and capabilities (Hart, 1995).
Education Harper (2016)	Used theoretical considerations as both the rationale undergirding the study and for implementation to justify, organize, and execute the research process.	Academic optimism is based on the three constructs of faculty trust, collective efficacy, and academic emphasis (Hoy, Tarter, & Hoy, 2006). As defined by Harper (2016), it is a set of beliefs comprised of three sub-constructs: (1) collective efficacy—the view that faculty can even teach the most challenging students; (2) faculty trust—the notion that faculty trust students and parents, and; (3) academic emphasis—the idea that faculty prioritize academics.
Health sciences (Kron et al., 2017)	The system was grounded in two theories: the theory of multimedia learning and the interactive instructional approach	Multimedia learning holds that people learn better through words and pictures than through either alone (Sorden, 2012). The interactive instructional approach emphasizes a dynamic relationship between the learner and the learning system, and it integrates system-based elements to engage behavioral, cognitive, and emotional activities of the learner (Domagk, Schwartz, & Plass, 2010).

Activity: Identifying the Potential Role of Theory/Conceptual Models

In Workbox 4.2.2, identify what role you see for theory or a conceptual model in your project, and explain how. Review the examples from Workbox Illustrations 4.2.1. Do you see this work as generating theory, constructing and testing theory, adapting an existing theory for a new sociocultural context, justifying an existing theory, or just using the theory? Are you taking an existing theory that has been developed and tested in one sociocultural group and seeking to adapt the theory for a different sociocultural group? Or, if using theory, do you see its use as an overall justification of the mixed methods project? Can you envision how to use theory in the mixed methods design, sampling, data collection, analysis, interpretation, and presentation of findings?

Workbox 4.2.2: Identifying the Potential Role of Theory or a Conceptual Model

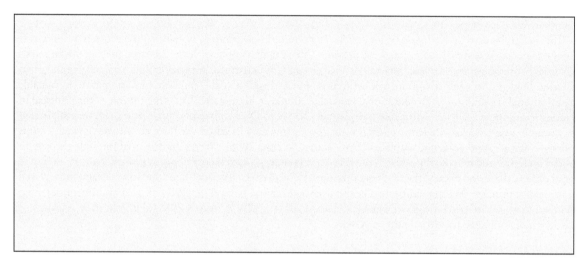

Identifying a Theoretical/Conceptual Model

As with many other aspects of the research design process, the best way to identify a theoretical/conceptual model for your MMR project is through reading the literature about other research projects in your field. A mixed methods workshop participant shared an efficient strategy. She advised using an online search engine, restrict the search to images, and then type in the topic of interest. The search yields figures of theoretical models (as well as unrelated media as well). But I can vouch for its effectiveness for an initial search that needs to be supplemented with reading of the original source material. You may also want to reflect on your personal inventory and how it can help identify a model. For example, my own experiences led me to take an interest in medical ethics and the model of shared decision making (Elwyn et al., 2012).

Many dissertations are expected to include a theory section that situates the research broadly. Moreover, major funding agencies, and specifically committees that review grants, typically expect for the author to articulate a specific theoretical or conceptual model, and illustrate how the model will be utilized (NIH Office of Behavioral and Social Sciences Research, 2018). These ideas weigh heavily in the minds of reviewers on committees empowered to assess project proposal quality and advise funding decisions. Hence, it is not just intellectual rumination to consider a model, but practical and critical to identify a theoretical model appropriate for the project. In Workbox 4.3, identify one or more theoretical/conceptual models that you *could* utilize in your project.

Workbox 4.3: Identifying a Specific Theoretical/Conceptual Model for Your Project

```




```

Identifying Strengths and Limitations of the Theoretical/Conceptual Model

In Workbox 4.4, consider what are the potential strengths in the application of the model or models chosen. For example, you note that the proposed theory has been used extensively in the field, and it is widely accepted. Or you feel that progress in the field has been "stuck" for use of the same models, and not developing or applying new models that could address the phenomenon you are interested in addressing, etc. Consider also the potential limitations in the application of the model or models you have chosen. For example, you note that while the proposed theory has been used in your field, it has never been used in your specific content area. Or you feel that the model only partially addresses the phenomenon of interest.

Workbox 4.4: Identifying Potential Strengths and Limitations of the Chosen Theoretical/Conceptual Model

Potential Strengths:

Potential Limitations:

PHILOSOPHICAL ASSUMPTIONS

Philosophical assumptions are beliefs and values about the nature of reality, as well as how one gains knowledge (Plano Clark & Ivankova, 2016). Researchers, regardless of the primary field—for example, business, education, health sciences, and many branches in the social sciences—work within a set of philosophical assumptions about how to do research. One of the most hotly debated issues in the field of MMR has been about the role of philosophical assumptions. As a result, debates about the philosophical underpinnings of MMR subsumed a significant amount of academic discussion in the first decade of publication of the *Journal of Mixed Methods Research*. For example, six editorials have been devoted to discussions about the paradigms in MMR (Fetters & Molina-Azorin, 2017b).

To put the philosophical debate in perspective, in some fields, such as the social sciences, these debates are at the forefront and will require a great deal of reading and thought. Students and scholars need to be prepared to defend their assumptions and position relative to the research. In other disciplines, such as the health sciences, there may be less emphasis, though this may be changing as the second edition of the *Best Practices for Mixed Methods Research in the Health Sciences* emphasizes pragmatism as an underlying philosophy of MMR in the health sciences (NIH Office of Behavioral and Social Science Research, 2018). Regardless of your disciplinary background, it is fair to say that every mixed methods researcher at a minimum needs to understand the fundamentals of the philosophical framing of MMR and consider how philosophical assumptions can impact MMR.

A decade of philosophical detente can be viewed from three perspectives (Plano Clark & Ivankova, 2016). First, qualitative and quantitative paradigms are fundamentally incompatible, and hence, MMR cannot be conducted. This viewpoint, sometimes called the incompatibility thesis, resonates among some critics, while others view that the field has continued to progress despite this critique. For example, David Morgan discussed the use of family resemblances to illustrate the need to tolerate the blurry boundary between qualitative and quantitative paradigms, while also appreciating the value of distinguishing between qualitative and quantitative research (Morgan, 2018). If you espouse this incompatibility thesis viewpoint, you have probably not purchased this workbook!

Second, Plano Clark and Ivankova (2016) illustrate that a single philosophical view can support work in mixed methods. There are multiple philosophical frameworks, pragmatism, participatory/transformative, critical realism, postmodernism, and yinyang, that mixed methodologists have articulated as relevant (Shannon-Baker, 2016; Fetters & Molina-Azorin, 2019). Third, Plano Clark and Ivankova (2016) identify dialectical pluralism as has been articulated by Johnson (2012) to be accepting of different philosophical stances that can coexist when conducting MMR.

Elements of Philosophical Assumptions

To fully understand how philosophical assumptions can influence your own MMR project, an understanding of the elements of philosophical assumptions is needed. An extensive literature has developed about this process. As time permits, delving into this literature is highly advised. As different individuals bring different levels of knowledge about philosophy to their projects, here, the discussion will focus on the most general ideas and, specifically, how they can apply. But be aware that there is much more to know than will be covered in this chapter. For further information about implications of these philosophical assumptions, see Plano Clark and Ivankova (2016). Moreover, Creswell and Plano Clark (2018) developed a useful table for comparing postpositivism, constructivism, transformative, and pragmatism. For purposes of the workbook, I review five dimensions of philosophical assumptions, namely ontology, epistemology, axiology, methodology, and rhetoric.

Ontology in Mixed Methods Research

The term *ontology* is a branch of metaphysics dealing with the theory of being. The word is derived from the Greek *ont* meaning "being" and *logia* meaning "science" or "reason." It is concerned with the nature of being or existing ("ontology," n.d.). Creswell and Plano Clark (2018) frame this as the question, "What is the nature of reality?" On one hand, there is a view that reality is objective and measurable. On the other hand, there is a view that reality is socially constructed by one's lived experience. A mixed methods view acknowledges both realities, one that is objective and measurable within certain contexts, and the other that perceptions of reality are strongly constructed by the one's lived experience.

Epistemology in Mixed Methods Research

The term *epistemology* is derived from the Greek words *epistēmē* meaning "knowledge" and *logos* meaning "science" or "reason" ("epistemology," n.d.). Epistemology thus refers to knowledge and know-how, as well as the nature, origin, and limits of human knowledge. It includes understanding of methods and validity as well as scope. Thus, mixed methods researchers need to ponder what kind of evidence is used to make claims about reality. Creswell and Plano Clark (2018) frame this as the question, "What is the relationship between the researcher and that which is being researched?"

Axiology in Mixed Methods Research

The term *axiology* is derived from the Greek words *axia*, meaning "worth" or value, and *logos*, meaning "science" or "reason" ("axiology," n.d.). Hence, it can be thought of as a theory of value. It refers to the study of value and valuation. In MMR context, axiology refers to the values researchers espouse for learning about reality. Creswell and Plano Clark (2018) frame this as the question, "What is the role of values?"

Methodology in Mixed Methods Research

The term *methodology* is derived from the Latin *methodologia* or French *méthodologie* ("methodology," n.d.). Methodology refers to the system of methods a mixed methods researcher employs when conducting research. It includes the data collection approaches used. Creswell and Plano Clark (2018) frame this as the question, "What is the process of research?"

The Rhetoric in Mixed Methods Research

The term *rhetoric* is derived from the Greek *rhētorikos* and means "eloquently expressed" ("rhetoric," n.d.). Fundamentally, it means to persuade. It is the language of argumentation. In MMR, it refers to how researchers write about their mixed methods studies. In recently published research, McKim (2017) for example illustrated that an integrated mixed methods approach to writing is viewed as having more value than writing only with quantitative language or qualitative language. Hence, the rhetoric refers to the science of writing effectively and persuasively. Creswell and Plano Clark (2018) frame this as the question, "What is the language of the research?"

Having reviewed these five elements, it is apropos to illustrate these elements for seven philosophical frameworks regarded as supportive of MMR: pragmatism, participatory/transformative, critical realism, postmodernism, yinyang, dialectical pluralism, and performative paradigm.

Mixed Methods Stances Relative to Postpositivism and Constructivism

The seven philosophical frameworks—pragmatism, participatory/transformative, critical realism, postmodernism, yinyang, dialectical pluralism, and performative paradigm—fit between the two poles of postpositivism, a philosophical foundation of quantitative research, and constructivism/interpretivism, a philosophical foundation of qualitative research. Figure 4.2 provides a visual illustrating this spectrum. Each can be characterized based on ontological, epistemological, axiological, methodological, and rhetorical facets.

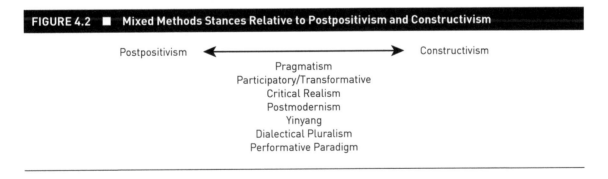

FIGURE 4.2 ■ Mixed Methods Stances Relative to Postpositivism and Constructivism

In the following, I draw from Plano Clark and Ivankova (2016), Shannon-Baker (2016), and Creswell and Plano Clark (2018) to consider each of these philosophical frameworks from the perspectives of ontology, epistemology, axiology, methodology, and rhetoric.

Postpositivism

Postpositivism generally characterizes the philosophical assumptions of a highly quantitatively oriented researcher. Ontologically, a postpositivist researcher assumes that there is a single reality to be proven or discovered. Epistemologically, the researcher assumes that knowledge is acquired from a distance and the observer acts independently. Axiologically, the researcher seeks to conduct research in an unbiased way and control the researcher's bias. Methodologically, the postpositivist researcher commonly applies deductive reasoning, for example, tests *a priori* theory. Rhetorically, the researcher follows a formal, structured, agreed-upon style, and often writes in third person.

Constructivism/Interpretivism

At the other end of the philosophical spectrum resides constructivism/interpretivism. Constructivism/interpretivism generally characterizes the philosophical assumptions of a highly qualitatively oriented researcher. Ontologically, the constructivist researcher assumes that there are multiple realities. Epistemologically, the researcher holds that knowledge is obtained by being close to participants and exploring their world. Axiologically, the researcher considers bias to be natural, to be something that should be discussed and used. Methodologically, the researcher tends to be more inductive and focused on building new patterns and theories. Rhetorically, the researcher prefers a more informal style that is less structured and often written in first person.

Philosophical Assumptions Supporting Mixed Methods Research

With no fewer than seven stances supporting MMR, the extreme differences seen between postpositivism and constructivism/interpretivism seem not to be so stark. That said, there are differences and variations as illustrated by each as follows.

Pragmatism

While others have followed in articulating utility of pragmatism, David Morgan was one of the first to offer a philosophical grounding for mixed methods research in the form of pragmatism (Morgan, 2007). Pragmatic views are common in applied sciences, for example, in health sciences (Curry & Nunez-Smith, 2015). Ontologically, the researcher assumes that there are multiple views of reality. Epistemologically, the researcher assumes that knowledge is gained iteratively using both independent and subjective interpretations. Axiologically, the researcher sees the role of values as useful in the construction of research questions and making conclusions. Methodologically, the researcher collects both qualitative and quantitative data. Rhetorically, the mixed methods researcher employs both writing styles.

Participatory/Transformative

The participatory/transformative framework, also referred to as "transformative/emancipatory" by Shannon-Baker (2016), can commonly be found in community-based participatory research or, as illustrated by Mertens (2007), transformative research and used by activist researchers. This work is often applied when working with marginalized or underprivileged communities. Ontologically, a participatory/transformative researcher assumes that there are diverse realities that are formed through sociopolitical forces. Epistemologically, the researcher holds that knowledge about reality is gained by collaborating with the marginalized or fringe community of interest. Axiologically, the researcher sees the value of both qualitative and quantitative inquiry for framing effective sociopolitical arguments. Methodologically, the researcher may use either carefully mapped-out designs that collect both qualitative and quantitative data, or collect qualitative and quantitative data iteratively in cycles to address salient sociopolitical topics. Rhetorically, the researcher uses a flexible style to illustrate and change oppression and injustice.

Critical Realism

Maxwell and Mittapalli (2010) present a case for critical realism as a philosophical stance for MMR. The researcher who works under the philosophical assumptions of critical realism ontologically views reality as having both a real world and a mental world. Epistemologically, knowledge is constructed by perceptions and perspectives of researchers. Hence, axiologically, the researcher's values are an integral part of the research. Methodologically, the researcher collects both qualitative and quantitative data to carefully consider context and attend to diversity in meaning and contextual influences. Rhetorically, there is a qualitative emphasis to describe context and personal views with quantitative findings used to support the findings.

Postmodernism

Hesse-Biber and Kelly (2010) illustrate relevance of postmodernism and its particular appeal for qualitatively driven mixed methods researchers. A postmodern researcher ontologically assumes that reality is chaotic, disordered, and unstructured. Epistemologically, the researcher assumes different forms of knowledge are equal, regardless of source, and through examining writings and narrative, social structures can best be understood. Axiologically, the researcher espouses that one's own views are important, but no more important than others' values. Methodologically, collection of qualitative and quantitative data are used to challenge existing discourses and stimulate innovative ways of thinking. Rhetorically, the researcher uses qualitative and quantitative structure as needed to critique the status quo.

Yinyang

Yinyang represents an Asian worldview only recently recognized in the literature as a philosophical system of thought supporting MMR (Fetters & Molina-Azorin, 2019). *Yin* with associations of the moon, feminine, dark, and wet fits with a qualitative approach, while *yang* with associations of the sun, male, light, and dry fits with a quantitative approach. When brought together, the resulting whole is greater that the individual parts as symbolized by the *taijitsu* symbol (Figure 4.3). The symbol includes two symbols in the shape of two teardrops together, or two fish swimming in a circle (Wang, 2012). The dark shape represents yin the qualitative, and the white shape represents yang the quantitative. Both shapes have a small dot of the opposite color indicating that each has a component of the opposite.

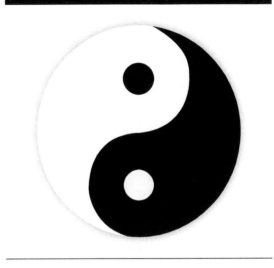

FIGURE 4.3 ■ The *Taijitu* Symbol

When influenced by yinyang philosophy, a researcher ontologically sees in the world a duality of reality as yin and yang that constitute a singular reality together. The qualitative and the quantitative are separate yet simultaneously interconnected and indivisible. Epistemologically, the researcher holds that knowledge comes from that represented by knowing both, and that each are necessary for understanding the oneness or holism of a phenomenon. Axiologically, the researcher values both and the synergism that comes from incorporating both the yin-qualitative and the yang-quantitative parts to understand a mutual interconnected whole. As within yin there exists yang, and within yang there exists yin—within the qualitative, there exists the qualitative, and within the quantitative, there exists the qualitative. Methodologically, the researcher recognizes that in any given investigation, the weighting of the qualitative and quantitative may be equal, or one may be more prominent than the other, though both the qualitative and quantitative are needed to provide an understanding of the whole. Rhetorically, the researcher supports flexibility in presentation with component parts being balanced, while accepting that one component may be more emphasized than the other.

Dialectical Pluralism

A dialectic stance as introduced by Greene (2007), further expanded by Greene and Hall (2010), and expounded as a meta-paradigm by Johnson (2015) provides a view of acceptance and embracing of multiple worldviews. The researcher espousing dialectical pluralism ontologically accepts that there are different approaches to constructing reality. Epistemologically, the researcher assumes that knowledge will be gained through respectful dialogue among different conceptualizations. Axiologically, the researcher values tolerance, acceptance, and equity. Methodologically, the researcher collects both qualitative and quantitative data to examine both convergence and divergence of the findings. Rhetorically, the researcher utilizes the language of both qualitative and quantitative disciplines.

Performative Paradigm

As articulated by Schoonenboom (2017), the performative paradigm provides a view to explore unknown created worlds. In research, through a cycle called a "mangle of practice" (p. 9) or rounds of feedback, the researcher incorporates feedback and adapts the research. While the ontology and epistemology of the performative paradigm stem from dialectical pluralism, the focus on action resembles pragmatism. Hence, when influenced by the performative paradigm, a researcher ontologically assumes multiple realities that can be known and researched differently, and are varied and changing. Epistemologically, the researcher holds that knowledge comes from multiple realities and can be understood in different ways. The temporary and created worlds arise from concepts given to them by researchers who frame them in a specific context in time. Axiologically, the researcher values the development of knowledge from a single reality that is pluralistic. Methodologically, the researcher seeks to create and explore new worlds in a process involving mangles or changes in understanding the trigger switching between the researcher's idea and the reality of the data. Rhetorically, the researcher's task is to articulate a better understanding of a created world. The researcher must speak about a specific concept in a specific context.

Having reviewed major philosophical assumptions that can influence researchers, I provide an example regarding my own position in Workbox Illustration 4.5.1. This box links back to Workbox Illustration 4.1.1 where I laid out a candid assessment using a personal inventory.

Workbox Illustration 4.5.1: Identifying Philosophical Assumptions Consistent With a Personal Worldview for a Mixed Methods Project

Based on the information provided in *Workbox Illustration 4.1.1*, it is clear that I have been influenced strongly by multiple philosophical frameworks. On one hand, my experience in Japan where I witnessed and learned firsthand how personal experiences shape one's worldview, one's values, and one's views about "rights and wrongs" fits well with social constructivism. This also provided my first exposure to a society embedded with yinyang thinking. On the flip side, my training in the basic and clinical sciences in medicine also illustrate for me the value of a postpositivistic stance. Over the decades of my career in medicine and social science, I have seen how advances in medical science based in postpositivism (seemingly invisible to many in the field) have led to greatly enhanced medical outcomes, for example, better survival for cancer patients and improvements in approaches to palliative care, to mention a few. Undoubtedly, both of these experiences led to my pursuit of master's degrees in epidemiology (quantitatively focused) and anthropology/ethics (qualitatively focused). Finally, my training in family medicine, where I routinely rely on the patients' history (words) and the results of medical testing (often numbers but also many results that are text based and descriptive) naturally lends to my embrace of pragmatism. My mutual respect for the differences and similarities of goals, values, methodological stances, and methodologies allows me to take a pluralist ontological stance and desire to learn from differences as is consistent with dialetical pluralism (Johnson, 2012).

Activity: Identifying Philosophical Assumptions Consistent With Your Worldview for Your Mixed Methods Project

Using Workbox Illustration 4.5.1, in Workbox 4.5.2, write what philosophical assumption(s) best fit(s) with your own personal worldview and why. You may have a clear sense based on the information above or previous knowledge. You may want to reflect back on your personal inventory to consider how your own experiences or particular theories may resonate with a particular philosophical stance. Similarly, you may be in a course where the instructor has assigned readings that will assist your thinking about your philosophical assumptions, especially if you are taking a research methods course for a specific field.

Workbox 4.5.2: Identifying Philosophical Assumptions Consistent With Your Worldview for Your Mixed Methods Project

Activity: Explaining How Philosophical Assumptions Fit Your Mixed Methods Project

In Workbox Illustration 4.6.1, I explain my own philosophical assumptions relative to participation in the MPathic-VR mixed methods medical education study (Kron et al., 2017) and provide an example for your reflection.

Workbox Illustrations 4.6.1: Explaining How Philosophical Assumptions Fit With the MPathic-VR Mixed Methods Medical Education Study

Ontology: I acknowledge both a scientific view of the world, that there are universal laws and principles, and objective realities in the physical and biological world. I also embrace a view of multiple realities as social constructions.

Epistemology: I view knowledge as derived through both processes of experimentation using objective measures, as well as through processes of living and knowing based on experience.

Axiology: I value the use of measurement and comparisons of outcomes informed by the science of statistics evidence of an effect of an intervention suffices for me to change my behavior as a family physician. But, I also value the meaning attached by humans to processes and phenomena in the world.

Methodology: I prioritize the use of methods that will answer the compelling questions I seek to answer, including both procedures to quantify aspects of a given phenomenon, as well as approaches useful for describing and understanding human experiences with a phenomenon.

Rhetoric: I respect both traditions of writing in third-person objective language, though I prefer the choice of writing in first and second person to attribute actions to the owners of those actions. I respect the differences in the preferred rhetoric among different fields, while also recognizing the perceived limitations from someone who does not self-affiliate with the conventions of that field.

In Workbox 4.6.2, explain why you see it as a good fit for your project idea. Try to think about the five levels of ontology, epistemology, axiology, methodology, and rhetoric.

Workbox 4.6.2: Explaining How Your Philosophical Assumptions Fit With Your Mixed Methods Project

Ontology:

Epistemology:

Axiology:

Methodology:

Rhetoric:

How Philosophical Assumptions Can Influence a Project

In the workbox below, I illustrate how social constructivism, postpositivism, and pragmatism can and do influence my thinking, a pattern most consistent with dialectical pluralism. This snippet is actually grounded in a true story as I was a Fulbright researcher in 1992 for 3 months in Japan when I conducted a series of qualitative interviews with physicians (Fetters, Elwyn, Sasaki, & Tsuda, 2000). This study was followed by a study led by a medical student I was supervising, Todd Elwyn, who distributed a survey built in part from the findings of the interview data (Elwyn, Fetters, Sasaki, & Tsuda, 2002).

Workbox Illustration 4.7.1: How Philosophical Assumptions Can Influence a Project

Philosophical framework: Dialectical pluralism (social constructivism and postpositivism)

1. **Research questions:** In formulating a cross-cultural perspective on physician approaches to cancer disclosure in another country, I might be interested in learning how sociocultural factors influence physician decision making about this question (social constructivism), but I would also be interested in larger patterns and predictors of specific cancer disclosure behaviors (postpositivism).

2. **Design:** In designing a mixed methods project, I might favor a qualitatively driven approach (social constructivism) and start with exploring sociocultural patterns and then follow this up with a quantitative strand of research to look at larger patterns (postpositivism).

   Note: This is called an exploratory sequential design as explained in Chapter 7

3. **Sampling:** For the initial qualitative strand, I might employ maximum variation sampling to get a full range of opinions (social constructivism), while for the subsequent quantitative strand I might use a power calculation to determine sample and utilize stratified random sampling to ensure my results are generalizable. (See Chapter 9 on sampling.)

4. **Data collection:** For the qualitative strand, I might propose depth interviews with 10-20 individuals and use saturation as my criteria cessation of data collection for the initial qualitative strand (social constructivism). I would then use these results to build a survey for use in the quantitative phase to measure the prevalence of the qualitatively identified patterns in a larger population (postpositivism).

5. **Analysis:** For the initial qualitative phase, I would conduct the data collection and analysis iteratively doing just a couple of interviews at a time, and reformulating my interview guide as the project progressed (social constructivism). For the subsequent quantitative component, I would identify usual practice of cancer communication, disclosing or not disclosing, and then look for predictors (postpositivism).

6. **Interpretation:** As I would be using a sequential design, I would complete my iterative data collection and iterative analysis of the qualitative strand first as I formulate a conceptual (idiographic) model (social constructivism). As the subsequent quantitative survey strand would be designed using the concepts from the qualitative strand, I would examine the quantitative data to confirm/disconfirm the formulated model (postpositivism). The broad, generalized findings may help move the conceptual model to become more nomothetic.

7. **Presentation:** I would publish initially the qualitative findings using thick, rich description of factors physicians consider in their cancer communication decision making (social constructivism), and then publish a second paper about the quantitative survey findings (postpositivism). Moreover, to emphasize the research used an overarching mixed methods approach, I would heavily reference the findings of the first paper in the second paper in both the introduction to the study and in the final discussion, where I would reconsider the survey findings relative to the extent they confirmed, expanded, disconfirmed, or contradicted the findings of the initial qualitative strand. Alternatively, the breadth of data might support a mixed methods paper where the qualitative and quantitative findings all came together about areas of commonality.

Activity: Identifying How Your Philosophical Assumptions Could Influence Your Project

As philosophical assumptions are central to your project, you should be able to articulate their relevance. Using as a reference Workbox Illustration 4.7.1, in Workbox 4.7.2, think of and record ways that your worldview could influence how you (will) conduct your project. Think of all the levels of the project, including the framing of the research questions, the design, sampling, data collection, analysis, interpretation, and presentation.

Activity: Identifying Potential Limitations of Your Philosophical Assumptions

As philosophical assumptions are central to your project, you must be able to not only articulate their relevance but also be prepared to defend your position. Using Workbox Illustration 4.8.1 as an example, in Workbox 4.8.2, record ways that your worldview could be viewed as a limitation regarding how you (will) conduct the project.

Workbox 4.7.2: Identifying How Philosophical Assumptions Could Influence Your Project

Philosophical framework:

1. **Research questions:**

2. **Design:**

3. **Sampling:**

4. **Data collection:**

5. **Analysis:**

6. **Interpretation:**

7. **Presentation:**

Workbox Illustration 4.8.1: Identifying Potential Limitations of Your Philosophical Assumptions

The risk of espousing social constructivism could be the critique that the qualitative data were not thick enough and not supplemented with the depth that a social constructivist would seek through other means of data collection—for example, observations, document analysis, contemporary or historical depictions in cinema, etc. The flip side could be criticism that forms a postpositivistic perspective that the methods could be more rigorous, or on a larger scale. Dialectical pluralism allows me to bridge the gap.

Workbox 4.8.2: Identifying Potential Limitations of Your Philosophical Assumptions

Application Activities

1. **Peer Feedback**. If you are working on your project as part of a class or in a workshop, please pair up with a peer mentor, and each spend about 5 minutes talking about your personal contexts. Rather than focus on the element that was easiest, focus on the component that was most difficult. If struggling with an element of the personal model (e.g., theory or philosophical), ask your instructor, advisor, or colleague about theory and philosophical stances in your field. If you are working independently, share your ideas with a colleague or mentor for each section.

2. **Peer Feedback Guidance**. As you listen to your partner, focus on learning and honing the valuable skills of critiquing. Help your partner refine the influences of personal models on their research. Help your partner focus on the level or area where your partner needs feedback the most.

3. **Group Debrief**. If you are in a classroom or large group setting, take volunteers to present their personal models. Reflect on how these same questions may play out in your own project.

Concluding Thoughts

Use this checklist to assess your progress in achieving the Chapter 4 objectives:

☐ I reflected about how my personal context is comprised of influences from my background, theoretical models, and philosophical assumptions.

☐ I identified how my own personal experiences, values, and training cumulatively have produced my personal background and how it impacts my research or evaluation project.

☐ I explored the value of theoretical models, learned a process for identifying one appropriate to my mixed methods project, and considered how to apply it.

☐ I examined multiple philosophical stances, considered my own, and considered how my assumptions can influence my MMR project.

☐ I discussed my worldviews with a partner to consider areas that were unclear, and I provided feedback to help my peer's consideration of the three levels of the personal contexts model.

Now that you have completed these objectives, Chapter 5 will help you frame the background, objectives, and questions for your MMR or evaluation project.

Key Resources

1. **FURTHER READING ON PERSONAL MODELS**

   - Finlay, L. (2002). "Outing" the researcher: The provenance, process, and practice of reflexivity. *Qualitative Health Research, 12*, 531–545. doi: 10.1177/104973202129120052.

   - Greene, J. C. (2007). *Mixed methods in social inquiry.* San Francisco, CA: Jossey-Bass.

   - Plano Clark, V. L., & Ivankova, N. V. (2016). How do personal contexts shape mixed methods research? In: *Mixed methods research: A guide to the field*. Thousand Oaks, CA: Sage.

2. **FURTHER READING ON THEORETICAL MODELS**

   - Imenda, S. (2014). Is there a conceptual difference between theoretical and conceptual frameworks? *Journal of Social Sciences, 38*, 185–195.

   - Nilsen, P. (2015). Making sense of implementation theories, models and frameworks. *Implementation Science, 10*, 53. doi:10.1186/s13012-015-0242-0

   - U.S. Department of Health and Human Services (2005). *Theory at a glance: A guide for health promotion practice* (2nd ed.). Washington, DC: National Cancer Institute, National Institutes of Health. NIH Pub. No. 05-3896.

3. **FURTHER READING ON PHILOSOPHICAL MODELS.**

   - Creswell, J. W., & Plano Clark, V. L. (2011). The foundations of mixed methods research. In *Designing and conducting mixed methods research* (2nd ed., pp 19–52). Thousand Oaks, CA: Sage.

   - Johnson, R. B. (2015). Dialectical pluralism. *Journal of Mixed Methods Research, 11*, 156–173. doi:10.1177/1558689815607692

   - Plano Clark, V. L., & Ivankova, N. V. (2016). How do personal contexts shape mixed methods research? In *Mixed methods research: A guide to the field*. Thousand Oaks, CA: Sage.

   - Shannon-Baker, P. (2016). Making paradigms meaningful in mixed methods research. *Journal of Mixed Methods Research, 10*, 319–334. doi: 10.1177/1558689815575861

DEVELOPING THE BACKGROUND, RESEARCH OBJECTIVES, AND RESEARCH QUESTIONS FOR A MIXED METHODS RESEARCH PROJECT

Experienced researchers recognize how the entirety of mixed projects emanate from the research questions, hypotheses, and specific aims. Devoting careful consideration and development of the research questions, hypotheses, and specific aims may seem a formidable task. This chapter and its activities will help you develop a concise summary of the overarching context for the project topic, elucidate a gap or problem from the literature justifying a mixed methods project, identify a primary objective to pursue in the project, and develop research questions appropriate for your mixed methods project. As a key outcome, you will develop the background information that can serve as a key component of a mixed methods research (MMR) proposal, protocol, and future manuscripts.

LEARNING OBJECTIVES

To help you articulate the rationale and focus of your MMR or evaluation project, the ideas and activities here will help you

- Provide a concise summary of the overarching context of your topic from the literature
- Elucidate a focused problem or gap from the literature that justifies a mixed methods project
- Identify a primary objective to pursue in your mixed methods project
- Develop research questions appropriate for your mixed methods project

DEVELOPING THE BACKGROUND OF MIXED METHODS RESEARCH AND EVALUATION PROJECTS

All published research projects, MMR projects included, are conducted within the context of a larger body of academic literature. For the purposes of this chapter, the **background** refers to the context of the project, usually some **gap in the literature**, and your study objective. You need to articulate the background for two reasons: first, to illustrate that the proposed work has not been done before, and second, to illustrate why addressing the identified research gap would matter.

SITUATING THE PROJECT IN THE BROADER LITERATURE OF THE FIELD

Four Levels in the Background

In the background section of publications in the social sciences, health sciences, and business, authors typically begin by situating the phenomenon of study in the broader literature. This first level gives an **overarching context**. In a short summary such as an abstract, this may involve only one or two lines. While highly dependent upon the field, the length in articles may range from one to several paragraphs or even pages. The following references to length are assuming about a 3,000 to 4,000 word paper.

The second level narrows or tapers specifically to ideas and literature for a specific context. The argumentation should focus on finding a gap or need in the literature. In an abstract or short summary, this may be only a sentence. In a longer paper, this will comprise only one or two paragraphs.

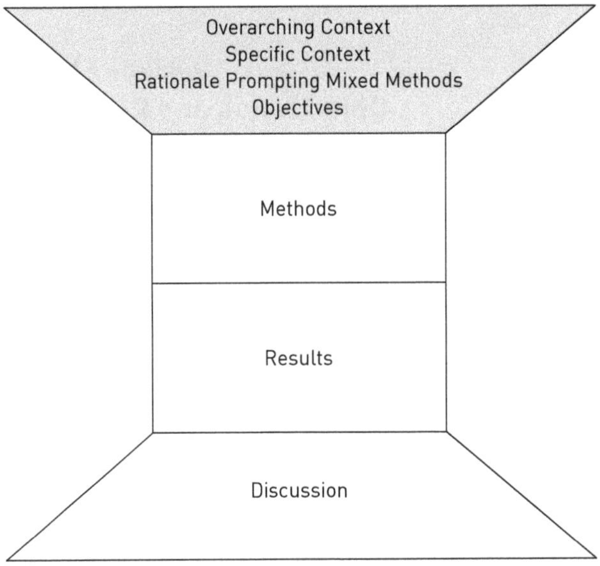

The third level tapers down to the specific scope or relevance of the research or evaluation project. In mixed methods studies, the written text will narrowly focus on the rationale for collecting both qualitative and quantitative research or evaluation study. In an abstract or short summary, it will be a single statement that may be organized as an extension of the second level. In a full article, this will comprise about a single paragraph that ideally will articulate the need for both the qualitative and quantitative data collection proposed (in the order appropriate for the project).

The fourth level becomes the narrowest, and it focuses on the project objectives or purpose. The bottommost point represents the focused MMR objective and research questions. In the study abstract or summary, there should be a clear statement about the purpose. Often it will be the same statement in the abstract and the background of the article.

Some researchers use the image of a funnel, or the top globe of an hourglass (Figure 5.1). As will be seen in Chapter 18, there is a **hourglass design model of writing**. This chapter concerns the broad top and how it narrows down to mixed methods project questions. Below the broad top, as will be shown in Chapter 18, the hourglass model has a narrowly focused section on the methods, a narrowly focused section on the results, and a base that is a mirror image of the top that begins narrowly, and then expands broadly. For now, your focus should be on the top background information.

FIGURE 5.1 ■ The Background Section

Overarching Context
Specific Context
Rationale Prompting Mixed Methods
Objectives

Methods

Results

Discussion

Example of the Four Levels

When constructing the research background, think of the purpose of your research. If your design is to focus on developing a new instrument by qualitative exploration, building, and testing quantitatively of a novel research instrument, the background section would broadly need to speak to the general context in the field as contained in the literature and justify the research. You would then consider the more narrowly related literature. For example, in one project, we were interested in measuring health care quality, but we were unable to find previous instruments in the languages needed for the study (Hammoud et al., 2012). By virtue of not being culturally and linguistically adapted, existing instruments were problematic. This then naturally led to qualitatively exploring what needed to be adapted (Abdelrahim et al., 2017; Killawi et al., 2014), and building content based on qualitative research, which led to a refined instrument that could be distributed.

Conducting a Literature Review

If you have completed the literature review activity of Chapter 3, it will be relatively easy to complete the worksheet. Highly experienced researchers who have published extensively know well the literature that informs their projects and require less time reviewing the literature, whereas novices will spend significant time conducting a literature review and absorbing the implications. As discussed in Chapter 3, the background section needs to answer relatively simple questions, "What is known about this particular topic already?" and "Why is there a gap or problem based on the existing literature?" By focusing on these two simple questions, it will make the work of developing the background of your MMR project much easier.

Activity: Developing the Mixed Methods Research Project Background Page

Using Workbox Illustration 5.1.1 example as a reference, complete Workbox 5.1.2, the background page. Bearing in mind the hourglass model of the MMR design, provide in the proposal sufficient information to justify the need for both the qualitative and quantitative strands.

The MPathic-VR example in Workbox Illustration 5.1.1 represents the second phase in a mixed methods program of research. The project involved experts from medical education, health sciences, business, psychology, computer science, and many others (Appendix 3). A substantive body of research illustrates that communication is the most important aspect of the doctor–patient relationship, yet educators face serious challenges in teaching medical communication. While virtual humans are a recent technological innovation for simulation in education, little previous research examines the utility of virtual human programming to teach communication skills. In this research, we posed mixed methods questions and examined them in an MMR trial (Kron et al., 2017).

Workbox Illustration 5.1.1: Title, Background, Objective(s), and Research Questions of the MPathic-VR Mixed Methods Medical Education Study*

Title: Teaching Advanced Communication Using a Virtual Human: A Mixed Methods Trial
Author(s): Kron, Fetters, Scerbo, White, Lypson, Padilla, Gliva-McConvey, Belfore II, West, Wallace, Guetterman, Schleicher, Kennedy, Mangrulkar, Cleary, Marsella, Becker
Context of Your Project: Communication is the most important component of the doctor-patient encounter. Communication between doctor and patient is a complex phenomenon with many different factors interacting simultaneously, so effective communication assessment and training are correspondingly complex, especially for the teaching of empathy. Teachers of doctor-patient communication would benefit from additional educational tools.
Gap in the Literature: Virtual humans are intelligent conversational agents with human appearance and the capacity to interact using a wide range of communication behaviors that one would expect in face-to-face conversations between humans. Despite the promise virtual humans offer for teaching empathy and advanced communication skills, evidence for the effectiveness of interventions to improve skills in a simulation is lacking. Moreover, evidence that skills from a virtual human training program transfer to a realistic clinical care scenario is missing. Researchers need to understand student attitudes toward such technology, and why they feel that way.
General Objective: The purpose of this research is to determine whether MPathic-VR is effective for teaching advanced communication skills, and why.
Qualitative, Quantitative, and Mixed Methods Research Questions: **Quantitative:** *Will students who are exposed to a virtual human computer simulation perform better in a clinically realistic scenario than students who are exposed to a computer-based learning module control?* **Qualitative:** *What are the experiences of medical students who use virtual human training to learn communication skills?* **Mixed methods research question:** *How do qualitative findings from students' reflective comments and responses to a quantitative attitudinal survey compare between students in the interactive virtual human intervention and students who take a computer-based learning module?*
Revised Title: *Using a Computer Simulation for Teaching Communication Skills: A Blinded Multisite Mixed Methods Randomized Controlled Trial*

*This example was written for illustrative purposes and does not necessarily reflect the full details and specifics of the actual project.
Source: Kron et al. (2017).

When working on the background section in Workbox 5.1.2, progressively, fill in the working title, context, gap/problem, general research objective(s), research questions, and revised title.

Workbox 5.1.2: Developing the Title, Background, Objectives, and Questions of the Mixed Methods Research Project Proposal

Title:
Author(s):
Context of Your Project:
Gap in the Literature:
General Objective(s):
Qualitative, Quantitative, and Mixed Methods Research Questions:
Revised Title:

DEVELOPING A WORKING TITLE

Developing a **working title** is a process (recall Figure 2.1). Almost invariably, people change their titles after working on their methods. Getting a title down helps think of a name for the project. Be as parsimonious as possible but still include the major topic addressed, participants, and location of project. You will want to convey that it is a mixed methods study by either including the words *mixed methods* in the title or language that speaks to including both qualitative and quantitative data collection. While *qualitative* as a word often appears in titles, *quantitative* appears less frequently. If you already know it (but you are not expected to at this point in the workbook), include wording that explains the specific type of mixed methods design you use. Don't worry about getting it perfect, but get something down so that you and others can critique and assess how well it reflects your proposal. Table 5.1 provides several examples of mixed methods titles from published research.

TABLE 5.1 ■ Examples of Mixed Methods Titles From Published Research	
Titles	**References**
Business	
Proactive Corporate Environmental Strategy and the Development of Competitively Valuable Organizational Capabilities	Sharma, S., & Vredenburg, H. (1998). Proactive corporate environmental strategy and the development of competitively valuable organizational capabilities. *Strategic Management Journal, 19*, 729–753.

(Continued)

TABLE 5.1 ■ (Continued)	
Titles	**References**
Business	
Combining Quantitative and Qualitative Methodologies in Logistics Research	Mangan, J., Lalwani, C., & Gardner, B. (2004). Combining quantitative and qualitative methodologies in logistics research. *International Journal of Physical Distribution & Logistics Management, 34*(7), 565–578.
Mixed Methods in International Business Research: A Value-Added Perspective	Hurmerinta-Peltomäki, L., & Nummela, N. (2006). Mixed methods in international business research: A value-added perspective. *Management International Review, 46*(4), 439–459.
Field of Education	
Exploring the Role of the Principal in Creating a Culture of Academic Optimism: A Sequential QUAN to QUAL Mixed Methods Study	Harper, W. A. (2016). *Exploring the role of the principal in creating a culture of academic optimism: A sequential QUAN to QUAL mixed methods study* (Dissertation). University of Alabama, Birmingham.
Students' Persistence in a Distributed Doctoral Program in Educational Leadership in Higher Education: A Mixed Methods Study	Ivankova, N. V., & Stick, S. L. (2007). Students' persistence in a distributed doctoral program in educational leadership in higher education: A mixed methods study. *Research in Higher Education, 48*(1), 93.
A Mixed-Methods Explanatory Study of the Failure Rate for Freshman STEM Calculus Students	Worthley, M. R., Gloeckner, G. W., & Kennedy, P. A. (2016). A mixed-methods explanatory study of the failure rate for freshman STEM calculus students. *PRIMUS, 26*(2), 125–142.
A Comparative Study of Behavioural and Emotional Problems Among Children Living in Orphanages in Ghana: A Mixed Method Approach	Boadu, O. S. (2015). *A comparative study of behavioural and emotional problems among children living in orphanages in Ghana: A mixed method approach* (Doctoral dissertation, University of Ghana).
Health-Related Example	
Using a Computer Simulation for Teaching Communication Skills: A Blinded Multisite Mixed Methods Randomized Controlled Trial	Kron, et al. (2017). Using a computer simulation for teaching communication skills: A blinded multisite mixed methods randomized controlled trial. *Patient Education and Counseling, 100*(4), 748–759. doi:10.1016/j.pec.2016.10.024
The Cultural Context of Teaching and Learning Sexual Health Care Examinations in Japan: A Mixed Methods Case Study Assessing the Use of Standardized Patient Instructors Among Japanese Family Physician Trainees of the Shizuoka Family Medicine Program	Shultz, C. G., Chu, M. S., Yajima, A., Skye, E. P., Sano, K., Inoue, M., Tsuda, T., & Fetters, M. D. (2015). The cultural context of teaching and learning sexual health care examinations in Japan: A mixed methods case study assessing the use of standardized patient instructors among Japanese family physician trainees of the Shizuoka Family Medicine Program. *Asia Pacific Family Medicine, 14*, 8. doi:10.1186/s12930-015-0025-4
Health-Related Quality of Life in Patients With Serious Non-specific Symptoms Undergoing Evaluation for Possible Cancer, and Their Experience During the Process: A Mixed Methods Study	Moseholm, E., Rydahl-Hansen, S., Lindhardt, B. O., & Fetters, M. D. (2017). Health-related quality of life in patients with serious nonspecific symptoms undergoing evaluation for possible cancer and their experience during the process: A Mixed methods study. *Quality of Life Research, 26*(4), 993–1006. doi:10.1007/s11136-016-1423-2

SUMMARIZING THE OVERARCHING CONTEXT

This describes the literature that informs your topic. It is the most general level of background. Based on the hourglass design model, you will want to focus on literature in the broader context. Depending upon the project topic and research focus, you might choose related cultural, economical, educational, political, or social aspects. In educational research, it might be the national scope of the general educational problem. In business, it might be some larger trends in the market. In health sciences research, the focus is often on the epidemiology of an illness or frequency of a problem. Taking this as an example, the title might include a statement about the morbidity and mortality of a selected disease.

You might choose to focus on a problem in health, health services, or health policy. You may select a particular level of focus, for example, individual level, organizational level, community, state, or global level (see Table 5.2). While developing the general statement may sound overwhelming, think about the reasons your audience will perceive your work to have relevance. For example, if your audience will be managers of medium-sized businesses, emphasize literature relevant to them. If your audience will be secondary school educators, highlight an issue of importance to them. If your audience were family medicine and primary care doctors, present a compelling statement about the magnitude of a problem that is important to primary care doctors.

TABLE 5.2 ■ Illustrations of Overarching Context and a Gap in the Literature			
Field	**Reference**	**Overarching Context**	**Gap in the Literature**
Business	Sharma and Vredenburg (1998). Proactive corporate environmental strategy and the development of competitively valuable organizational capabilities. *Strategic Management Journal, 19*, 729–753.	World Commission on Environment and Development has challenged the business community to provide evidence on how and why corporations should incorporate environmental concerns into strategic decision making relative to economic performance.	The arguments linking environmental responsiveness to organizational capabilities and performance have been theoretical, and empirical evidence is needed to demonstrate that investments in environmental practices can yield tangible monetary benefits.
Education	Harper (2016). *Exploring the role of the principal in creating a culture of academic optimism: A sequential QUAN to QUAL mixed methods study* (Dissertation). University of Alabama, Birmingham.	Principals are held accountable for the academic achievement of their students.	Research linking academic optimism and high achievement in low socioeconomic middle schools is needed because the most commonly cited studies have focused on elementary and high schools.
Health services	Kron et al. (2017). Using a computer simulation for teaching communication skills: A blinded multisite mixed methods randomized controlled trial. *Patient Education and Counseling, 100*(4), 748–759. doi:10.1016/j.pec.2016.10.024	Communication is the most important component of the doctor–patient encounter.	Despite the promise virtual humans offer for teaching empathy and advance communication skills, evidence for the effectiveness of interventions to improve skills in a simulation is lacking.

IDENTIFYING A PROBLEM IN THE LITERATURE

This describes the specific problem the literature informs and illustrates why your particular project is justified. It is a subcategory of the literature reviewed in the overarching background. Most research teams seek to make a difference with their findings. When considering the research design, think how the project could address the identified problem. That is, how could the current situation improve if there were research findings you hope to generate? What type of difference might you expect?

Writing a Justification Statement

Many participants in workshops and my graduate course on MMR have found "model scripts" to be useful in writing their justification statements. Workbox 5.2 provides scripts of various forms of rationales for mixed methods projects that can be grounded to a deficit in the literature. The rationale may be characterized as a "gap" or "deficiency." You might note that the existing literature has limitations or that previous research has been primarily theoretical. In setting up a mixed methods study, point out issues that are problematic from both a qualitative and quantitative perspective. If you have completed Chapter 3 on literature review, list the key limitations, gaps, and problems identified to justify the study.

Workbox 5.2: Justification Statement
Scripts Relative to a Gap or Problem in the Literature That
Can Be Used in a Mixed Methods Research Project

Gap in the Literature:

"Despite the magnitude of [the problem], previous research has only addressed [fill in the blank], and has not addressed [fill in the gap to address]."

Limitation in the Literature:

"While previous research has examined [fill in the blank with the general topic], the previous studies have had limitations. These limitations can be summarized as [write in the limitations identified]."

Previous Literature Has Been Theoretical:

"The arguments linking [insert topic] to [insert topic] have been theoretical to date. Consequently, empirical research integrating [qualitative perspective] and [quantitative perspective] is needed to advance the field of [enter field name]."

Justification Statement Pointing Out the Need for Mixed Methods Research:

"The range of attitudes about [insert topic] and the experiences/perspectives of these [insert topic/relationship] key stakeholders have been neglected."

Your Justification Statement:

CREATING GENERAL RESEARCH GOALS/OBJECTIVES

This section pushes you to define the purpose, goal, and/or objectives you seek to pursue based on the gaps/problem identified above. The preference for inclusion of the language of purpose, goals, and objectives depends on your academic culture and your own field. While closely related, purpose refers to the desired or intended outcome. The **goal** may be considered the result or achievement sought through the research and may be considered by some a subcategory of a purpose. In contrast, **objectives** often refer to the specific measurable outcomes sought through the research. In deciding precise language, seek advice from mentors and other colleagues. Table 5.3 provides examples and variations from business, education, and health sciences.

Remember, link the purpose/goal/objectives to the positive outcome you hope to achieve. So, if there is a gap in information needed by policy makers, the objective of the research is to assess the [magnitude, prevalence, or other quantitative measure] and to provide insight into the nature of the [experiences/perspectives or other qualitative descriptor] of those who have been affected by these policies to inform a new policy, or policy revision.

In doing a mixed methods project, it is logical to include both deductive reasoning and inductive reasoning. For example, you test relationships between variables deductively and explore participant perspectives inductively.

TABLE 5.3 ■ Examples of Purpose Statements From Empirical Studies in Business, Education, and Health Sciences Research	
Field	**Research Goal/Objective/Purpose**
Business	"The objective of this article is to examine the validity of the hypothesized linkages between environmental responsiveness strategies and the emergence of competitively valuable organizational capabilities" (Sharma & Vredenburg, 1998, p. 730).
Education	"The purpose of this sequential QUAN → QUAL mixed methods research study was to understand how principals in Alabama middle schools created a culture of academic optimism that promoted high student achievement. The goal of the first quantitative strand was to identify how different dimensions of academic optimism predicted student achievement. Based on the statistical results of the quantitative strand of the study, a representative sample of principals from high-achieving schools was selected for follow-up interviews using a maximal variation sampling strategy. The goal of the second qualitative strand was to identify strategies by which principals created a culture of academic optimism and thus indirectly contributed to increased student achievement" (Harper, 2016, p. 6).
Health Services	The study goal is "the creation and study of practical, innovative methods to help learners master the complexity of healthcare communication, and develop excellent communication skills that will meet current and future competency-oriented accreditation standards" (Kron et al., 2017, p. 749).

CRAFTING MIXED METHODS RESEARCH QUESTIONS

This describes the process of framing the research objectives into research questions appropriate for your topic.

Identifying Qualitative Research Questions

Qualitative research questions typically focus on a single phenomenon or concept. They usually start with a question. For example, the words, *what, how,* or *why* are commonly found at the beginning of qualitative questions. The objective is often to explore. Thus, qualitative questions often include language such as *explore, discover, understand, describe,* or *report.* See Table 5.4 for some commonly used questions in qualitative research.

TABLE 5.4 ■ Common Qualitative Research Questions
What is the meaning of [the phenomenon of interest] to these individuals?
What are the patterns found relative to [the phenomenon of interest]?
What is the nature of relationships between [one phenomenon of interest] and [another phenomenon of interest]?
What does this population value relative to [the phenomenon of interest]?
How does this population value [the phenomenon of interest]?
Why does this population value [the phenomenon of interest]?
What issues relative to [the phenomenon of interest] are important?
How are these issues relative to [the phenomenon of interest] important?
Why are these issues relative to [the phenomenon of interest] important?
What are barriers and facilitators relative to [the phenomenon of interest]?

Identifying Quantitative Research Questions and Hypotheses

Quantitative research questions can be stated as questions or as hypotheses. Researchers intensively trained in basic sciences frequently conduct their studies using specific hypotheses. Other disciplines may favor the research question format. If you look at several articles from your field (review the articles found in Chapter 3), this will give you a hint about general expectations. Consult with your instructor, mentor, or senior colleague about which approach would be preferred in your field. When formulating quantitative research questions, researchers frequently use verbs to suggest causality. For example, the language of these questions or hypotheses may include *cause, affect, impact, associate, correlate* or *relate.* Researchers typically state explicitly their independent and dependent variables. Table 5.5 has commonly used language of quantitative questions or hypotheses.

TABLE 5.5 ■ Common Quantitative Research Questions
How many of [the phenomenon of interest]?
How much of [the phenomenon of interest]?
How often does [the phenomenon of interest] occur?
What size is [the phenomenon of interest]?
What is the association between [one phenomenon of interest] and [another phenomenon of interest]?
What is the correlation between [one phenomenon of interest] and [another phenomenon of interest]?
Is intervention [one] more effective than intervention [two]?
How does previous experience/exposure predict [the phenomenon of interest]?

Identifying Mixed Methods Research Questions

The MMR question ideally will reflect a linkage between the qualitative and quantitative strands of the study. It is preferable to be explicit but at least be implicit that qualitative and quantitative data are to be collected. If there is a sequential component to the project, in most cases, name the components in the order collected. That is, if there will be an initial quantitative assessment followed by a qualitative assessment, describe the quantitative component before the qualitative component. If the qualitative and quantitative data were collected and analyzed at roughly the same time, indicate the component that most strongly frames the analysis.

For example, in the MPathic-VR study that involved a comparison of virtual human interaction compared with a computer-based learning module for teaching advanced communication skills to medical students in a mixed methods randomized controlled trial, the analysis initially examined specific quantitative questions obtained from when students participated in the educational simulation (Kron et al., 2017). Hence, this section is listed first (see Workbox Illustration 5.1.1). This was followed by mixed methods data collection, including attitudinal responses about specific domains, as well as qualitative comments elicited after the simulation exercise was completed—together these addressed the study's mixed methods question.

In the health sciences and some other fields, especially where investigators are trained primarily in quantitative methods, investigators may choose to state hypotheses rather than questions for quantitative data collection. Below is an alternative representation of the MPathic-VR study using two hypotheses and an MMR question:

> To examine whether MPathic-VR is useful for teaching advanced communication skills, the investigators developed and tested the following hypotheses: 1) students randomized to learn with MPathic-VR would improve their communication performance after engaging in a communication scenario, receiving feedback on their performance, and then applying the feedback in a second run-through of the scenario; and 2) knowledge acquired through MPathic-VR would be resilient (i.e., students would incorporate learned materials into their manner of communication), and that the performance of MPathic-VR-trained students assessed in a subsequent advanced communication objective structured clinical exam (OSCE) would be scored higher than students trained with a conventional, widely used multimedia, computer-based learning (CBL). The investigators also asked the mixed methods research question, how do qualitative findings from students' reflective comments and responses to an attitudinal survey compare for the MPathic-VR and the CBL experiences (Kron et al., 2017, p. 750)?

From the field of business, the Sharma and Vredenberg (1998) study was designed to examine the validity of hypothesized linkages between environmental responsiveness strategies and the emergence of competitively valuable organizational capabilities. The authors described their plans for the study based on a two-phase design:

> The first phase of the study involved comparative case studies through in-depth interviews in seven firms in the Canadian oil and gas industry to ground the resource-based view of the firm within the domain of corporate environmental responsiveness. This study was intended to examine linkages between environmental strategies and the development of capabilities, and understand the nature of any emergent capabilities and their competitive outcomes. The exploratory study was conducted longitudinally over a period of 18 months using the same cohort of respondent companies and managers. The second phase involved testing the emergent linkages through a mail survey-based study of the Canadian oil and gas industry. (p. 730)

While the authors did not explicitly state research questions, their questions can be inferred based on the above passage. For example, their statements could have been reframed as questions: "What are the linkages between environmental strategies and the development of capabilities?" (qualitative); "What is the nature of emergent capabilities and their competitive outcomes?" (qualitative); and "Are the discovered linkages associated when examined in a larger population using a mail survey-based study of the Canadian oil and gas industry?"(quantitative).

Contrast these two approaches with an approach from educational research. In Harper's (2016) MMR examining the linkage between academic optimism and high-performing middle schools, he sought to understand how middle school principals created a culture of academic optimism to promote high academic achievement. He states,

> The overarching research question that addressed an overall study content aim was: How do principals create a culture of academic optimism that fosters high academic optimism in high and low socioeconomic status Alabama middle schools? . . . The quantitative research questions in Strand I were (a) What is the relationship between academic optimism in Alabama middle schools and student achievement in math and reading? (b) What is the relationship between the three dimensions of academic optimism (faculty trust, collective efficacy, and academic emphasis) and student achievement in math and reading? The qualitative research question in Strand II was: What strategies do principals use to create a culture of academic optimism that

fosters high student achievement in Alabama middle schools? Three subquestions were posited to help explore and explain the quantitative results from Strand I: (a) What strategies might account for the unusually strong association of academic emphasis with levels of academic achievement? (b) What strategies do principals use to develop faculty trust? (c) What strategies do principals use to develop collaborative efficacy? (pp. 8–9)

This passage illustrates the use of an overarching research question and specific research questions, both for the initial quantitative strand and for the subsequent qualitative strand.

Activity: Developing Mixed Methods Research Questions

Based on the examples provided above as a reference and in consultation with mentors or colleagues in your field regarding preferred approaches, use Workbox 5.3–5.5, to develop one or more research questions appropriate for your project.

If the mixed methods project will involve an initial quantitative strand of research, followed by a qualitative strand of work, then Workbox 5.3 provides a script you can use.

Workbox 5.3: Mixed Methods Research Question Example When Initial Quantitative Assessment Is Followed by a Qualitative Assessment

How are the initial quantitative results collected by [specify the data collection procedure] explained by the subsequent qualitative results collected by [specify the data collection procedure]?

Your question:

If the mixed methods project will involve an initial qualitative strand of research, followed by a quantitative strand of work, then Workbox 5.4 provides a script you can use.

Workbox 5.4: Mixed Methods Research Question Example When Initial Qualitative Assessment Is Followed by a Quantitative Assessment

How does exploring with the initial qualitative results [specify the data collection procedure] become validated/expanded upon by the subsequent quantitative results [specify the data collection procedure]?

Your question:

If the mixed methods project will involve essentially simultaneous collection of a qualitative strand of research and a quantitative strand of work, then Workbox 5.5 provides a script you can use. If the work of the qualitative strand weighs more heavily than the quantitative strand, or would provide better framing of your work, use the first script. If the work of the quantitative strand weighs more heavily than the qualitative strand, or would provide better framing of your work, use the second script.

Workbox 5.5: Mixed Methods Research Question Examples When Simultaneous Quantitative Assessment and Quantitative Assessment Are Conducted

How are the qualitative findings collected by [specify the data collection procedure] further understood when compared with the simultaneously conducted quantitative findings collected by [specify the data collection procedure]?

Or,

How are the quantitative findings collected by [specify the data collection procedure] further understood when compared with the simultaneously conducted qualitative findings collected by [specify the data collection procedure]?

Your question:

REFINING THE TITLE OF THE MIXED METHODS PROJECT

Developing the MMR project title is an iterative process—after developing a clearer focus of the MMR questions, you are now ready to revise the project title (recall Figure 2.1). For example, when designing the study, if the order of data collection changed from what was originally developed, it will be logical to rewrite the title to reflect **project procedures** temporally. The title should be parsimonious but still include the major topic addressed, participants, and location of project. Check to see that the title conveys that you conducted a mixed methods study, that is, if you included the words *mixed methods* in the title, or language implying inclusion of both qualitative and quantitative data collection. Table 5.4 has examples of qualitative questions and language, while Table 5.5 has language found commonly in quantitative questions. While *qualitative* as a word often appears in titles, *quantitative* appears less frequently. If you know the design you will use, add it now. Remember, most researchers revise their project titles multiple times. It is important to write something down so that you and others can critique the title and allow it to benefit from constructive criticism. By iteratively working on and reconsidering the title, you will be able to refine it.

Application Activities

1. **Peer Feedback.** If working on this project as part of a class or in a workshop, pair up with a peer mentor, and spend about 5 minutes each talking about the background sheet. Rather than talking about the broader context, *focus discussion on the mixed methods research objectives and questions*. Your partner should help you focus on methodological issues. Take turns talking about each person's project and giving feedback. As you talk about it, make a candid assessment to yourself as to where to focus energy to improve the mixed methods question.

2. **Peer Feedback Guidance.** When listening to your partner, hone your critiquing skills. The goal is to help refine the research questions. Specifically, has your partner raised objectives and questions that reflect the work of both qualitative and quantitative research? Is there a mixed methods question bringing together both the qualitative and quantitative strands? Does the ordering of the questions make sense?

3. **Group Debrief.** If in a classroom or large group setting, have volunteers present their topics, general objectives, and MMR questions.

Concluding Thoughts

Use this checklist to assess your progress in achieving the Chapter 5 objectives:

☐ I summarized the overarching context about the topic from the literature with depth and breadth appropriate for my mixed methods project.

☐ I found a focused problem or gap from the literature that justifies my mixed methods project.

☐ I identified a primary objective to pursue in my mixed methods project.

☐ I developed research questions appropriate for my mixed methods project.

☐ I reviewed my Chapter 5 outputs with a peer or colleague to refine my mixed methods objectives and questions.

Now that you have completed these objectives, Chapter 6 will help you identify data sources for your research or evaluation project.

Key Resources

1. **SUGGESTION FOR WRITING A COMPREHENSIVE LITERATURE REVIEW**

   - Onwuegbuzie, A. J., & Frels, R. K. (2016). *Seven steps to a comprehensive literature review: A multimodal and cultural approach.* London, UK: Sage.

2. **SUGGESTION FOR FURTHER READING ABOUT MIXED METHODS RESEARCH SYNTHESIS LITERATURE REVIEWS**

   - Heyvaert M., Hammes K., & Onghena P. (2017). *Using mixed methods research synthesis for literature reviews.* Thousand Oaks, CA: Sage.

3. **SUGGESTION FOR FURTHER READING ON META-INTEGRATION**

   - Frantzen K. K., & Fetters M. D. (2015). Meta-integration for synthesizing data in a systematic mixed studies review: Insights from research on Autism Spectrum Disorder. *Quality and Quantity*, 1–27.

4. **SUGGESTION FOR WRITING THE BACKGROUND SECTION, PURPOSE STATEMENTS, AND MIXED METHODS RESEARCH QUESTIONS**

   - Creswell, J. W., & Plano Clark, V. L. (2011). Introducing a mixed methods research study. In *Designing and conducting mixed methods research*. Thousand Oaks, CA: Sage.

   - Plano Clark, V. L., & Badiee, M. (2010). Research questions in mixed methods research. In A. Tashakkori & C. Teddlie (Eds.), *SAGE handbook of mixed methods in social & behavioral research* (2nd ed., pp. 275–304). Thousand Oaks, CA: Sage.

   - Plano Clark, V. L., & Ivankova, N. V. (2016). Why use mixed methods research? Identifying rationales for mixing methods. In *Mixed methods research: A guide to the field*. Thousand Oaks, CA: Sage.

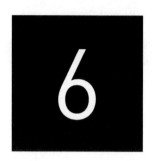

IDENTIFYING DATA SOURCES FOR A MIXED METHODS PROJECT

The ability to use a variety of qualitative and quantitative data collection procedures attracts many researchers to mixed methods projects. Success in your mixed methods project demands your identification of both qualitative and quantitative procedures, even if this feels like a mundane task. This chapter and its activities will help you appraise the main categories of data procedures and data sources, discern how different types of data can be used in mixed methods projects, identify qualitative and quantitative data sources, and develop a data sources table delineating the qualitative and quantitative data sources, the procedure/instruments to be used, the target participants, and any comments for further consideration. As a key outcome, you will complete a data sources table that can be used in a research protocol or manuscript.

LEARNING OBJECTIVES

The concepts and activities of this chapter will help you to

- Consider the main categories of data procedures and data sources
- Illustrate how different types of data can be used in your mixed methods project
- Identify qualitative data sources that you could use in your mixed methods project
- Identify quantitative data sources that you could use in your mixed methods project

WHAT IS A DATA SOURCES TABLE?

A **data sources table** is a matrix or graphic that identifies potential information sources for use in mixed methods projects. A refined table can be used in a publication about your study as illustrated in a previous publication about methodology for building a website to promote colorectal cancer screening (see Table 1 in Fetters, Ivankova, Ruffin, Creswell, & Power (2004)).

Why Have a Data Sources Table?

When teaching mixed methods, I find people encounter difficulty fully integrating their projects until they distinguish the qualitative and quantitative data sources. Many people have not considered fully data sources they *could* use, or for collected data, whether it is qualitative or quantitative. I fondly call completing the data sources table a "**brain stretch**," as the activity seeks to stretch and expand thinking about information you could use. Quantitatively oriented researchers often have limited understanding about the breadth of qualitative procedures that *could* be used in mixed methods projects. Moreover, qualitatively oriented researchers may lack awareness of available measures and datasets. Ensuring data collection procedures fit with the research questions and hypotheses in a proposal, dissertation, or paper for publication provides another reason to complete a data sources table. By proactively thinking about data collection sources and procedures, research questions can change as data collection strategies evolve or expand. A natural phenomenon, research questions, aims, and designs often develop iteratively.

DATA COLLECTION PROCEDURES

Johnson and Turner (2003) identified six major data collection procedures: observations, interviews/focus groups, documents, audiovisual/media, questionnaires, and secondary datasets. Additional potential sources include secondary datasets, biological/medical/engineering, and physical sciences–produced information. Figure 6.1 illustrates these major sources of potential data. The elongated lateral triangular boxes for each source illustrate that the amount of qualitative and quantitative data collected lies on a continuum. The thicker the corresponding depth on the spectrum, the more that type of data has been collected; and the thinner the depth, the less that type of data has been collected.

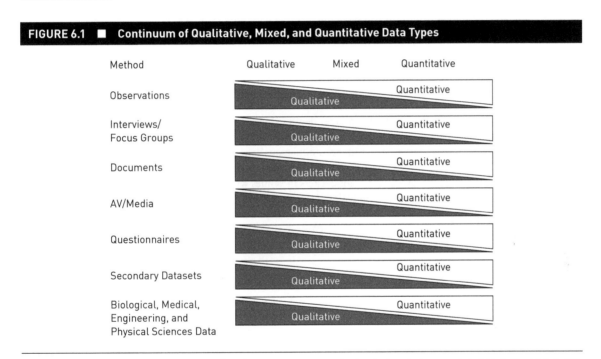

FIGURE 6.1 ■ Continuum of Qualitative, Mixed, and Quantitative Data Types

Source: Adapted from Johnson, B., & Turner, L. A. (2003). Data collection strategies in mixed methods research. In A. Tashakkori & C. Teddlie (Eds.), *Handbook of mixed methods in social and behavioral research* (pp. 297–319). Thousand Oaks, CA: Sage.

Intramethod and Intermethod Data Collection

Methodologists distinguish between intramethod and intermethod data collection procedures (Johnson & Turner, 2003). *Intramethod* data collection involves the gathering of qualitative and quantitative data using one data collection procedure. For example, questionnaires often include both close-ended and open-ended questions. *Intermethod data collection* involves two or more procedures. For example, conducting both qualitative focus groups and a structured survey with close-ended questions would be an intermethod approach.

Observations

Observations are a particularly valuable tool for understanding behaviors (Angrosino, 2007). While often thought of as a qualitative approach due to the particularly rich history and development in anthropology, observations can occur over the entire qualitative, mixed, and quantitative spectrum. Qualitative observations are used to create "thick description" using words. Quantitative observations involve examining for predetermined categories of information. For example, in work to advance computational instruction in the classroom, Dragon et al. (2008) sought to identify physical behaviors linked to emotional states and identify linkages between emotional states and student learning. They used quantitative observations by recording student usage of intelligent tutors. In primary care research to understand the actual content and physician behaviors in outpatient offices, observers recorded on a checklist physician behaviors every 30 seconds (Callahan & Bertakis, 1991). Observations are conducive to mixed data collection using a combination of qualitative descriptive language as well as quantitative close-ended language.

Interviews

Interviews are a mainstay in the social and behavioral sciences (Brinkman & Kvale, 2014). Interviews are often considered primarily a qualitative approach, but they can be completely structured for pure quantitative data collection alone. Interviews can be with individuals or with a group, for example, when there are two or more people present, and there are special procedures to follow (see further discussion below). The spectrum of interviews can include completely unstructured, semistructured, a mix of open-ended questions with close-ended questions, or a series of close-ended questions only. In narrative research, an unstructured interview approach may be guided only by encouraging the subject to tell his or her story. In semistructured interviews, the interviewer will have a series of questions, often 3–5 main questions, planned for the interview. In any interview approach, some structured questions may be added. For example, the interviewer may ask demographic questions, for example, age, gender, level of education, number in household, etc. Completely structured interviews are less common, but they commonly occur around election season. Pollsters collect information in a structured format about a candidate for office. They use key demographic variables determined to be predictors of a voting pattern, as well as the interviewee's current choice of a candidate.

Group Interviews

Group interviews involve a researcher interviewing two or more people together. Focus group interviews, a common format, are conducted with a particular focus using specific procedures (Morgan, 1997). Additional group interview variations include dyadic interviews with two interviewees (Morgan, 2016; Morgan, Ataie, Carder, & Hoffman, 2013), and mini-focus groups with 3 to 4 participants (Krueger & Casey, 1994). In the typical focus group, the interviewer uses a semistructured interview guide to produce qualitative data (transcripts). Fully structured group interviews are not common, but they can occur in public settings such as college classrooms or other public venues. For example, participants may use smartphones (or clickers in venues wired for the technology) to send responses to a website that summarizes the responses for discussion. Instructors or researchers project the results in the classroom, allowing for the data to be discussed, to illustrate variations in opinions. If the discussions are audiorecorded they produce mixed data, both the quantitative data collected from the participants and the ensuring discussion.

Documents

Various documents are potential data sources for mixed methods researchers. Documents are very diverse sources of information. These can include purely textual information, such as the content of subject or researcher diaries or journals, letters, public documents, memos, policy and procedures, forms, proceedings of meetings or conferences, the language used on online Web discussion forums, blogs, text messages, or social media narratives on Facebook or many other platforms. Historical documents, school archives, and medical records can also serve as document sources. Within any individual document, one might find qualitative, mixed, or quantitative data sources.

Audiovisual Media

Audiovisual or media of various types can also serve as qualitative, mixed, or quantitative data (Prosessor, 2011). Examples of source materials include videos, photographs, drawings, sounds, or other recordings, such as music. Business researchers could use a series of commercials in media to assess marketing trends. For education researchers, a multitude of sources, classroom drawings, photos of class layouts, student learning assessments, videos of class-based work, etc., are available to classroom instructors. The health sciences have a large variety of potential sources, such as images from radiography, computed tomography scanning, heart sounds, or other types of scans that manifest as wave forms, for example, brain waves on an electroencephalogram. These raw sources of data often require some kind of interpretation. For example, video data can be extracted through researcher observations and rendered as qualitative, mixed, or quantitative data.

Questionnaires

Researchers in mixed methods studies often use questionnaires or surveys (DeVellis, 2012). These instruments of data collection can conceivably fall along the spectrum between qualitative and quantitative, but most frequently contain structured items with close-ended choices, or open choices when the respondent replies with a specific number. In business, education, health sciences, and sociobehavioral sciences, examples can include opinion surveys, attitudinal assessments, cognitive tests, aptitude tests, or psychological tests. Researchers often employ a strategy of qualitative and quantitative data collection in a single instrument. This type of intramethod data collection may produce a relatively limited volume of qualitative data and will be used as supplemental material to explain answers on other parts of the instrument, or to explore new questions that a researcher would like to pose.

Secondary Datasets

Though not considered by Johnson and Turner (2003), yet another source of data used increasingly by researchers is secondary datasets. One could arguably lump these data sources into the documents category, but there are some distinguishing features. Secondary datasets often have been collected specifically with the intent of analyzing the information for other research interests. In business, researchers frequently use marketing and sales data. In education, researchers may make use of the Early Childhood Longitudinal Study (National Center for Education Statistics). (See Case Study 6.1.) Many businesses are now scrambling to survive in the era of "big data." While a widely accepted definition is still elusive, Gartner (n.d.) defines big data as "high-volume, high-velocity and/or high-variety information assets that demand cost-effective, innovative forms of information processing that enable enhanced insight, decision making, and process automation." Big data also sometimes includes a fourth V (veracity), to address trust and uncertainty (*MIT Technology Review*, 2013). Ward and Barker (2013) define it as, "Big data is a term describing the storage and analysis of large and or complex data sets using a series of techniques including, but not limited to, NoSQL, MapReduce and machine learning" (p. 2).

The challenge of how to include big data in MMR is one of the important and rapidly evolving challenges of the field (Mertens et al., 2016). This information can be either structured or unstructured. However, data mining of large qualitative databases has similarly emerged among some researchers. Secondary datasets, like all the other data sources, can have varying amounts of quantitative mixed, and qualitative data. The drive to use "big data" is pouring into health care to help make better decisions (Swain, 2016). In the health sciences, researchers may access Medicare claims or other health insurance data. The Health and Retirement Study in the United States has for over 20 years collected information health and economic well-being of adults over the age of 50 (University of Michigan, 2018). Once collected, such information can also be used in a secondary way. That is, while the data were collected with another primary purpose, the data can also be used to address secondary interests.

CASE STUDY 6.1
THE EARLY CHILDHOOD LONGITUDINAL STUDY

The Early Childhood Longitudinal Study (ECLS) program of research involves three longitudinal studies examining child development, school readiness, and early school experiences. The "birth cohort" comprises a sample of children born in 2001, who were followed from birth through entry into kindergarten. The "kindergarten class" cohort is followed from kindergarten through the eighth grade and was started in the 1998–1999 sample of children. The "kindergarten cohort" represents a sample of children from kindergarten through the fifth grade and was

started in 2010–2011. The ECLS provides researchers a database with information about children's status at birth, and other points in their growth trajectory, early childhood transitions, early education programs, and children's growth and experiences through eighth grade. The database has information about relationships between multiple entities including family, school, and individual variables relative to development, early learning, and school performance (2018).

Biological, Medical, Engineering, and Physical Sciences Data

While still emerging, a small number of mixed methods researchers have begun to use biological, engineering, medical, and physical sciences data. Biological markers or biomarkers can be defined as "a distinctive biological or biologically derived indicator (as a biochemical metabolite in the body) of a process, event, or condition (as aging, disease, or exposure to a toxic substance)" ("biomarker," n.d.). In public health, sputum, cheek swabs, etc. have become a common source of data in testing. Medicine has a qualitative, quantitative, and mixed methods data from a variety of sources, for example, blood tests, brain scans, heart tracing, etc. Using data outputs from research and development in engineering information sciences has begun to find traction as well (Venkatesh, Brown, & Bala, 2013). Finally, data from environmental measures, for example, air quality indicators, have found a place in mixed methods studies as well (Schulz et al., 2011). These types of data will assuredly find increasingly prominent roles in MMR.

ELEMENTS OF A DATA SOURCES TABLE

The elements of a data sources table, as demonstrated in the Workbox Illustrations 6.1.1 and 6.2.1, and activity Workboxes 6.1.2 and 6.2.2, include four columns of information. In the first column, the general type of data collection procedure can be found (for types, see Figure 6.1). The second column contains the heading "Who/What" to stimulate consideration about participants in the project, or what kind of data will be collected. In the third column, you will record how many of the procedures or intervention will be conducted. This column can be completed with the number of participants, the number of observations, the number of datasets, etc. The final column is not structured for a specific type of data, but it is there for you to list any comments that could be helpful as you think about your project. For example, to access a database you might record the name of a person who you need to talk with for permission. Alternatively, you may want to keep a note to yourself that you need to conduct a power analysis to determine the quantitative data collection sample size, or you might make a note to check with your advisor regarding how you will determine the qualitative data sample size.

Completing Your Data Sources Tables

You can complete the data sources tables in a variety of ways. You might choose to fill them out one at a time as you read an overview chapter first of qualitative data collection procedures (fill out Workbox 6.1.2) and then an overview chapter of quantitative data collection procedures (fill out Workbox 6.2.2). Alternatively, if you are in a workshop, you may fill these sections in as you proceed through the lecture material of each type. You may also complete the data sources tables bit-by-bit over the course of several weeks.

How to Complete a Data Sources Table
When Using One Data Collection Procedure

While some researchers question whether using only one form of data collection qualifies as MMR, I always ask, "Are you collecting both open-ended and closed-ended data?" You may want to refer above to the discussion on intramethod data collection. One of the most common questions involves using a survey with some open-ended questions that are used to "supplement" quantitative answers. If you are using a single data collection procedure, list it in both tables. For example, in a mixed data collection survey with closed- and open-ended questions, you would list the survey in both tables. The number of participants will most likely be the same or slightly less (due to nonresponse in the qualitative section). In the corresponding line of the qualitative data sources table, list how many questions you will have. In the comment box, you might mention which other questions in the survey it corresponds with. Alternatively, you might use interviews to collect both qualitative and quantitative data, for example, collecting demographic information as part of the interview process rather than using a separate form. The primary type, who/what, how many, and comments boxes can all be filled in to reflect your procedures.

Qualitative Data Sources Table Example:
The MPathic-VR Mixed Methods Medical Education Study

Workbox Illustration 6.1.1 presents an example from the MPathic-VR mixed methods medical education study (Kron et al., 2017). Before the trial of our virtual human intervention versus control with a computer-based learning module, we needed written feedback on scripts to optimize the language and credibility. As the scenarios involved cultural dilemmas, we sought out cultural content experts, including a Salvadoran woman and her husband, Latino physicians, an lesbian, gay, bisexual, transgender, and queer or questioning (LGBTQ) advocate, and senior oncology nurses. Only a small number of participants were needed to ensure realistic approaches. After the trial, we administered posttrial surveys to medical students in all arms of the study to collect posttrial reflective essays about their experience using the system. Controversy for the team to solve involved how long to make the essays and whether to have all students reflect about the same issue or a different issue. As a third potential source of data, the project team collected video recordings of students in the trial that were recorded as part of the analytics of their facial expressions for nonverbal behaviors. In each case, the target population of participants was the entire class of students. As noted, there are significant challenges relative to the analysis of video recordings that were beyond the scope of the project. In short, this data sources table summarized *potential* sources of data that were used or could have been used in the MPathic-VR mixed methods trial.

Workbox Illustration 6.1.1: Potential Qualitative Data Sources Table From the MPathic-VR Mixed Methods Medical Education Study

General Type?	Who/What?	How Many?	Comments
Written feedback on scripts	Cultural content experts	n = 2	Cultural content expert and Salvadoran husband–wife pair
	Lay Salvadoran woman and husband	n = 2	
	Latino physician	n = 1	Two oncology nurses
	LGBTQ advocate	n = 1	
	Oncology nurses	n = 2	
Posttrial self-reflective essays	Medical students in both arms of trial	All participants	Need to be of sufficient length, but not too long
			Due to number of students, can use several questions
Videotapes	Medical students in intervention arm of trial	All participants	Analysis will be challenging.

Sources: Kron et al. (2017) and Fetters, M.D. and Kron, F.W. (2012–15). *Modeling Professional Attitudes and Teaching Humanistic Communication in Virtual Reality (MPathic-VRII).* National Center for Advancing Translational Science/NIH 9R44TR000360-04.

Activity: Completing Your Qualitative Data Sources Table

Having conducted a "brain stretch" about your topic, consider all the different types of data that could be collected or that you could access. In the first box "General Type?," list all the different types of qualitative data that *could* be used or have already been collected in your mixed methods project. To think systematically, reference Workbox Illustration 6.1.1. You might choose individual interviews, focus group interviews, or field observations. Perhaps you anticipate having diaries of participants or essays from a classroom where you observe. Alternatively, you may have logs from a workplace where you observe. Record the number of participants that you would include for this data collection strategy. Especially among researchers who received their primary training in a quantitative tradition, the tendency is to considerably overestimate the number of participants that would be needed in qualitative data collection. Regardless, writing down some estimates will allow you to start a dialogue about how many participants or documents you will likely need. The final column, "Comments," is space to write down any issues that might affect the data collection. Perhaps it is doubts about access to the population, concerns about informed consent procedures, privacy issues, or uncertainty about how you would analyze the information.

Workbox 6.1.2: Your Potential Qualitative Data Sources Table

General Type?	Who/What?	How Many?	Comments

Quantitative Data Sources Table Example: The MPathic-VR Mixed Methods Medical Education Study

The MPathic-VR mixed methods medical education study illustrates use of multiple quantitative data sources (Kron et al., 2017). Before the trial of the virtual human intervention versus control with a computer-based learning module, we needed to ensure that all medical students, both those in the intervention arm and those in the control arm, had similar baseline knowledge about fundamentals of communication. Since the trial would target all the medical students in a class, from piloting we chose graduate students as a comparable population, information noted in the comments section. This pilot work required few, only eight, individuals. Based on their performance on a presimulation quiz, a passing score indicated that the questions were useful for assessing baseline knowledge about communication prior to the trial. Actual scores on two virtual human training modules—one on intercultural communication and a second on interprofessional communication—served as another source of data. As these scores would be available only from medical students randomized into the trial, this information is recorded in the "Who/What?" column. A third source of quantitative data would be scores on an attitudinal survey. In this case, the "Who/What?" would be all students in both the intervention and control arms. Under the "How Many" header, all students would be eligible. As noted under the "Comments" header, the students randomized to the control arm had a specific question about virtual human interaction. Finally, to assess a critical outcome to assess if skills learned during the virtual human simulation would transfer to a clinically realistic scenario, we collected data from scoring during an objective structured clinical examination (OSCE). OSCE refers to terminology in the field of medical education where actors or real patients play the role of a person with a particular medical condition or concern. Students from the entire class can participate in the OSCE with a formative (participate and then receive feedback to learn) or evaluative (assess if the student has adequate skills) purpose. In this research, a real concern was to ensure that the OSCE instructors would evaluate medical students in the same way. Hence this concern was noted in the table.

Workbox Illustration 6.2.1: Potential Quantitative Data Sources Table Example From the MPathic-VR Mixed Methods Medical Education Study

General Type?	Who/What?	How Many?	Comments
Communications skills knowledge quiz	Graduate students: Students will pilot surveys, assess item function/ refinement.	n = 8	Avoid medical students in the study sites, graduate students' equivalent skills in learning challenging material.
Scores on intercultural communication and scores on interprofessional skills module	Medical students in the intervention arm	All students in intervention arm	
Attitudes about the educational experience questionnaire	Medical students in the intervention and control arms	All students	One question about interactivity is not relevant to controls.
OSCE performance evaluation	Scaled data from medical students in the intervention and control arms	All students	Need to calibrate the standardized patient instructors (the people who assess student performance) across all sites

Sources: Kron et al. (2017) and Fetters, M.D. and Kron, F.W. (2012–15). *Modeling Professional Attitudes and Teaching Humanistic Communication in Virtual Reality (MPathic-VRII).* National Center for Advancing Translational Science/NIH 9R44TR000360-04.

Activity: Completing Your Quantitative Data Sources Table

Use Workbox 6.2.2 to record quantitative data sources you *could* collect or have already collected. Quantitative data could come from any of the sources listed in Figure 6.1 that you are measuring or counting. For example, quantitative data in an education project might include scores on exams or quizzes. In business, quantitative data might include productivity reports, sales, benchmarks, or any other metrics used such as a customer satisfaction survey. In health sciences research, it could include compliance or completion of a particular service. For "Who/What?," you should list who would actually participate, for example, adult males and females, or what you would include, for example, scores or rankings. The question "How many?" triggers thinking about the number of participants you anticipate recruiting for data collection, or the number of scores that you anticipate would be collected. Researchers who have received training primarily in the qualitative tradition may not know how to determine sample size for the quantitative component and may need to conduct a power analysis in consultation with an expert with those skills. The "Comments" column provides space to record any issues that you think might be necessary to consider. In the study, you may have concern about particular feasibility issues that can be recorded. A challenge might be funding and how much would be paid to compensate individuals. Any of these ideas, or others as deemed important by you, would be appropriate for this box.

Workbox 6.2.2: Your Potential Quantitative Data Sources Table

General Type?	Who/What?	How Many?	Comments

Application Activities

1. **Peer Feedback.** Having filled in ideas about data collection in the qualitative and quantitative data sources tables, review your data sources tables with a peer mentor or several colleagues. If in a classroom or workshop, share the table with other students. If part of a learning group, or research lab, project the data sources tables on a screen for discussion. Ascertain the viability of including each in the project and need to revise the study purpose and research questions.

2. **Peer Feedback Guidance.** Apply the concepts learned critiquing the ideas of others. Do the proposed data sources seem reasonable? Have the participants chosen resonate as an appropriate group or source of information for exploring the research questions? Does the sample size seem appropriate? Do the purpose statement and research questions need adjustment?

3. **Group Debrief.** If you are in a classroom or large-group setting, volunteers can present their qualitative and quantitative data sources tables. Individually, reflect on how approaches identified by others could be used in your project.

Concluding Thoughts

Use this checklist to assess your progress in achieving the Chapter 6 objectives:

☐ I reviewed the main categories of data collection procedures and data sources.

☐ I explored how different types of data can be used in my mixed methods project.

☐ I identified potential qualitative data sources for my mixed methods project.

☐ I identified potential quantitative data sources for use in my mixed methods project.

☐ I reviewed my Chapter 6 output with a peer or colleague to refine my project focus.

Now that you have completed these objectives, Chapter 7 will help you choose among core mixed methods designs for use in your research or evaluation project.

Key Resources

1. **FURTHER READING ON DATA COLLECTION STRATEGIES**

- Creswell, J. W. (2003). *Research design: Qualitative, quantitative, and mixed methods approaches*. Thousand Oaks, CA: Sage.
- Johnson, B., & Turner, L. A. (2003). Data collection strategies in mixed methods research. In A. Tashakkori & C. Teddlie (Eds.), *Handbook of mixed methods in social and behavioral research* (pp. 297–319). Thousand Oaks, CA: Sage.

2. **FURTHER READING ON FOCUS GROUPS AND DYADIC INTERVIEWS**

- Morgan, D. L. (1997). *The focus group guidebook* (Vol. 1). Thousand Oaks, CA: Sage.
- Morgan, D. L. (2016). *Essentials of dyadic interviewing*. New York, NY: Routledge.

3. **FURTHER READING ON CONDUCTING OBSERVATIONS**

- Angrosino, M. (2007). *Doing ethnographic and observational research*. Thousand Oaks, CA: Sage.

4. **FURTHER READING ON THE USE OF INTERVIEWS**

- Brinkman, S., & Kvale, S. (2014). *Interviews: Learning the craft of qualitative research interviewing* (3rd ed.). Thousand Oaks, CA: Sage.

5. **FURTHER READING ON THE USE OF AUDIOVISUAL MEDIA**

- Prosessor, J. (2011). Visual methodology: Toward a more seeing research. In N. K. Denzin & Y. S. Lincoln (Eds.), *The Sage handbook of qualitative research* (4th ed., pp. 479–496). Thousand Oaks, CA: Sage.

6. **FURTHER READING ON DEVELOPING SURVEYS AND SCALES**

- DeVellis, R. F. (2012). *Scale development: Theory and applications* (3rd ed., Vol. 26). Thousand Oaks, CA: Sage.

7. **FURTHER READING ON USING DOCUMENTS QUANTITATIVELY**

- Krippendorff, K. (2013). *Content analysis: An introduction to its methodology* (3rd ed.). Thousand Oaks, CA: Sage.

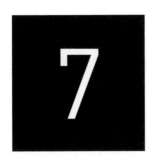

CREATING PROCEDURAL DIAGRAMS OF CORE MIXED METHODS RESEARCH DESIGNS

A mixed methods design provides a framework for organizing multiple aspects of mixed methods research and evaluation studies. Understanding core mixed methods designs and creating a figure for your study can seem challenging as it necessitates an understanding of fixed and emergent designs and core mixed method designs and their applications. This chapter and its activities will help you situate your mixed methods planning along the spectrum of fixed and emergent designs, distinguish between three core mixed methods designs, choose a core design for your mixed methods project, and draw a procedural diagram to represent your mixed methods study. As a key outcome, you will choose a design, core or expanded, and draw a procedural diagram.

LEARNING OBJECTIVES

The ideas presented here will help you

- Situate your research design planning along the spectrum of fixed and emergent designs in mixed methods research (MMR)

- Distinguish between the three core MMR designs and their features

- Recognize conventional notations used to draw and present mixed methods design figures

- Choose a core design for use in your project, or in a phase of your project

- Draw a draft of your chosen design using a template

GETTING STARTED BY CHOOSING A MIXED METHODS DESIGN

The reasons you will mix qualitative and quantitative methods reflects the research questions you are asking. If you have not already done so, consider completing Chapter 5 to help you develop or refine your qualitative, quantitative, and mixed methods project questions. The research designs you will use reflect both your research questions and reasons for mixing. Moreover, it will be helpful to have in mind both qualitative and quantitative data sources you can use in your mixed methods research (MMR) or evaluation study. If you have not identified potential data sources, you should consider completing Chapter 6.

SPECTRUM OF FIXED AND EMERGENT MIXED METHODS RESEARCH DESIGNS

As indicated in Figure 7.1, designs can fall on a spectrum from fixed to emergent (Creswell & Plano Clark, 2018a). Among mixed methods researchers, some take the position that the steps or phases of a mixed methods study should be planned in advance. With a fixed design, the mixed methods researcher can carefully consider the intent of the study and approaches to integration during all dimensions of the research enterprise. With emergent designs, the steps of the mixed methods study emerge as the study is conducted, the results are understood, and then the next step becomes clearer. The rationale goes that until one obtains results of one step or phase of the study, it will be very difficult to consider what should occur next until the results are seen (Creswell & Plano Clark, 2018b). I find that many projects have elements of both. When researchers conduct fixed designs, they anticipate that it will be difficult to plan every detail, and that they can adapt as the need arises. On the flip side, when researchers conduct emergent designs, they also have some sense about what will come next. Particularly in programs of study that extend over years where one project builds on a previous project, there almost certainly will be an element of emergence. Lucero et al. (2016) in a community-based participatory research project initially planned to do multiple case studies, and then distributed a survey, but based on how the project evolved, they actually started the survey while still in the course of conducting their initial case study. Most funding agencies require a clear research design and implementation strategy. Moreover, dissertations also require students to have a fully conceptualized plan that makes emergent elements clear. Finally, **human subjects review** boards will want these elements clear as well. Hence, the Mixed Methods Workbook will help prepare you to become as detailed as you can in your planning, but accept that you will need to adapt as circumstances dictate.

FIGURE 7.1 ■ Spectrum of Structure Between Fixed Design to Emergent Design

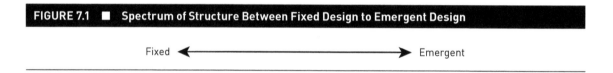

Fixed ⟵————————————————⟶ Emergent

THREE CORE MIXED METHODS DESIGNS

Creswell and Plano Clark (2018b) have identified 15 different design typologies offered by various authors since 1989. The activities in this chapter of the Mixed Methods Workbook follow and expand upon the three **core mixed methods designs**, as these have gained significant popularity and traction (Creswell & Plano Clark, 2018b). This choice to use these core designs is intentional, as these designs are conceptually simple and very popular. For any given course or field, the design terminology may vary regarding the preferred language, approaches, and design typologies that are presented by the author or preferred by an instructor. In the interest of inclusivity, some of the other more popular naming conventions will be included.

Intent and Timing as Elements in Design Naming

At the simplest level for core designs, naming conventions draw upon intent, and for sequential designs, the additional element of timing. Creswell and Plano Clark (2018b) refer to these as core designs, though there have been variations in the naming that have evolved over time (p. 59). For a **convergent mixed methods research design**, the primary intent is *comparison* of the two types of data, and the timing of data collection and analysis, while often roughly at the same time, can also be asynchronous. When one form of data collection and analysis comes first and the results are used in the following phase of data collection and analysis, the design name has intent and sequential elements. There are two core variations in sequential designs with naming conventions that vary by the intent of the *qualitative* data collection. For an **explanatory sequential mixed methods research design**, there is initial quantitative data collection and analysis to examine trends or associations in a study population, and the *intent of subsequent qualitative data collection is to explain* the initial quantitative findings. In an **exploratory sequential mixed methods research design**, the initial *intent of the qualitative data collection and analysis is to explore* a phenomenon, and the subsequent quantitative data collection is to utilize some aspect of the qualitative findings to examine trends or associations in a study population.

Increasingly, researchers from various fields are integrating MMR and evaluation procedures with additional research applications, methodological approaches, or theoretical frameworks. Hence, there are combinations of underlying core mixed methods design or combinations of core mixed methods designs with other research applications, methodological approaches, or theoretical frameworks. These combinations variably have been called advanced frameworks, advanced designs (Creswell, 2015), advanced applications (Plano Clark & Ivankova, 2016a), and complex applications (Creswell & Plano Clark, 2018b). As the evolution in language reflects a lack of consensus, and in my view remains problematic, I prefer the rhetoric of "scaffolded mixed methods designs" to refer to this group of designs. **Scaffolded mixed methods research designs** are research strategies or plans that collect and analyze both qualitative and quantitative data, are built with a core design or combination of core designs, and typically are integrated with another methodology and/or theory/ideology. Popular examples that are presented in Chapter 8 include general scaffolded mixed methods design, scaffolded experimental (intervention) designs, scaffolded mixed methods case study designs, scaffolded mixed methods participatory-social justice designs, scaffolded mixed methods program evaluations, and scaffolded mixed methods website/mobile app (application used in mobile devices) designs.

How to Choose a Mixed Methods Design

While choosing a design seems daunting, based on your MMR questions, the data sources you want to collect for your mixed methods study, and intent, you will find choosing a core design template for constructing your mixed methods design figure is relatively easy if you complete the activity in Workbox 7.1.

Activity: Choosing a Mixed Methods Design

To choose your mixed methods design, you will want to consider the intent foremost but also the relative timing of when your qualitative and quantitative data interface. By completing the activity in Workbox 7.1, you will be able to identify your design, and then choose a template for creating a figure for your project. If you will have a scaffolded design (i.e., complex design, advanced framework), you will want to choose a template for the first phase, the main phase, or create a template for each phase.

Workbox 7.1: Choosing a Mixed Methods Research Design

1. Have you identified potential qualitative and quantitative data sources for your mixed methods study?

    - If yes, continue to Question 2.

    - If no, go to Chapter 6, identify QUAL and QUAN data sources, and go on to Question 2.

2. Will you collect and analyze both QUAL and QUAN data with the primary intent of comparing the two types of data?

    - If yes, refer to Workbox Illustration 7.2.1 and use it as a guide to complete the convergent design template Workbox 7.2.2.

    - If no, continue to Question 3.

3. If you will collect and analyze:

    - Quantitative data initially to examine trends or associations in a study population, then collect and analyze qualitative data to explain the quantitative data, you should refer to Workbox Illustration 7.3.1 and use it as a guide to complete the explanatory design template Workbox 7.3.2.

    - Qualitative data initially to explore a phenomenon first, then collect and analyze quantitative data to examine trends or associations in a study population, you should refer to Workbox Illustration 7.4.1 and use it to complete the exploratory design template Workbox 7.4.2.

    - Both types of data in multiple stages or using a scaffolded mixed methods research study design with a specific application, methodological, or theoretical framework, you should diagram either the first phase, the main phase, or create each phase. If unclear, keep this focus in mind and go back to Question 2.

My core mixed methods research design(s) will be:

The *first question* requires you to simply decide whether you will be collecting and analyzing both qualitative and quantitative data. If you have not identified both qualitative and quantitative data sources, you need to go to Chapter 6, and then return to this activity.

The *second question* has you consider when the data will be interfacing with each other for comparison. If you will be conducting the analytics separately and synchronously (almost assuredly your results will not be available at exactly the same time), and then bringing the findings together, you will be using a convergent design. If your answer is yes, then you will use a convergent design template Workbox 7.2.2. If your answer is no, then you will continue to Assessment 3.

The *third question* has you consider the intent and timing of the collection of your qualitative and quantitative methods. If you will be collecting and analyzing quantitative data initially to assess trends in a larger population, and then collecting and analyzing qualitative data afterwards with a smaller sample, you will use the explanatory sequential mixed methods design template Workbox 7.3.2. If you will be collecting and analyzing qualitative data initially to explore a topic in depth with a smaller number of individuals, and then collecting and analyzing quantitative data afterwards with a larger sample, you will use the exploratory sequential mixed methods design template Workbox 7.4.2.

If you will be collecting and analyzing both types of data in multiple stages or phases, you may need to use a scaffolded MMR study design (a.k.a., advanced design or framework or complex design) as per Chapter 8. If you will be conducting a multistage/multiphase or scaffolded (advanced framework, advanced design, complex framework) mixed methods design, choose either the first phase, the main phase, or create each phase using the templates in this chapter.

If you are planning to use an emergent design, you may feel uncertain about which template to use. To start your emergent design mixed methods study, you will at least need to commit to your first step of data collection. If you have committed to collecting and analyzing both qualitative and quantitative data in you first step, then use Workbox 7.2.2 Convergent Design Template. If your first phase will be to collect and analyze quantitative data, then you should choose Workbox 7.3.2. Explanatory Sequential Design Template. If your first phase will be to collect and analyze qualitative data, then choose Workbox 7.4.2.

With an emergent design, regardless of your first step, you could choose to conduct subsequent qualitative data collection and analysis or subsequent quantitative data collection and analysis. For now, leaving the bottom half of your template empty is completely acceptable. You can add further information as it becomes clearer. In fact, committing to your first phase may help the planning for your second phase.

Complete Workbox 7.1 by writing in your core MMR design(s).

GUIDELINES FOR DRAWING PROCEDURAL DIAGRAMS FOR MIXED METHODS STUDIES

Ivankova, Creswell, and Stick (2006) developed a 10-step guideline for drawing procedural diagrams for mixed methods studies. These can be seen in Figure 7.2. In drawing a procedural diagram, you should bear in mind these recommendations. I advise that you follow the instructions as you refer to the relevant illustration and complete your own template.

One caveat about these recommendations is in order. The fourth, using uppercase or lowercase letters to design the relative priority, remains controversial for at least two reasons: (1) When designing a study, the researcher may anticipate one component to have a greater priority, but in fact, after the study is complete, it may not prove to be true (Teddlie & Tashakkori, 2006). It is possible that in a negative trial, the reasons elucidated in a qualitative study after the trial may provide more valuable information than a negative trial itself. (2) Using the distinction may denigrate one methodology relative to the other, for example, a QUAN + qual demarcation may imply that the qualitative research was less valuable and could unintentionally be implied or construed as suggesting qualitative methodology is not on equal methodological standing as quantitative methodology.

Convergent Mixed Methods Research Design

A convergent design occurs when both the qualitative and the quantitative data are collected and analyzed at roughly the same time. Some authors refer to this as "concurrent parallel," "concurrent," or "triangulation" design (Creswell & Plano Clark, 2018b). A strong, but not completely agreed upon rationale for the language of convergent is the implication that the findings come together. Concurrent suggests only that the research

FIGURE 7.2 ■ Guidelines for Drawing Procedural Diagrams for Mixed Methods Studies
1. Give a title to the diagram.
2. Choose either a horizontal or a vertical layout for the diagram.
3. Draw boxes for the quantitative and qualitative stages of data collection, data analysis, and interpretation of the study results.
4. Use uppercase or lowercase letters to design the relative priority of the quantitative and qualitative data collection and analysis.*
5. Use single-headed arrows to show the flow procedures in the design.
6. Specify procedures for each stage of the quantitative and qualitative data collection and analysis.
7. Specify expected products or outcomes of each procedure in quantitative and qualitative data collection and analysis.
8. Use concise language for describing the procedures and products.
9. Make your diagram simple.
10. Limit your diagram to a single page.

Source: Reprinted from Ivankova et al. (2006) with permission of SAGE Publishing, Inc.

*This recommendation remains controversial.

is being conducted simultaneously, and parallel implies that the two streams of research never come together. Triangulation is viewed as problematic for multiple reasons. Particularly problematic has been the use of triangulation in so many ways as to be confusing. Another reason is the nautical use of triangulation to identify an exact location that indirectly implies multiple strands must confirm each other. The reasons for collecting and analyzing data using a convergent design are several fold. Collecting data at the same time is efficient if you will have limited access to subjects, or if it is prohibitive for time or financial costs to make recurrent trips into the field. Moreover, collecting and analyzing the data at the same time may be useful for ensuring the collected data are tightly linked relative to a particular moment in time.

The relevance of these questions can be considered in the intervention study assessing the benefit of a virtual reality program to teach communications skills by Kron et al. (2017), where the investigators evaluated the experiences of students taking both the intervention and control modules. Although not referred to as a convergent design, a convergent design for evaluation was embedded into the overarching mixed methods experimental design (this will be discussed more in Chapter 8). They collected 7-point Likert scale attitudinal ratings about student experiences and reflective essays immediately after 210 students in the intervention arm took the virtual reality training, or 211 medical students in the control arm took the state-of-the-art computer-based learning module (Kron et al., 2017). As the students had just completed the training, collecting the data immediately afterwards was efficient, and the quantitative and qualitative data were linked temporally.

For a convergent MMR design, Creswell and Plano Clark (2018b) point out four key questions to consider (pp. 184–185): (1) Will the two samples include different or the same individuals? (2) Will the samples be the same size? (3) Will the same concepts be examined? (4) Will the data be collected from independent sources or from a single source?

These can be considered in light of the Kron et al. (2017) study examining the effectiveness of exposure to virtual reality program for improving communication skills: (1) The researchers used the full sample of 421 medical students from all three medical schools. (2) All participating medical students answered the quantitative attitudinal questions and reflection essays, but there was a comparison of virtual reality – exposed students—210 from the intervention and 211 from the control arm—exposed to a computer-based learning module. (3) The quantitative attitudinal survey had 12 items using a 7-point Likert scale relative to the constructs of clarity, purpose, utility, and likelihood to recommend the module to others. The qualitative reflective essays were designed to be comparable. But the authors also recognized that having more than 200 qualitative responses from the same question for the reflective essay of each arm of the trial would be unnecessary, so the students were randomized to four different open-ended questions (two about interactivity were not given to the control module students). This allowed for saturation for each qualitative question but avoided too many responses that would be redundant, unnecessary, and restrictive. (4) The data were collected using the same source, and at the same time in an online survey that was programmed into both learning modules.

Workbox Illustration 7.2.1: Convergent Mixed Methods Research Design From the MPathic-VR Mixed Methods Medical Education Study in the Health Sciences Field

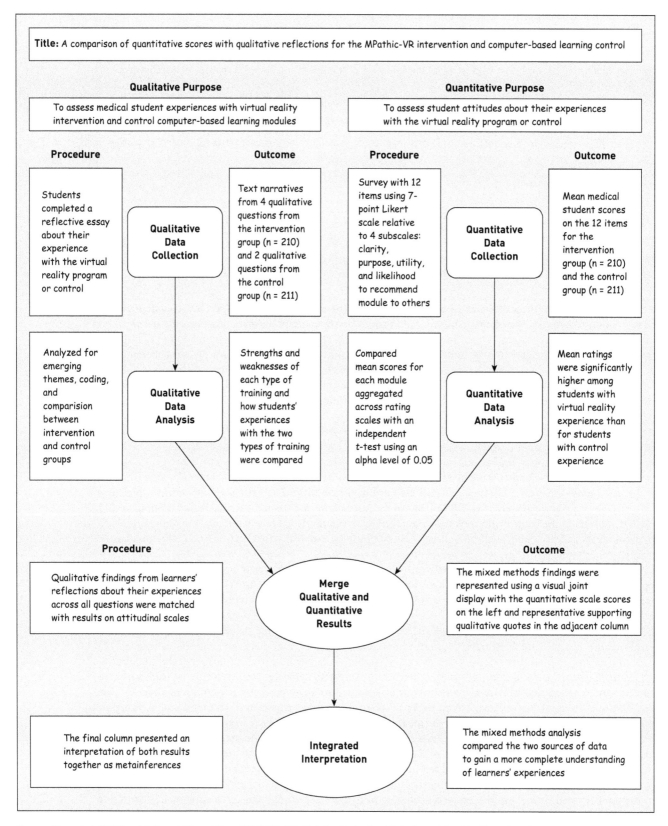

Title: A comparison of quantitative scores with qualitative reflections for the MPathic-VR intervention and computer-based learning control

Qualitative Purpose

To assess medical student experiences with virtual reality intervention and control computer-based learning modules

Quantitative Purpose

To assess student attitudes about their experiences with the virtual reality program or control

Procedure

Students completed a reflective essay about their experience with the virtual reality program or control

Qualitative Data Collection

Outcome

Text narratives from 4 qualitative questions from the intervention group (n = 210) and 2 qualitative questions from the control group (n = 211)

Procedure

Survey with 12 items using 7-point Likert scale relative to 4 subscales: clarity, purpose, utility, and likelihood to recommend module to others

Quantitative Data Collection

Outcome

Mean medical student scores on the 12 items for the intervention group (n = 210) and the control group (n = 211)

Analyzed for emerging themes, coding, and comparision between intervention and control groups

Qualitative Data Analysis

Strengths and weaknesses of each type of training and how students' experiences with the two types of training were compared

Compared mean scores for each module aggregated across rating scales with an independent t-test using an alpha level of 0.05

Quantitative Data Analysis

Mean ratings were significantly higher among students with virtual reality experience than for students with control experience

Procedure

Qualitative findings from learners' reflections about their experiences across all questions were matched with results on attitudinal scales

Merge Qualitative and Quantitative Results

Outcome

The mixed methods findings were represented using a visual joint display with the quantitative scale scores on the left and representative supporting qualitative quotes in the adjacent column

The final column presented an interpretation of both results together as metainferences

Integrated Interpretation

The mixed methods analysis compared the two sources of data to gain a more complete understanding of learners' experiences

Sources: Kron et al. (2017) and Fetters, M.D. and Kron, F.W. (2012–15). *Modeling Professional Attitudes and Teaching Humanistic Communication in Virtual Reality (MPathic-VRII).* National Center for Advancing Translational Science/NIH 9R44TR000360-04.

Activity: Developing a Convergent Mixed Methods Research Design

In Workbox 7.2.2, complete each section. This would be a good time to use a pencil with an eraser if you still have such an archaic tool lying around! The order you complete the figure is not critical, but you may want to begin by filling in completely the section with which you are most comfortable. You may also want to refer to Figure 7.2 for guidance. For each box enter your purpose, data collection and analytic plans, or your outcomes. For the purpose statements, you may want to reflect above to the different rationales for conducting research. If you have completed the Workboxes from Chapter 5, you may want to review to the research questions you posed. For the data collection, be as specific as possible regarding the number of participants and the data collection approach you will use. If you have completed Chapter 6 on data sources, you should refer to the procedures you identified. For the outcomes, try to anticipate what information you will receive. Your own example may differ from the template as it has been written based on a completed study. You may choose to use present or future tense. Finally, anticipate what integrating the two types of data will produce relative to merged results. In light of the possible need to deviate from your proposed design, recall you can update your design figure at any time in the future. I advise students to use the Template Workboxes to develop the overall picture, and then create the design electronically using software (I typically use PowerPoint).

Workbox 7.2.2: Convergent Mixed Methods Research Design Template

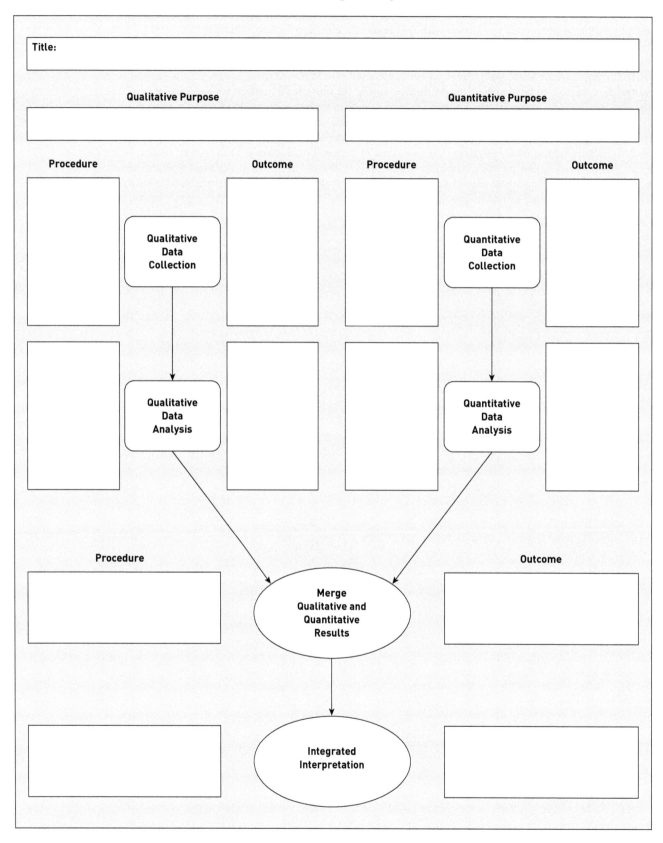

EXPLANATORY SEQUENTIAL MIXED METHODS RESEARCH DESIGN

An explanatory sequential mixed methods design occurs when the investigator first collects and analyzes quantitative data with a large subject population to examine trends, prevalence of ideas or behaviors, etc. Subsequent to the collection of the quantitative data, the researcher seeks to explain findings from the quantitative assessment by conducting and analyzing qualitative data, usually from a smaller number of subjects.

For example, in his research, to understand how principals can improve student achievement by improving school culture (Workbox Illustration 7.3.1), Harper (2016) identified 26 of Alabama's 218 middle schools deemed eligible for inclusion by examining high (n=21) and low (n=5) categories of student achievement that he then further stratified by high, medium, and low socioeconomic status. Based on his analysis, he found academic emphasis, a dimension of academic optimism, was a significant predictor of academic achievement. He then collected qualitative data to explain these findings through interviews with 11 principals of the schools in the larger study.

For an explanatory sequential MMR design, Creswell and Plano Clark (2018b) point out five key questions to consider (p. 185): (1) Will the same or different individuals be used in both samples? (2) Will the samples be the same size? (3) What quantitative results will be followed up on? (4) How will follow-up participants be selected? (5) How should the emerging follow-up phase be described for institutional review board (IRB) approval?

To apply these questions, consider Harper's (2016) study on exploring academic optimism and student achievement (Workbox illustration 7.3.1). (1) He used 26 schools in the Phase I survey that involved 334 teachers in these schools. (2) Phase II involved interviews involved 11 principals selected from among 18 high achieving middle schools. (3) Harper followed up on the significant predictor of academic achievement, namely the academic emphasis dimension of academic optimism in the follow-up interviews. (4) Harper selected follow-up participants using purposeful, maximum variation sampling based on different levels of socioeconomic status, geographic location, and a broad range of academic optimism scores (p. 86). (5) Harper submitted an IRB amendment after the analysis of the first quantitative phase was completed.

Workbox Illustration 7.3.1: Explanatory Sequential Mixed Methods Research Design Example From the Field of Education

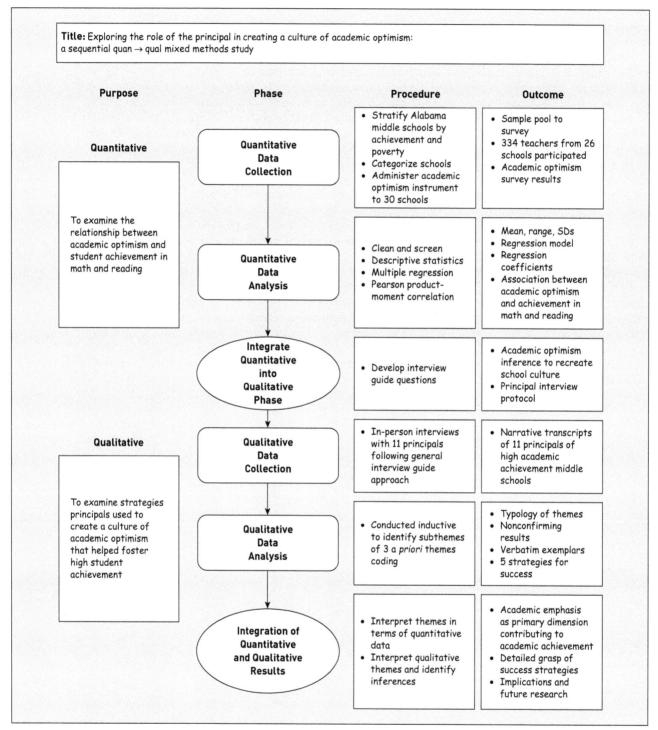

Title: Exploring the role of the principal in creating a culture of academic optimism: a sequential quan → qual mixed methods study

Purpose	Phase	Procedure	Outcome
Quantitative	**Quantitative Data Collection**	• Stratify Alabama middle schools by achievement and poverty • Categorize schools • Administer academic optimism instrument to 30 schools	• Sample pool to survey • 334 teachers from 26 schools participated • Academic optimism survey results
To examine the relationship between academic optimism and student achievement in math and reading	**Quantitative Data Analysis**	• Clean and screen • Descriptive statistics • Multiple regression • Pearson product-moment correlation	• Mean, range, SDs • Regression model • Regression coefficients • Association between academic optimism and achievement in math and reading
	Integrate Quantitative into Qualitative Phase	• Develop interview guide questions	• Academic optimism inference to recreate school culture • Principal interview protocol
Qualitative	**Qualitative Data Collection**	• In-person interviews with 11 principals following general interview guide approach	• Narrative transcripts of 11 principals of high academic achievement middle schools
To examine strategies principals used to create a culture of academic optimism that helped foster high student achievement	**Qualitative Data Analysis**	• Conducted inductive to identify subthemes of 3 a *priori* themes coding	• Typology of themes • Nonconfirming results • Verbatim exemplars • 5 strategies for success
	Integration of Quantitative and Qualitative Results	• Interpret themes in terms of quantitative data • Interpret qualitative themes and identify inferences	• Academic emphasis as primary dimension contributing to academic achievement • Detailed grasp of success strategies • Implications and future research

Source: Harper (2016, p.210) with adaptations by the *Mixed Methods Research Workbook* author.

Activity: Developing an Explanatory Sequential Methods Research Design

In Workbox 7.3.2, complete each section. The order you complete the figure is not critical, but you may want to begin by filling in completely the section with which you are most comfortable. You may also want to refer to the Figure 7.2 guidelines. For each box enter your purpose, data collection and analytic plans, as well as your outcomes. For the purpose statements you may want to reflect above to the different rationales for conducting research. If you have completed the Workboxes from Chapter 5, you may want to review the research questions you posed. For the data collection, be as specific as possible regarding the number of subjects and the data collection approach you will use. If you have completed Chapter 6 on data sources, you should refer to the procedures you identified. For the outcomes, try to anticipate what information you will receive. Your own example will differ from the template as it has been written based on a completed study. You may choose to use present or future tense. Finally, anticipate what integrating the two types of data will produce relative to merged results.

If you are using an emergent design, it is acceptable to fill out only the first phase of the design. But for your peer mentoring, you should begin considering what you think you might find from the first phase, and where that will take you in the subsequent phase.

Workbox 7.3.2: Explanatory Sequential Mixed Methods Research Design Template

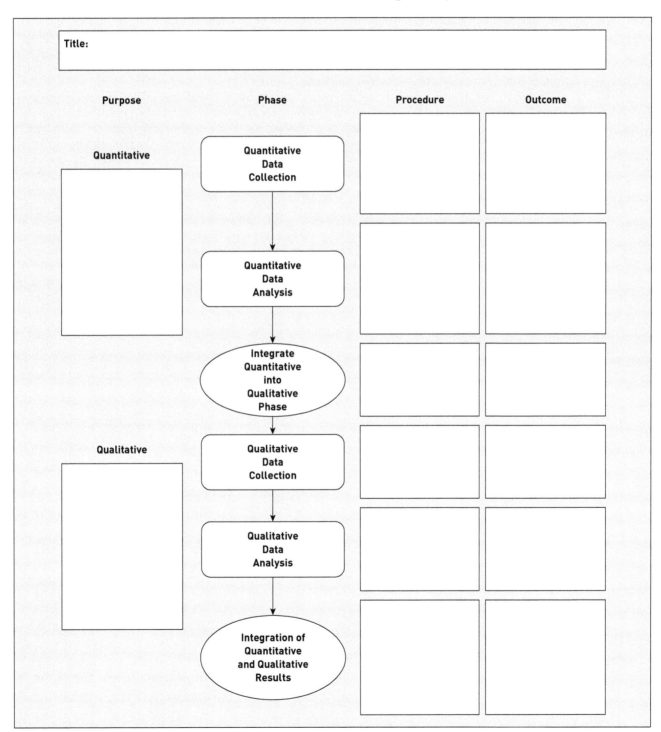

EXPLORATORY SEQUENTIAL MIXED METHODS RESEARCH DESIGN

An exploratory sequential mixed methods design occurs when the investigator first collects and analyzes qualitative data to explore a phenomenon of interest with a small number of participants. Based on the findings, the researcher then collects and analyzes data from a larger sample of participants to determine the trends and patterns in a representative sample.

For example, Sharma and Vredenburg (1998) conducted 19 in-depth interviews with executives in the Canadian oil and gas industry to develop 7 case studies and hypotheses about linkages between corporate environmental responsiveness to organizational capacity and performance that they then tested with a mail survey with responses from 99 corporations. Hence initial qualitative findings were used for item development and hypothesis generation that could be tested subsequently (Workbox Illustration 7.4.1).

For an exploratory sequential MMR design, Creswell and Plano Clark (2018b) point out five key questions to consider (p. 185): (1) Who and how many individuals should be included in the quantitative follow-up phase? (2) How should the emerging follow-up phase be described for IRB approval? (3) What qualitative results will be used to inform the quantitative data collection? (4) In the survey development-variant, how do you do a good instrument? (5) How do you convey the rigor-development variant?

To examine these questions in an actual study, consider Sharma and Vredenburg's (1998) investigation that examined corporate environmental strategy and the development of competitively valuable organizational capabilities (Workbox Illustration 7.4.1). (1) The authors targeted 110 companies and called each company to identify the names of the CEO or a member of the top management team more likely to respond, the manager responsible for environmental affairs, a crude oil production and/or refinery manager, divisional supervisors, a drilling supervisor, and a marketing manager. They mailed questionnaires to 3–5 people per company and used faxes and telephone calls after two weeks to obtain a 90% (99 of 110) response rate by company based on responses from 162 individuals. (2) Information on the IRB was not provided. (3) The qualitative results with additional information from the literature identified 11 dimensions that were used to develop the survey items and the hypotheses for testing. (4) In this survey variant, the authors' 95-item, 7-point Likert scale instrument had three constructs: (a) environmental strategies, (b) organizational capability, and (c) competitive benefits. The instrument was vetted with key informants and pretested with 25 oil and gas industry managers. The authors assessed reliability, conducted data diagnostics to ensure no violations of regression assumptions, and conducted factor analysis. (5) The authors conveyed the rigor of their steps through narrative and three tables to illustrate the items for each construct and the associated Cronbach's coefficient alpha.

Workbox Illustration 7.4.1: Exploratory Sequential Mixed Methods Research Design From Business

Title: Proactive Corporate Environmental Strategy and the Development of Competitively Valuable Organizational Capabilities

Purpose	Phase	Procedure	Outcome
Qualitative			
• To ground the applicability of the resource-based view of corporations within the domain of environmental responsiveness through the use of comparative case studies	**Qualitative Data Collection**	• Phase I: Interviews with executives of 7 companies • Literature review • Phase II: 2-5 brief interviews each with 27 execs. over 1.5 yrs • Document analysis	• Phase I: Transcripts from 19 interviews • Literature review provided theory-base • Phase II: Transcripts from multiple longitudinal interviews with 27 execs.
	Qualitative Data Analysis	• Constant comparative analysis • Create interview summaries • Comparative case study analysis	• 11 environmental-strategy dimensions • Two case types, proactive (n = 2) or reactive (n = 5) • Two hypotheses for testing in quantitative phase
	Integrate Qualitative into Quantitative Phase	• Developed instrument • Pilot tested survey • Assessed psychometrics using data diagnostics tests and factor analysis	• Survey with 95-items using 7-point Likert-scale • Most reliability constructs (Cronbach's coefficient alpha) in excess of 0.80
Quantitative	**Quantitative Data Collection**	• Mail survey administered to total population of Canadian oil and gas companies with annual sales revenues in excess of $20 million	• Closed-end survey responses from 99 corporations (response rate 90%) • Responses included 2-5 executives per company for total of 162 surveys completed
• To assess linkages between corporate environmental responsiveness to organizational capacity and performance observed during the case studies through a mail survey	**Quantitative Data Analysis**	• Tested two hypotheses using multivariate regression	• 20% of corporate capability explained by environmental responsiveness • Proactive respons-iveness did not negatively impact competitiveness
	Integration of Qualitative and Quantitative Results	• Relationships identified qualitatively using case study approach were tested quantitatively based on survey findings of target corporations	• Proactive-responsiveness strategies relative to ecological issues were associated with unique organizational capabilities and firm competitiveness

Source: Sharma and Vredenburg (1998). Procedural diagram created by the *Mixed Methods Research Workbook* author.

Activity: Developing an Exploratory Sequential Methods Research Design

In Workbox 7.4.2, complete each section. The order in which you complete the figure is not critical, but you may want to begin by filling in completely the section with which you are most comfortable. You may also want to refer to the Figure 7.2 guidelines. For each box, enter your purpose, data collection, and analytic plans, as well as your outcomes. For the purpose statements you may want to reflect above to the different rationales for conducting research. If you have completed the Workboxes from Chapter 5, you may want to review the research questions you posed. For the data collection, be as specific as possible regarding the number of subjects and the data collection approach you will use. If you have completed Chapter 6 on data sources, you should refer to the procedures you identified. For the outcomes, try to anticipate what information you will receive. Your own example will differ from the template as it has been written based on a completed study. You may choose to use present or future tense. Finally, anticipate that integrating the two types of data will produce relative to merged results.

If you are using an emergent design, it is acceptable to fill out only the first phase of the design. But for your peer mentoring, you should begin considering what you think you might find from the first phase and where that will take you in the subsequent phase.

Workbox 7.4.2: Exploratory Sequential
Mixed Methods Research Design Template

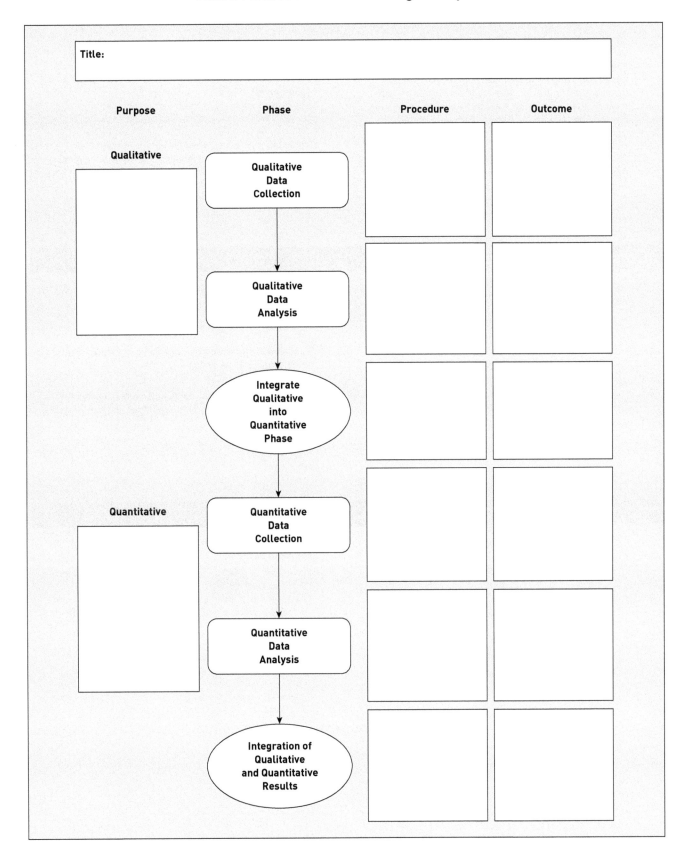

Application Activities

1. **Peer Feedback**. If you are working on your project as part of a class or in a workshop, pair up with a peer mentor, and one of you spend about 5 minutes talking about your mixed methods design figure. Take turns talking about your design and giving feedback. The helpful parts to discuss are those that you struggled with the most. In particular, focus on the intent and timing, as these are the areas that are often most challenging, and the areas that a partner in a mixed methods course will likely have the greatest interest. If you are working independently, share your design with a colleague or mentor.

2. **Peer Feedback Guidance**. As you listen to your partner, continue learning and improving the valuable skills of critiquing. Your goal is to help your partner refine the mixed methods figure. What section or area does your partner need feedback the most? Are there any sections that don't make sense, or seem infeasible? Does the chosen design make sense?

3. **Group Debrief**. If you are in a classroom or large group setting, take volunteers to present their diagrams. Reflect on how these same issues may play out in your own project. Consider using a projector to display several figures, have the author present the design, and have others critique and ask questions of the presenter.

Concluding Thoughts

Use this checklist to assess your progress in achieving the Chapter 7 objectives:

☐ I considered the spectrum of fixed and emergent designs in MMR and chose one for my mixed methods project.

☐ I compared the three core MMR designs and can articulate the essential features of each.

☐ I reviewed and can recognize conventional notations used to draw and present a mixed methods design figure.

☐ I chose a core design for use in my project or in a phase of my project.

☐ I drafted a drawing of my design.

☐ I reviewed my core design with a peer or colleague to confirm/revise my design.

Now that you have completed these objectives, Chapter 8 will help you consider relevance of a scaffolded design for your mixed methods project.

Key Resources

1. **FURTHER READING ON RESEARCH DESIGNS**

   - Creswell, J. W., & Plano Clark, V. L. (2018). Core mixed methods designs. In *Designing and conducting mixed methods research* (3rd ed.). Thousand Oaks, CA: Sage.

   - Curry, L., & Nunez-Smith, M. (2015). *Mixed methods in health sciences research: A practical primer.* Thousand Oaks, CA: Sage.

   - Johnson, R. B., & Christensen L. (2017). *Educational research: Qualitative, quantitative and mixed approaches* (6th ed.). Thousand Oaks, CA: Sage.

   - Plano Clark, V. L., & Ivankova, N. (2016). *Mixed methods research: A guide to the field.* Thousand Oaks, CA: Sage.

2. **FURTHER READING ON DRAWING MIXED METHODS RESEARCH DESIGNS**

   - Morse, J. M. (2003). Principles of mixed methods and multimethod research design. In A. Tashakkori & C. Teddlie (Eds.), *Handbook of mixed methods in social and behavioral research* (pp. 89–208). Oxford, UK: Oxford University Press.

   - Morse, J. M. (2015). Issues in qualitatively-driven mixed-method designs: Walking through a mixed-method project. In S. Hesse-Biber & R. B. Johnson (Eds.), *The Oxford handbook of multimethod and mixed methods research inquiry* (pp. 206–224). Thousand Oaks, CA: Sage.

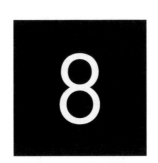

8

CONSTRUCTING PROCEDURAL DIAGRAMS OF SCAFFOLDED MIXED METHODS DESIGNS THAT EXPAND UPON CORE DESIGNS

Scaffolded mixed methods designs, also sometimes called advanced frameworks, complex designs, or intersected designs, are plans that involve the collection and analysis of both qualitative and quantitative data, are built with a core design or combination of core designs, and are typically integrated with another design and/or theory or ideology. The opportunities raised by the use of scaffolded mixed methods designs may be exciting and intriguing as you consider how these expanded designs can be built with core designs and linked together with other designs, theories, or ideologies. This chapter and its activities will help you examine features that define these types of designs, differentiate among three categories of scaffolded designs, recognize variations in how to diagram these designs, deconstruct a series of exemplar designs, and develop a procedural diagram of the project's scaffolded mixed methods design as appropriate. As a key outcome, you will draw a procedural diagram of your mixed methods study.

LEARNING OBJECTIVES

The concepts and activities presented here will help you

- Describe features of scaffolded mixed methods designs and recognize language other methodologists have used for this group of designs

- Differentiate between three categories of scaffolded mixed methods designs: (1) mixed methods integrated in multiple stages or phases; (2) mixed methods integrated with another methodology; and (3) mixed methods integrated with a theory

- Recognize variations researchers have used to diagram scaffolded mixed methods designs

- Deconstruct a scaffolded mixed methods design into its underlying core mixed methods design elements

- Develop a scaffolded mixed methods procedural diagram for your project

MIXED METHODS DESIGNS BEYOND CORE DESIGNS

If you came into my office or one of my workshops, you might request assistance drawing your procedural diagram because your design is more complicated than the core design templates you examined in Chapter 7. You might inquire about using mixed methods procedures in a program of research with multiple phases, to use mixed methods in research in combination with another design like an intervention, for building and refining a mobile device app, or in conjunction with a theory.

I would explain to you two critical issues. First, mixed methodologists have designed procedures for building or expanding upon the core mixed methods designs by linking core mixed methods designs as phases or stages of research. Conceptually, these core designs are building blocks or 'Legos' that can be used together to create expanded mixed methods research (MMR) designs. Second, mixed methodologists have developed procedures that can integrate mixed methods procedures (1) through a series of core designs, (2) with other designs, or (3) with theoretical/ideological frameworks (Plano Clark & Ivankova, 2016). In these designs, one finds an underlying structure or skeleton comprised of one more of the core mixed methods designs.

What to Call the Categories of Expanded Mixed Methods Designs

Collectively, designs expanding or building upon core design procedures have been called different names, e.g., advanced designs (Creswell, 2015), advanced applications (Plano Clark & Ivankova, 2016), or most recently, complex applications/designs (Creswell & Plano Clark, 2018). The disadvantage of the rubric of advanced designs or applications is that each implies that core designs are basic or simple. Still, in discussion of advanced applications, Plano Clark and Ivankova (2016, p. 137) progressed the field by creating categories of advanced applications they describe as "intersected" with (1) another primarily qualitative or quantitative method, (2) another methodological approach, and (3) theory or ideology. But as a rubric, I find intersecting invites confusion due to its potentially positive nuances, for example, *overlap* or *pierce*, and negative nuances, for example, *divide* or *cut*. Grounded in the conceptualizations of Nastasi and Hitchcock (2016), Creswell and Plano Clark (2018) used "complex applications/designs" as a rubric for these designs, but I find this choice may invite confusion for two reasons. First, the term *complex* like *advanced* suggests that core designs are basic, simple, or not complex. More importantly, researchers have begun integrating complexity theory and MMR to yield mixed methods complexity designs (Koopmans, 2017; Poth, 2018b). While the conceptualization of a category of these other types of designs is highly useful, to avoid potential confusion, I believe an alternative rubric is needed.

SCAFFOLDED MIXED METHODS DESIGNS DEFINED

I advise the language of **scaffolded mixed methods designs**. Scaffolded mixed methods designs are research strategies or plans that collect and analyze both qualitative and quantitative data, are built with a core design or combination of core designs, and are typically integrated with another application, methodology or theory in accordance with the categories developed by Plano Clark & Ivankova (2016). The rationale for the rubric scaffolded is that it underscores mixed methods procedures as providing a foundation, an infrastructure, a skeleton, a grid work, or lattice work, that is, the underlying structure for expanding mixed methods designs.

Other methodologies, for example, interventions, can be built on a mixed methods design infrastructure. Mixed methods designs can provide an underlying structure for theory, for example, complexity theory, and mixed methods procedures can provide an infrastructure for survey development. Just as vertebrates have an underlying skeleton not usually obvious without radiological viewing, scaffolded mixed methods designs feature mixed methods as a "backbone" that is not obvious unless viewed with the mixed methods lens.

A transformative design, participatory, or action mixed methods design can have one or more underlying mixed methods designs and possibly even another methodology (e.g., interventional design), while also being integrated with a theoretical framework. A case study can be built based on a single, or combination of, mixed methods core design(s). Hence, when mixed methods procedures occur with other methods, methodologies, and/or theories/ideologies, the concept of scaffolding expresses how mixed methods provide an infrastructure for the study.

Developing a Procedural Diagram of Your Scaffolded Mixed Methods Study Design

As discussed in Chapter 7, a procedural diagram provides an overview on a single page of your MMR or evaluation. The examples presented in this chapter are highly diverse, and you should feel free to choose elements from any or even develop your own. For each design's procedural illustration, I will point out noteworthy elements. As studies become more complex, it does become more challenging to include all of the details provided for core designs in Chapter 7, Workbox Illustrations 7.2.1, 7.3.1, and 7.4.1. If you are at the stage where you are writing up your findings for publication in a manuscript or your dissertation, you may prefer a more or less parsimonious procedural diagram depending upon your needs. The Choosing a Procedural Diagram Workbox 8.1 provides a list of the workbox illustrations in this chapter that you can choose to guide your procedural diagram development.

Workbox 8.1: Choosing a Procedural Diagram to Emulate From Among Seven Types of Scaffolded Mixed Methods Designs

Your Choice	Design Categories	Type of Scaffolded Mixed Methods Design	Corresponding Illustration
☐	Multistage/ multiphase) designs	Multistage mixed methods design	Workbox Illustration 8.4.1
☐	Methodological	Mixed methods intervention/trial design	Workbox Illustration 8.5.1
☐		Mixed methods case study design	Workbox Illustration 8.6.1
☐		Mixed methods evaluation design	Workbox Illustration 8.7.1
☐		Mixed methods survey development design	Workbox Illustration 8.8.1
☐		Mixed methods interactive-user-centered design	Workbox Illustration 8.9.1
☐	Theoretical	Mixed methods community-based participatory design	Workbox Illustration 8.10.1

Activity: Choosing a Workbox Illustration for Creating a Procedural Diagram of Your Scaffolded Mixed Methods Study Design

If you are considering a scaffolded design, you are now ready to develop a procedural diagram. In Workbox 8.1, choose the type of scaffolded design you are planning to use. Review the checklist for creating a procedural diagram (Workbox 8.2) and the procedural diagram template (Workbox 8.3). Once you understand the exemplar choices and the overall creation process, you can choose from the Workbox Illustrations 8.4.1 to 8.10.1 and emulate features of the procedural diagram from the chosen workbox illustration. You will find it informative to read the study description. Complete the workbox activity after identifying the underling core mixed methods design, as this will help you consider your own diagram. As time permits, review all seven procedural diagram examples, as each has interesting variations that you could incorporate into your procedural diagram regardless of the specific type of scaffolded design you are planning.

Workbox 8.2: Checklist for Creating a Mixed Methods Scaffolded Design Procedural Diagram

☐ Create a title for your procedural diagram

☐ Decide whether you prefer a top-to-bottom vertical look or a left-to-right horizontal look

☐ Fill in the big picture ideas first, and gradually add detail

☐ Identify your underlying core design(s)

☐ Complete the components of the procedural diagram template easiest for you first

☐ Draw with boxes, circles, and arrows—the core designs

☐ Create a box for each type of data collected, the analysis, and results, and label the data collection box with QUAL, QUAN, or mixed methods

☐ Add labels adjacent to the QUAL, QUAN, or mixed methods boxes

☐ Complete the expected outcomes box

☐ Insert your analytical approach

☐ Add labels to indicate your phases, specific aims, research questions, and/or hypotheses in the margins

☐ Populate the missing areas you skipped

☐ Clarify your procedures and update your choices

☐ Edit your procedural diagram and boxes to optimal size

☐ Edit for aesthetic appearance

STEPS FOR CREATING A SCAFFOLDED PROCEDURAL DIAGRAM FROM THE BEGINNING

Having reviewed one or more Workbox Illustrations (8.4.1 to 8.10.1), begin drawing your own procedural diagram. Review Workbox 8.2 to help guide your creative process. Remember, the process is not linear. Because these diagrams are even more complex than core design diagrams, you will likely (most certainly) need to write multiple drafts. Check off the steps as you complete them to your satisfaction. Remember you can always come back after a few steps and will almost certainly need to. After making some progress, share with a peer mentor, colleague, or dissertation advisor.

The following 15 steps will assist your building a procedural diagram.

1. *Create a title for your procedural diagram.* This helps you keep focus on your study. If you have a particular theoretical/ideological perspective, you can add this, for example, "a transformative mixed methods design." Be sure to include the type of the particular design in the study title.

2. *Decide whether you prefer a top-to-bottom vertical look or a left-to-right horizontal look.* If working directly in the Workbook, I advise starting with the vertical format (portrait), but if using a drawing program (e.g., Microsoft PowerPoint), I advise using horizontal (landscape). More complicated designs tend to go top-to-bottom, though some authors choose to go left-to-right, then come back right-to-left, and then again left-to-right (See Workbox Illustration 8.5). Be creative! You may want to reference guidelines in Chapter 7, Figure 7.2, to inform the conventions in your design, and to structure your design procedural diagram. Organize the diagram to optimize understanding of the reader.

3. *Fill in the big picture ideas first, and gradually add detail.* Ironically, the big picture details may be the most difficult, but it is the best place to start. If you add detail but are uncertain about your choice, leave a question mark.

4. *Identify your underlying core design(s).* If your scaffolded MMR design involves more than one core design, if needed, complete relevant core design templates in Chapter 7.

5. *Complete the components of the procedural diagram template easiest for you first.* You will find it most efficient to complete the information you already have committed to. In workshops, I often find people have identified the methods that they want to use, for example, interviews, surveys, document analysis, observations, secondary dataset, etc. Add this information first. The more difficult information requires estimating how much of each type of data will be collected. A common mistake for researchers less familiar with qualitative methodology is to overestimate the number of participants.

6. *Draw with the boxes, circles, and arrows—the core designs.* Generally, it is easiest if you go in chronological order. When working sequentially, the latter box of your core design may well become your initial box(es) for a second core design. You may choose to use circles to denote points of integration. Review Figure 7.2 for Ivanakova et al.'s (2006) recommended steps for drawing a design.

7. *Create a box for each type of data collected, the analysis, and results.* Add QUAL, QUAN, or mixed methods to denote if the data collected will be qualitative, quantitative, or mixed methods.

8. *Add labels adjacent to the QUAL, QUAN, or mixed methods boxes.* Use the explicit type of data collection and sample size (e.g., interviews, n = 20). If you haven't decided yet, leave the number out, or write a guestimate with a question mark.

9. *Complete the expected outcomes box.* Of course, you do not know exactly what your research will find, but you should have a general idea. Having projected outcomes really helps supervisors and colleagues, and especially reviewers of grant applications.

10. *Insert your analytical approach.* Envisioning your products or outcomes may help you decide (see Workbox Illustration 8.8.1). You will learn more about mixed methods analytical procedures later in Chapters 13–15.

11. *Add labels to indicate your phases, specific aims, research questions, and/or hypotheses in the margins.* You should now add in the margins your study phase, aims, questions, and hypotheses (see study phases in Workbox Illustration 8.8.1). You may be able to use or adapt the MMR questions/hypotheses you developed in Chapter 6.

12. *Populate the missing areas you skipped.* Gradually add in the more difficult boxes or text based on your further reading or consultation with others.

13. *Clarify your procedures and update your choices.* Iteratively add and update your choices. Check with others to determine if you have included sufficient detail for the reader of the implementation matrix to understand your qualitative, quantitative, and mixed methods integration procedures.

14. *Edit your procedural diagram and boxes to proportionate size.* As you add more information to the procedural diagram, you may find that one section takes up an inordinate amount of space. For example, the data collection label may seem very long. You will find yourself editing and re-editing to shorten. If using a drawing program on a computer, you can use the grouping function to move whole sections.

15. *Edit for aesthetic appearance.* As a final step, edit the procedural diagram to be aesthetically appealing. The diagram will receive a lot of interest, and by having visual appeal, it is much easier to engage others. Do you have consistent capitalization and punctuation? Are all sections within a single column similarly formatted? You will be able to use this diagram in your grant proposal, manuscripts, or dissertation (or some iteration in all of the above, if lucky!).

Workbox 8.3: Drawing a Procedural
Diagram of Your Scaffolded Mixed Methods Study

Title:

OVERVIEW OF SEVEN WORKBOX ILLUSTRATIONS

The sections below present three categories of scaffolded mixed methods design types: (1) multistage (multiphase) mixed methods designs; (2) mixed methods integrated with another methodology; and (3) mixed methods integrated with a theory/ideology (Plano Clark & Ivankova, 2016). Each section reviews the fundamental features, recommends other selected studies in the literature that might be of interest, and identifies noteworthy procedural elements. Among the design examples included in this chapter, some align more closely to the system of notations for mixed methods studies presented in Chapter 7 than others. As the field of MMR is still changing rapidly, emulate features you see as strengths, rather than focusing on limitations.

1. FUNDAMENTALS OF A GENERAL MULTISTAGE FRAMEWORK

A mixed methods multistage (multiphase) study refers to the use of a series of mixed methods core designs, and/ or scaffolded mixed methods designs, for a sustained program of research conducted over an extended period of research. These designs can incorporate elements of one or more core design(s), or be scaffolded mixed methods designs. Authors have used the language of multistage (Fetters, Curry, & Creswell, 2013) or multiphase (Creswell & Plano Clark, 2011) without a clear distinction. In full recognition that it is an arbitrary choice, for purposes of this workbook, the language of multistage implies a larger enterprise or degree of activity than a phase. I will favor use of *multistage* unless the authors of described studies have chosen *multiphase*.

Example of a Mixed Methods Multiphase Explanatory Sequential Study Design From the Field of Education

Tsushima examined perspectives of secondary school Japanese teachers of English as a foreign language, relative to concordance of their teaching and testing practices and their speaking-focused course objectives (Tsushima, 2012, 2015). She conducted a three-phase, explanatory sequential design (Workbox Illustration 8.4.1). In Phase I, she conducted a survey of secondary school Japanese teachers of English as a foreign language. To obtain a more in-depth view of classroom organization, teaching, and testing, she used two data collection integration approaches of building for additional data collection and connecting her sample with teachers from the previous phase for qualitative observations and term exam qualitative analysis. In Phase III, she built from Phase II findings an interview guide and interviewed teachers for greater insight into classroom teaching and assessment. She merged all the information in her final analysis.

Noteworthy Diagram Elements

The design flows in a vertical format top-to-bottom and effectively demonstrates the concomitant qualitative data collection. The use of circles illustrates points for integration during implementation of the research—in the upper circle for building data collection tools, and the bottom circle for merging data together for analysis.

Workbox Illustration 8.4.1: Example of a Mixed Methods Multiphase Explanatory Sequential Study Design From the Field of Education

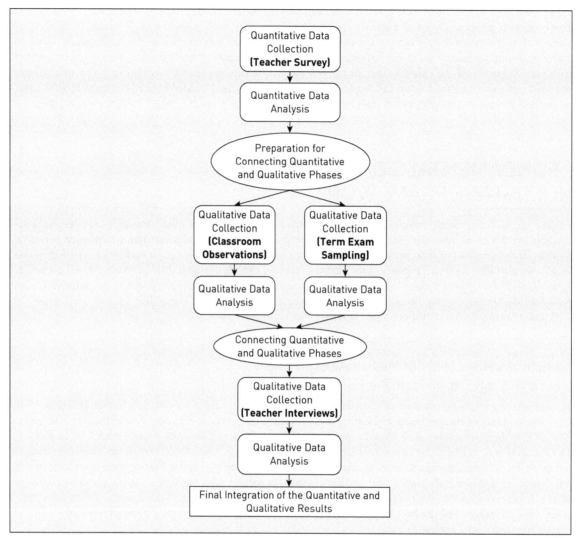

Source: Tsushima, R. (2015). Methodological diversity in language assessment research: The role of mixed methods in classroom-based language assessment studies. *International Journal of Qualitative Methods, 14,* 104–121. doi:10.1177/160940691501400202 with permission of SAGE Publications.

Workbox 8.4.2: What Underlying Core Design(s) Can Be Found in the Mixed Methods Multiphase Explanatory Sequential Study Design of Workbox Illustration 8.4.1, and Why?

Core mixed methods design:

Explanation:

(See explanation in Table 8.1.)

Programs of Mixed Methods Research

When starting a research project, it seems difficult just to imagine two or even three phases of data collection, analysis, and perform data merging. But there are examples of sustained lines of research using mixed methods procedures for each project. For example, Crabtree et al. (2011) reported on their experience of continuous funding in the health sciences where one funded program built on a previously funded program, and how, when completed, the most recently completed research became a springboard for the next study (Case Study 8.1). In total, the investigators successfully built upon, and sustained, major funding for six investigations for improving primary care practice. Ultimately, they called this an emergent longitudinal mixed methods developmental collaborative design. While the series of funded investigations emerged over time, the individual grants were comprised of more specific design plans. This case study illustrates using a combination of fixed designs during funded studies and emergent strategies over the course of multiple studies (Figure 8.9).

CASE STUDY 8.1

THE LINKAGE OF MULTIPLE MIXED METHODS RESEARCH STUDIES IN A PROGRAM OF RESEARCH: AN EXAMPLE FROM A 15-YEAR DEVELOPMENTAL PROGRAM OF RESEARCH ON PRIMARY CARE PRACTICE TRANSFORMATION

In 2011, Crabtree and colleagues published their experience in sustained, funded research on primary care practice transformation. The underlying idea of practice transformation is that real improvements in clinical performance relative to delivery of preventive services such as immunizations to preventable infectious diseases (e.g., flu vaccination to prevent influenza, human papilloma vaccination to prevent cervical cancer), behavior changes to prevent later disease, illness, or injury

(e.g., smoking cessation, promotion of seatbelt use), early identification of conditions when still highly treatable (e.g., breast and colorectal cancer screening), and reducing progression of chronic conditions (e.g., diabetes or high blood pressure) require fundamental changes in the way doctors provide clinical care. Over the course of 15 years, Crabtree and colleagues used MMR in six funded studies to understand and intervene successfully to improve practice.

FIGURE 8.1 ■ Linking Multiple Studies in an Emergent Longitudinal Mixed Methods Developmental Collaborative Design

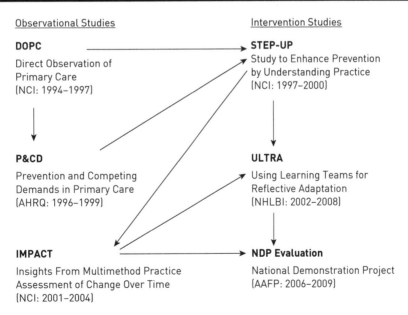

Source: Crabtree, B. F., Nutting, P. A., Miller, W. L., McDaniel, R. R., Stange, K. C., Jaén, C. R., & Stewart, E. (2011). Primary care practice transformation is hard work: Insights from a 15-year developmental program of research. *Medical Care, 49*, S28. doi:10.1097%2FMLR.0b013e3181cad65c with permission of Lippincott Williams & Wilkins.

2. FUNDAMENTALS OF MIXED METHODS DESIGNS INTEGRATED WITH ANOTHER METHODOLOGY

The first category of scaffolded design occurs when mixed methods are integrated with another methodology as a mixed methods intervention/experiment or mixed methods case study (Plano Clark & Ivankova, 2016). In education, the health sciences, and many other fields, researchers rely on interventional or experimental designs to examine associations, causality, and effect size. The scaffolded MMR designs presented here include (a) mixed methods experimental (intervention) design (Workbox Illustration 8.5.1) and (b) mixed methods case study design (Workbox Illustration 8.6.1). Mixed methods procedures can be incorporated into interventional designs or trials before, during, or after the trial data collection as an important source of information. Similarly, mixed methods procedures can be incorporated into case study designs through the collection of a variety of different types of available qualitative and quantitative data about a bounded-phenomenon of interest (Yin, 2014). Another possible scaffolded methodology is action research. Conducted as mixed methodology, it is focused on finding solutions of practical importance for social change through empowerment and emancipation for a specific group (Ivankova, 2015). Due to space constraints, an example is beyond the scope of this chapter.

Mixed Methods Experimental/Interventional Designs

In a mixed methods experimental study design, the overarching purpose is to conduct an experiment or intervention (O'Cathain, 2018). The addition of mixed methods into the trial is a modification of the well-established procedures for conducting a trial. Hence, the naming convention features *mixed methods* modifying *experimental*. In the mixed methods literature, authors often speak of embedding qualitative research into the experimental design prior to the trial, during the trial, or after the trial.

Mixed Methods Scaffolded Into a Quasi-Experimental Intervention From Education

The intersection of a quasi-experimental intervention onto mixed methods scaffolding using an education example can be seen in Workbox Illustration 8.5.1 by Kong, Mohd Yaacob, and Mohd Ariffin (2016). To develop and test a three-dimensional (3-D) textbook to teach architecture to fifth-grade elementary students, the authors conducted a two-phase study. In the Phase I, exploratory phase, they conducted a qualitative case study. They conducted interviews with fifth graders, teachers, administrative staff, and the project architect, as well as observations in the Green School in Bali, Indonesia. This allowed them to understand the child–environment interaction and develop an initial description of the 3-D architectural textbook. In an intermediate phase, they constructed a physical model of the 3-D textbook and defined variables for testing in Phase II. In Phase II, the investigators implemented a quasi-experimental design with qualitative data collection embedded as observations during the intervention and interviews after the study. Students completed instruments pre- and postintervention about pro-environmental knowledge, attitudes, and behaviors as measures of their environmental education. Initial qualitative in-depth interviews and qualitative observations led to the development of the intervention and testing quantitatively by checking pre/postintervention assessments. While this was occurring, the investigators conducted qualitative observations. This led to a posttrial qualitative phase used to explain the findings of the trial based on posttrial interviews.

Noteworthy Diagram Elements

This example illustrates the use of a case study as the qualitative data collection procedure in Phase I (see also discussion on mixed methods case study designs). While both Phases I and II are portrayed left-to-right, there is a dotted line traversing back to the left that identified the intermediate phase that then moves further to the intervention as it begins on the left. The structure of Phases I and II horizontally allows for portrayal of integration of all the data in the final oblong rectangle on the right, as arrows from both Phase I and Phase II lead into it.

Workbox Illustration 8.5.1: Example of
Quasi-experimental Mixed Methods Study Design

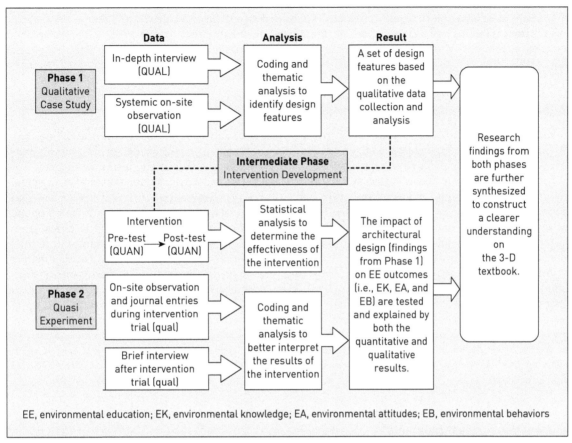

EE, environmental education; EK, environmental knowledge; EA, environmental attitudes; EB, environmental behaviors

Source: Kong, S. Y., Mohd Yaacob, N., & Mohd Ariffin, A. R. (2016). Constructing a mixed methods research design: Exploration of an architectural intervention. *Journal of Mixed Methods Research*, 1–18. doi:10.1177/1558689816651807 with permission of SAGE Publications.

Workbox 8.5.2: What Underlying
Core Design(s) Can Be Found in the Mixed Methods Quasi-experimental
Design of Workbox Illustration 8.5.1, and Why?

Core mixed methods designs:

Explanation:

(See explanation in Table 8.1)

Mixed Methods Case Study Designs

A mixed methods case study design involves the use of mixed methods to study a case. Another iteration is a mixed methods design with an embedded case study (Guetterman & Fetters, 2018). The mixed methods case study refers to utilizing one or more core mixed methods design(s) that provide(s) scaffolding for a research investigation, collecting and analyzing both qualitative and quantitative data to examine a well-bounded phenomenon, that is, clarifying the unit of analysis to have clear criteria for what/who will be included in the case (Yin, 2014).

Mixed Methods Case Study From Medical Education

Workbox Illustration 8.6.1 illustrates the intersection of a case study with mixed methods scaffolding (Yin, 2014). Shultz et al. (2015) conducted a mixed methods case study using a convergent design. The authors' purpose was to examine the perceived acceptability and impact of a standardized patient–instructor program that trained Japanese family medicine physician trainees in female breast and pelvic examinations and male genital and prostate examinations. In this intrinsic case study, that is, the case was chosen as it is unique and thus important (Guetterman & Fetters, 2018), the residents who participated in the educational program bound the case. The qualitative data sources included standardized patient–instructor and resident feedback about the training and follow-up semi-structured interviews 1–2 years later with the trainees and clinic staff in their home institution. The quantitative data were the trainees' self-assessments of their own sensitive examination performance. The researchers collected and analyzed all of the qualitative and quantitative data and then compared the qualitative and quantitative findings. They examined the extent that the findings from each phase of data collection corroborated or contradicted the findings from the other. The data were collected over two waves, but brought together for analysis at the same time. In the first wave, the authors used qualitative text from instructor feedback, as well as qualitative reflections of the residents while in the United States. In the second wave, the authors conducted assessments of resident physicians during actual patient care in Japan involving qualitative semi-structured interviews, staff semi-structured interviews, and quantitative resident self-assessments.

Noteworthy Diagram Elements

The procedural diagram illustrates the relationship between educational activities and mixed methods data collection. Moreover, it illustrates different time points for data collection, though a unique aspect of this study is that the data were all merged at the same time, thus precluding its categorization as a sequential design.

Workbox Illustration 8.6.1: Example of a Mixed Methods Case Study Design Used in Medical Education

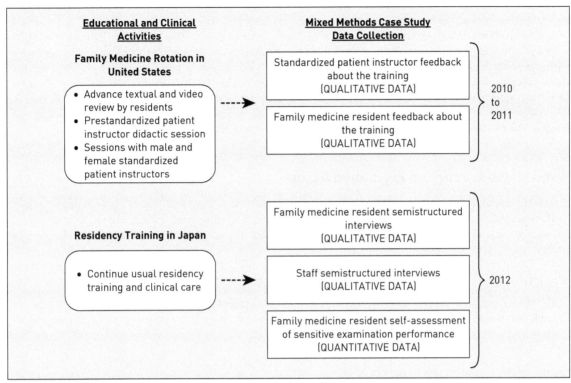

Source: Shultz, C. G., Chu, M. S., Yajima, A., Skye, E. P., Sano, K., Inoue, M., . . . Fetters, M. D. (2015). The cultural context of teaching and learning sexual health care examinations in Japan: A mixed methods case study assessing the use of standardized patient instructors among Japanese family physician trainees of the Shizuoka Family Medicine Program. *Asia Pacific Family Medicine, 14*, 8. doi:10.1186/s12930-015-0025-4 with permission of BioMed Central Publications.

Workbox 8.6.2: What Underlying Core Design(s) Can Be Found in the Mixed Methods Case Study in Workbox Illustration 8.6.1, and Why?

Core mixed methods designs:

Explanation:

(See explanation in Table 8.1)

3. FUNDAMENTALS OF METHODS DESIGNS INTEGRATED WITH OTHER DESIGNS

The third category of scaffolded design occurs when mixed methods are integrated with a specific application such as a mixed methods evaluation, survey development, or an interactive user-centered design for development of websites or apps (Plano Clark & Ivankova, 2016). Mixed methods procedures can be used as part of an evaluation design where the overarching purpose is assessment or appraisal of the value, impact, or effectiveness of a project or service. Mixed methods procedures are core to both survey development and interactive user-centered designs utilized for the construction of online or mobile platform websites or applications/apps (Alwashmi, Hawboldt, Davis, & Fetters, 2019). When multiple combinations of mixed methods procedures are used in a series of studies or in a program of research, this can be described as a mixed methods multiphase or multistage design.

Mixed Methods Program Evaluation Design

A mixed methods program evaluation study refers to a rigorous research approach using one or more core mixed methods design(s) scaffolded into the assessment or appraisal of the merit, value, impact, worth, or effectiveness of a socially constructed system. Creswell and Plano Clark (2018) characterize mixed methods evaluation designs as thus:

> In large-scale evaluation projects, there are multiple objectives, numerous phases, and multiple investigators, all of which push the use of core mixed methods designs into a complex application. Typical phases include needs assessment, theory development and adaptation, program development and testing, and assessment of the program's impact through outcomes and processes. (p. 131)

Mixed methods evaluation procedures can be used in a variety of fields, such as business, education, and health care.

The intersection of mixed methods program evaluation study with underlying mixed methods scaffolding can be illustrated by examining Workbox Illustration 8.7.1. To evaluate a model integrating screening and exercise, the Healthy Exercise, Eating and Lifestyle Program model (HEELP) was implemented in primary schools in Canberra, Australia, by Cochrane and Davey (2017). They conducted a mixed methods evaluation to determine the effect of the program on measures of body status and physical performance as the primary outcome measure in 25 schools. Additional quantitative data collection to measure the effect of HEELP was implemented to assess if changes were sustained 6 months after the intervention. In Years 3 and 4 of the study, mixed data collection questionnaires, with structured and some open responses, were distributed to parents/guardians of participating children to assess major constructs of child enjoyment and benefit from the program, influence of the HEELP intervention on the child and family, use of diary and home activities, communication, and program aspects that were not liked by the child and family. The qualitative assessment begun in year 3 was used to elucidate perceptions and practices of schools to understand how the school environment supported healthy exercise and eating, lifestyle education, and involvement in after-school services. This involved semi-structured interviews and field observations at the schools. The quantitative analysis used a random effects model to estimate the true effect and heterogeneity in the entire population of studies. For a 6-month post-HEELP follow-up, they used repeated measures, analysis of variance, and paired t-tests to compare changes in measures over time. Qualitative thematic analysis, which they termed as an explanatory/confirmatory analysis, was used to examine the impact and value to the school, as well as corroboration of findings from direct measurements of children and parental surveys.

Noteworthy Diagram Elements

This study illustrates collection of mixed biometrics data and mixed survey data that are used together in the initial 2 years of the study, followed by qualitative analysis. This diagram effectively illustrates the longitudinal aspects of this program evaluation over the course of 4 years. By showing different years, the visual helps depict how the qualitative data collection occurred much later in the study.

Workbox Illustration 8.7.1: Example of a Program Evaluation Mixed Methods Study Design*

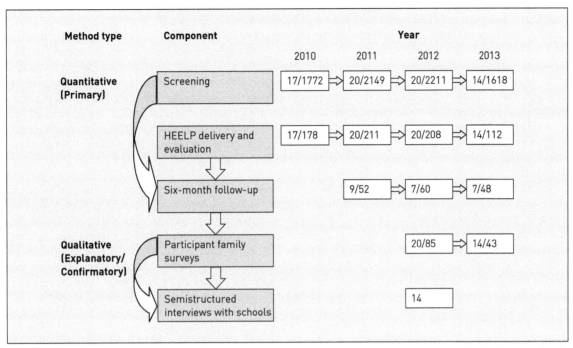

*Numbers in boxes represent number of schools/individual participants or respondents included in each component for the given year. HEELP: Healthy Exercise, Eating, and Lifestyle Program

Source: Cochrane, T., & Davey, R. C. (2017). Mixed-methods evaluation of a healthy exercise, eating, and lifestyle program for primary schools. *Journal of School Health, 87,* 823–831. doi:10.1111/josh.12555 with permission of American School Health Association.

Workbox 8.7.2: What Underlying Core Design(s) Can Be Found in the Mixed Methods Evaluation Study in Workbox Illustration 8.7.1, and Why?

Core mixed methods designs:

Explanation:

(See explanation in Table 8.1)

Mixed Methods Survey (Instrument) Development Design

A mixed methods survey development design refers to utilizing a combination of qualitative and quantitative data collection and analysis procedures scaffolded into the tool development, e.g., pilot and cognitive testing, and psychometrics and performance testing. The overarching purpose is the development of a robust survey. Creswell and Plano Clark (2018) describe the exploratory sequential design as a three-phase design, and Creswell, Fetters, and Ivankova (2004), based on review of studies in the health sciences, referred to this process as an instrument development design. The very common exploratory sequential mixed methods design for survey development typically involves three phases. A rigorous mixed methods survey study design involves a first phase of qualitative data collection and analysis to explore the phenomenon of interest, a second phase of instrument development and refinement using both quantitative pilot testing and qualitative data collection, and a third phase of deployment and quantitative data collection. The exploratory sequential mixed methods design may also involve a two-phase model. For example, a project might involve an initial qualitative phase to build a model that is then validated in a second phase using secondary dataset analysis of a large quantitative data base.

A survey development study integrated with mixed methods scaffolding can be seen in the study in Workbox Illustration 8.8.1. To explore the ecological context of how teacher education influence affects South Korean educators' professional development, Hwang (2014) used an exploratory sequential mixed methods design. In Phase I, the qualitative data collection involved 21 interviews with South Korean educators from three national universities of education. In Phase II, Hwang then created an online questionnaire with 10 demographic questions and 7 questions about South Korean teacher educators' work and concerns that had been raised in the interviews during the initial qualitative phase. Hwang additionally incorporated six 5-point Likert scale questions, anchored by strongly disagree "1" to strongly agree "5," that were written as statements to confirm the qualitative findings for a multilevel context (i.e., institutional context, national context, global context, and for student teachers, and school teachers and colleagues). The online survey was piloted with 39 teachers from 13 educational institutions. In Phase III, the instrument was again distributed, and the authors conducted analysis of their 164 responses.

Noteworthy Diagram Elements

This is a highly detailed procedural diagram. Study flow follows a vertical, top-to-bottom course. An interesting aspect is the depiction of the study subjects in the arrowed box on the left. This information is often included under the methods, though in this case, it was effective. A possible shortcoming of this diagram is the lack of a connection between the products of each step with the next box in the vertical trajectory, that is, the final column of products appears to be the final step. This could have been improved by adding into each of the product boxes a short phrase about what was done with the product. The figure could have been enhanced further with more information about the methods, data collection procedures, and products for Phase III.

Workbox Illustration 8.8.1: Example of a Mixed Methods Survey Development Design

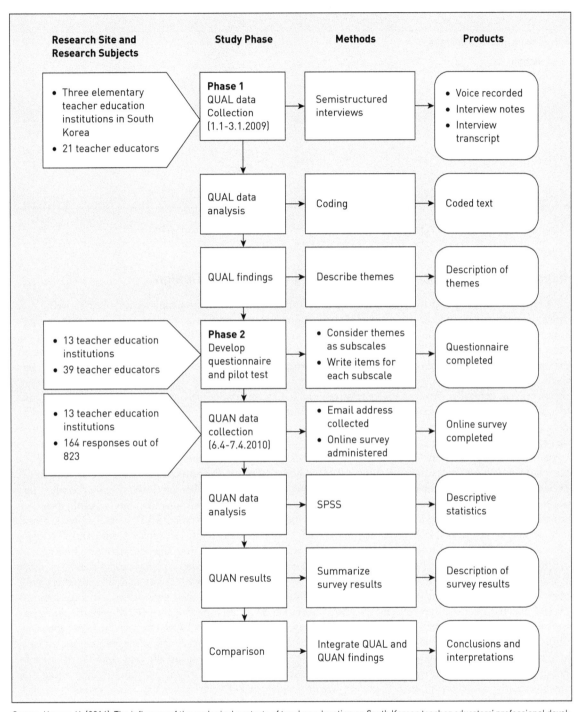

Source: Hwang, H. (2014). The influence of the ecological contexts of teacher education on South Korean teacher educators' professional development. *Teaching and Teacher Education, 43,* 1–14. doi:10.1016/j.tate.2014.05.003 with permission of SAGE Publications.

Workbox 8.8.2: What Underlying Core Design(s) Can Be Found in the Mixed Methods Survey Development Design in Workbox Illustration 8.8.1, and Why?

Core mixed methods designs:

Explanation:

(See explanation in Table 8.1)

Mixed Methods Interactive User-Centered Website/App Design

Along with the arrival of the Internet era and an explosion in the development of websites, as well as the advent of smartphones and the use of mobile applications or just "apps," has come an explosion of individuals using mixed methods procedures to develop websites and apps, as well as testing them using mixed methods procedures. While somewhat similar to development of a survey instrument, app and website development are much more of an iterative and continuous process. Alwashmi et al. (2019) describe this as an iterative convergent mixed methods design. While a mixed methods survey instrument creates a data collection tool that may have future versions, generally, surveys became relatively static data collection instruments. In contrast, websites, and especially apps, are under constant change based on usage patterns and user needs. In these cases, there is often heavy reliance on qualitative methods, more so than instrument development with scales that require more intensive psychometric development.

An interactive user-centered design using mixed methods procedures was employed to develop a hybrid website and smartphone app for weight management using mixed methods procedures (Morrison et al., 2014; Yardley et al., 2012). The authors developed an online intervention called Positive Online Weight Reduction (POWeR) that provides a flexible, nonprescriptive approach to weight management that encourages autonomy and adoption of healthy behaviors with the intent of maintaining long-term weight management (Workbox Illustration 8.9.1). Over a 12-week period, a new session became available to users each week. Each session offered "tools" to support participants developing self-regulatory skills. The development and testing were published in two articles. The first phase involved iterative development and qualitative testing (Yardley et al., 2012). The authors interviewed 25 people about their experiences with weight management. They then combined the results of these interviews with theory to design the intervention followed by in-depth, think-aloud cognitive testing of 16 people to elucidate their perceptions about the intervention and materials. For the intervention (Workbox Illustration 8.9.1), each participant selected personal eating and physical activity plans and goals for three initial Web-based sessions of the POWeR intervention (Morrison et al., 2014). Subsequently, the participants were asked to download the POWeR Tracker app, while maintaining access to the Web-based POWeR intervention. The study procedures and materials were initially pilot-tested with one user. During the intervention, the investigators monitored participants over a 4-week period and required them to complete daily quantitative self-report measures of goal engagement using the POWeR Tracker app. At the end of each week, the investigators conducted semistructured telephone interviews to elucidate each participant's experiences of using POWeR on the Web and the POWeR Tracker app. Usage of Web and app versions including when, how long, and in what order particular pages or screens were viewed were recorded automatically for each participant. The investigators measured motivation, self-efficacy, awareness, and achievement for eating and physical activity goals using 3-item scales. The investigators reported their quantitative and qualitative findings contiguously and drew inferences from the two sources of information in the discussion.

Noteworthy Diagram Elements

This diagram portrays the complex procedures needed to develop the app in this study. The longitudinal nature of the data collections is represented well. Moreover, the procedural diagram illustrates the trial. This allows the reader to surmise data collection pre-, during, and posttrial.

Workbox Illustration 8.9.1: Example of MMR Scaffolded Into a Hybrid Mobile Application and Website

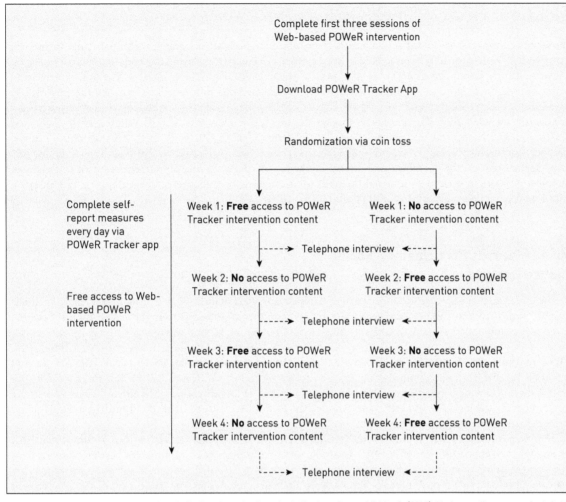

Source: Morrison, L. G., Hargood, C., Lin, S. X., Dennison, L., Joseph, J., Hughes, S., . . . Michie, S. (2014). Understanding usage of a hybrid website and smartphone app for weight management: A mixed-methods study. *Journal of Medical Internet Research, 16,* e201. doi:10.2196/jmir.3579 with permission of *Journal of Medical Internet Research.*

Workbox 8.9.2: What Underlying Core Design(s) Can Be Found in the Mixed Methods User-Centered Interactive Design in Figure 8.9.1, and Why?

Core mixed methods designs:

Explanation:

(See explanation in Table 8.1.)

4. FUNDAMENTALS OF MIXED METHODS DESIGNS INTEGRATED WITH A THEORETICAL/IDEOLOGICAL FRAMEWORK

The second category of scaffolded design occurs when mixed methods are integrated with a particular theoretical framework (Plano Clark & Ivankova, 2016). This category often occurs in mixed methods social justice designs. Researchers may emphasize diversity, equity, and inclusion in studies seeking social justice when there is an expressed interest to minimizing injustice. They use mixed methods procedures to enhance the findings, so as to bolster their credibility and increase the impact of the research. Mixed methods participatory-social justice designs include CBPR (DeJonckheere, Lindquist-Grantx, Toraman, Haddad, & Vaughn, 2018) (Workbox Illustration 8.10.1) and transformative approaches (Mertens, 2007, 2009, 2010, 2015). Transformative mixed methods, community-based participatory research, and action research (Ivankova, 2015) all have an underlying social agenda that can be combined with mixed methods procedures. While beyond the scope of this chapter, complexity theory integrated with mixed methods is an emerging area that researchers are using in innovative mixed methods studies (Koopmans, 2017; Poth, 2018a, 2018b).

Mixed Methods Participatory-Social Justice Designs

The mixed methods participatory-social justice study design refers to utilizing one or more core mixed methods design(s) scaffolded into and guided theoretically, by a commitment to incorporating the voices and collaboration of the population under research, usually with the intent of promoting fairness where there is inequity or discrimination. This category includes transformative mixed methods as pioneered by Donna Mertens (2007, 2009, 2010, 2015), and mixed methods community-based participatory research as popularized by Israel, Eng, Schulz, and Parker (2012) that has been examined in an extensive review by DeJonckheereet al. (2018). The use of social justice implies that these designs inherently seek to promote equity and reduce disparities. Moreover, they imply a strong requirement for the inclusion of participants who are the focus of research to be involved in the actual planning, implementation, analysis, and dissemination.

The intersection of a CBPR study with an underlying mixed methods scaffolding can be illustrated with an example (Workbox Illustration 8.10.1). To study partnership practices, and linkages between the practices and changes in health status and disparities outcomes, Lucero et al. (2016) conducted a community-based participatory study using a mixed methods approach. In their research design, the authors proposed a convergent MMR design structure, but in their actual study, they used an iterative approach with case study data collection occurring in parallel to instrument development, recruitment, and refinement. The authors also combined indigenous theory and transformative theory. Their approach involved initial qualitative data collection through a case study. They further employed cognitive debriefing interviews that influenced the quantitative instrument development. They then used a convergent design to conduct the Web-based survey and qualitative case studies. After intramethod analysis, that is, quantitative data analysis in accordance with usual statistical procedures, and qualitative data case series analysis, the authors compared the data with intent of validation. Through analysis of trust and governance, they illustrated the potential to incorporate community cultural values and improve quality of life.

Noteworthy Diagram Elements

An interesting contribution of this diagram is their illustration of the "proposed" and "actual" design figure. In the figure, they illustrate how they added selection measures, cognitive debriefing, and how this influenced sequential implementation rather than a more "fixed" implementation. In their revised design representing the actual procedures, there was "cross-talk" early, as they used information from the first case study conducted prior to the Web-based survey. Ultimately, the data collection and analysis were completed for both the Web-based survey and case studies, before the full data from each source were compared and merged with an intent of validating the findings from two sources.

Workbox Illustration 8.10.1: Example of a Community-Based Participatory Research Design

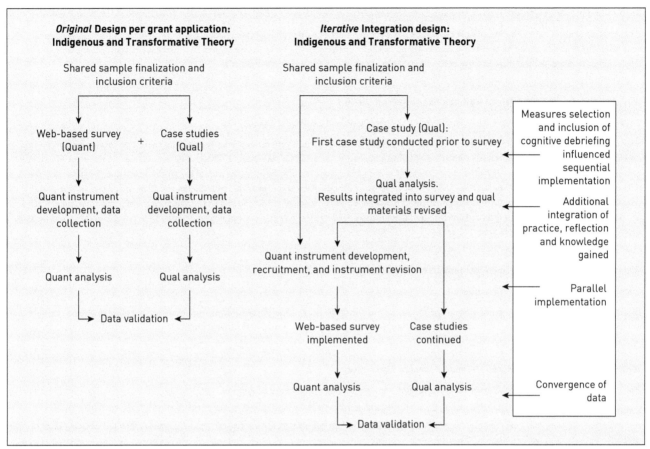

Source: Lucero, J., Wallerstein, N., Duran, B., Alegria, M., Greene-Moton, E., Israel, B., . . . Pearson, C. (2016). Development of a mixed methods investigation of process and outcomes of community-based participatory research. *Journal of Mixed Methods Research, 12*, 55–74. doi:10.1177/1558689816633309 with permission of SAGE Publications.

Workbox 8.10.2: What Underlying Core Design(s) Can Be Found in the Mixed Methods Community-Based Participatory Research Study in Workbox Illustration 8.10.1, and Why?

Core mixed methods designs:

Explanation:

(See explanation in Table 8.1.)

TABLE 8.1 ■ Underlying Core Design Answers for Workboxes 8.4.2 to 8.10.2

Workbox Illustration 8.4.1 Mixed Methods Multiphase Explanatory Sequential Study Design

Core mixed methods design: Explanatory sequential mixed methods design with two subsequent phases of qualitative data collection

Explanation: Initial data collection occurred with use of a survey. Based on the findings, the researcher then collected and analyzed qualitative information based on qualitative observations and text analysis of the term examinations. In a subsequent qualitative phase, those findings helped build an interview guide to collect further qualitative information from teachers.

Workbox Illustration 8.5.1 Mixed Methods Experimental Design.

Core mixed methods designs: Exploratory sequential, convergent, and explanatory sequential

Explanation: A pretrial qualitative case study was followed by qualitative data collection during the trial as on-site observations and journal entries, followed then by a posttrial qualitative evaluation designed to help explain the study findings. The core design of the first phase was exploratory sequential, as the qualitative data collection and analysis were used to develop the actual model for testing in the intermediate phase, as well as the variables for testing in the Phase II mixed methods quasi-experimental trial. During the trial, there is a convergent component because qualitative data, as observations and journal entries, were collected and analyzed at approximately the same time. There is a posttrial explanatory sequential component, as the qualitative findings were useful for helping to develop an expanded understanding and explain the quantitative findings from the trial.

Workbox Illustration 8.6.1 Mixed Methods Case Study Design

Core mixed methods design: Convergent

Explanation: Even though there was a 1-year gap between the data collection in the United States and the data collection in Japan, the data were all compared at essentially the same time, indicating that the underlying core design is convergent.

Workbox Illustration 8.7.1 Mixed Methods Program Evaluation

Core mixed methods designs: Explanatory sequential, convergent, and explanatory sequential

Explanation: Initial collection and analysis of biometric quantitative data led to a survey with mixed quantitative and qualitative data collection and analysis. Hence, initially collected quantitative data were then explored in a mixed methods survey. The simultaneous QUAN and QUAL data collection would be a convergent design. The authors then conducted two phases of qualitative data collection in sequence, qualitative interviews that fed into qualitative observations. The qualitative data collection in the last two steps were collected sequential to the convergent phase to explain the convergent findings, hence explanatory sequential. (This last step could be called a convergent explanatory sequential mixed methods design, as this conveys the convergent phase followed by qualitative phase to explain findings.)

Workbox Illustration 8.8.1 Mixed Methods Survey Design

Core mixed methods design: Exploratory sequential

Explanation: The instrument development work followed a classic model of initial qualitative exploration, pilot testing, and then quantitative field testing with a larger population. (Some might argue it is a multiphase design with an overarching exploratory sequential design and an intervening convergent design from the qualitative and quantitative piloting before the final quantitative assessment.)

Workbox Illustration 8.9.1 Mixed Methods User-Centered Mobile Application and Website Design

Core mixed methods designs: Exploratory sequential and convergent

Explanation: The development work involved extensive exploratory research that was then evaluated using a combination of mixed methods. Hence the initial aspect would be considered exploratory sequential design, while the subsequent procedures involved longitudinally collecting both the quantitative usage patterns and measures, as well as qualitative interviews that were repeated equally over 4 weeks. (This design could arguably be called an exploratory sequential, convergent design.) Recent authors describe also the iterative convergent mixed methods design (Alwashmi et al., 2019).

Workbox Illustration 8.10.1 Mixed Methods Community-Based Participatory Research Design

Core mixed methods designs: Exploratory sequential and convergent

Explanation: The originally proposed mixed methods design was a convergent design, but the authors allowed the design to emerge as the study developed. They added an initial exploratory sequential mixed methods core design, as the initial case study was used to build the instrument.

Application Activities

1. **Identification of Core Designs.** Use a marker or multicolor pen to outline the core designs for Workbox Illustrations 8.4.1 to 8.10.1. Discuss with a partner, or in the classroom, how others have classified the core mixed methods design components in the diagrams.

2. **Peer Feedback**. If you are working on your project as part of a class or in a workshop, pair up with a peer mentor, and take 5 minutes talking and critiquing your mixed methods design procedural diagram. Quickly present your plan, and then discuss areas that you struggled with the most. In particular, focus on identifying the underlying core design(s). Gradually incorporate all the major components of your project. If you are working independently, share your scaffolded mixed methods design with a colleague or mentor.

3. **Peer Feedback Guidance**. As you listen to your partner present, hone the valuable skills of critiquing. Your goal is to help your partner refine the mixed methods procedural diagram. Can you find the underlying core mixed methods design(s)? Is it clear what kind of other design or application the mixed methods scaffold supports?

4. **Group Debrief**. If you are in a classroom or large group setting, take volunteers to present their scaffolded diagrams. Discuss the underlying core mixed methods design(s). Consider using a projector to display several figures, have the author present the design, and have others critique and ask questions of the presenter.

Concluding Thoughts

Use this checklist to assess your progress in achieving the Chapter 8 objectives:

☐ I can describe the concept of scaffolded mixed methods designs and the language other methodologists have used for this group of designs.

☐ I can differentiate between three categories of scaffolded mixed methods designs: (1) mixed methods integrated in multiple stages or phases; (2) mixed methods integrated with another methodology; and (3) mixed methods integrated with a theory/ideology.

☐ I can recognize variations researchers have used to diagram scaffolded mixed methods designs.

☐ I can identify core components in scaffolded mixed methods designs.

☐ I developed a draft of a scaffolded mixed methods procedural diagram for my project.

☐ I reviewed my Chapter 8 design considerations and diagram with a peer or colleague to refine my project.

Now that you have completed these objectives, Chapter 9 will help you strategize for sampling in your MMR or evaluation project.

Key Resources

1. **FURTHER READING ABOUT SCAFFOLDED MIXED METHODS RESEARCH DESIGNS (COMPLEX APPLICATIONS/DESIGNS, ADVANCED APPLICATIONS)**

   - Creswell, J. W., & Plano Clark, V. L. (2018). *Designing and conducting mixed methods research* (3rd ed.). Thousand Oaks, CA: Sage.
   - Plano Clark, V. L., & Ivankova, N. V. (2016). *Mixed methods research: A guide to the field*. Thousand Oaks, CA: Sage.

2. **FURTHER READING ABOUT DESIGNS AND THEORETICAL FRAMEWORKS**

Action Research Design

   - Bradbury, H. (2015). *The SAGE handbook of action research* (3rd ed.). Thousand Oaks, CA: Sage.
   - Ivankova, N. V. (2015). *Mixed methods applications in action research: From methods to community action*. Thousand Oaks, CA: Sage.

Case Study Design

   - Guetterman, T. C., & Fetters, M. D. (2018). Two methodological approaches to the integration of mixed methods and case study designs: A systemic review. *American Behavioral Scientist, 62*(7), 900–918. https://doi.org/10.1177/0002764218772641
   - Yin, R. K. (2014). *Case study research: Design and methods* (5th ed.). Thousand Oaks, CA: Sage.

Interactive User-Centered Design (Website/Mobile Device App Development)

   - Alwashmi, M., Hawboldt, J., Davis, E., & Fetters, M. D. (2019). The iterative convergent design for mHealth usability testing: Mixed methods approach. *JMIR Mhealth Uhealth. 7*(4):e11656) doi:10.2196/11656
   - Holtzblatt, K., & Beyer, H. (2016). Contextual design: Design for life. *Interactive Technologies* (2nd ed.). Burlington, MA: Morgan Kaufmann.

- Holtzblatt, K., Burns Wendell, J., & Wood, S. (2005). *Rapid contextual design: A how-to guide to key techniques for user-centered design*. San Francisco, CA: Morgan Kaufmann.

Intervention Design

- Nastasi, B. K., & Hitchcock, J. H. (2016). *Mixed methods research and culture-specific interventions: Program design and evaluation*. Thousand Oaks, CA: Sage.
- O'Cathain, A. (2018). *A practical guide to using qualitative research with randomized controlled trials*. Oxford, UK: Oxford University Press.

Participatory/Social Justice/Transformative

- Israel, B. A., Eng, E., Schulz, A. J., & Parker, E. (2012). *Methods for community-based participatory research for health* (2nd ed.). San Francisco, CA: Jossey-Bass.
- Mertens, D. M. (2009). *Transformative research and evaluation*. New York, NY: Guilford Press.

Program Evaluation Design

- Burch, P., & Heinrich, C. J. (2015). *Mixed methods for policy research and program evaluation*. Thousand Oaks, CA: Sage.
- Mertens, D. M., & Wilson, A. T. (2012). *Program evaluation theory and practice*. New York, NY: Guilford Press.

Survey Development

- Andres, L. (2012). *Designing & doing survey research*. Thousand Oaks, CA: Sage.
- DeVellis, R. F. (2016). *Scale development: Theory and applications* (4th ed.). Thousand Oaks, CA: Sage.
- Onwuegbuzie, A. J., Bustamante, R. M., & Nelson, J. A. (2010). Mixed research as a tool for developing quantitative instruments. *Journal of Mixed Methods Research, 4*, 56–78. doi:10.1177/1558689809355805

9

INTEGRATING THROUGH SAMPLING IN MIXED METHODS RESEARCH

Sampling strategies are integral to qualitative, quantitative, and mixed methods data collection. The need to under-stand and choose among various sampling strategies can seem a formidable challenge when preparing for data col-lection. This chapter and its activities will help you examine differences in the intent and process for qualitative and quantitative sampling strategies, recognize the range of qualitative and quantitative sampling strategies available for mixed methods projects, consider sampling strategies that impact mixed methods projects, relate how sampling strategies are linked to mixed methods designs, and outline a sampling plan for your project. As a key outcome, you will complete a comprehensive data sampling plan.

LEARNING OBJECTIVES

This chapter introduces sampling in mixed methods research (MMR) and evaluation, so that you will

- Examine the major differences in sampling intent and process for quantitative and qualitative sampling strategies
- Recognize the range of quantitative sampling strategies available for a mixed methods project
- Appraise the range of qualitative sampling strategies available for a mixed methods project
- Consider sampling choices that impact conduct of mixed methods projects
- Relate how sampling strategies are closely linked to the mixed methods design
- Outline a plan for sampling in your mixed methods project

WHY SAMPLING MATTERS

Mixed methods researchers must identify participants for inclusion in research involving original data collection. A **sample** is a subset of the population from which participants are selected for enrollment into the study. The **sampling strategy** refers to the approach used to identify participants for inclusion in the study. Quantitative researchers use very different sampling strategies from qualitative researchers. Mixed methods researchers must become comfortable with the sampling procedures of both methodologies, as these have implications for research quality when using mixed methods methodology. While quantitative researchers typically use large sample sizes, qualitative researchers use smaller sample sizes.

Johnson (1998), an anthropologist, summarized the critical nature of sampling in the context of new statistical procedures and technology:

> [I]t is critical to remember the connection between theory, design (including sampling), and data analysis from the beginning, because how the data were collected, both in terms of measurement and sampling, is directly related to how they can be analyzed. (p. 153)

HOW TO MAKE DECISIONS ABOUT SAMPLING

This chapter is organized to help you consider thoroughly the choices you will make relative to sampling for your mixed methods project. Referencing Workbox Illustration 9.1.1 and completing Workbox 9.1.2 provides the means for accomplishing this end. In addition, you will have figures and additional work activities that will help support the choosing and clarifying of your mixed methods sampling approach in a comprehensive and robust way. Curry and Nunez-Smith (2015, p. 217) have developed a mixed methods sampling algorithm that you may find helpful as well.

Workbox Illustration 9.1.1: Sampling Choices From Business, Education and Health Sciences Examples

Sampling Consideration	Business Example (Sharma & Vredenburg, 1998)	Education Example (Harper, 2016)	Health Sciences Example (Kron et al., 2017)
Target/study population(s):	Single industry context: Firms in the Canadian oil and gas industry	Middle school teachers	Second-year medical students transitioning to 3rd year Standardized patient instructors (SPIs) assessing students
Sampling timing:	Asynchronous: Case studies conducted separately from survey	Asynchronous: Surveys and interviews done at different times	Synchronous: Timing of sampling within medical student and within SPIs
Sampling relationships:	Enlarged: From the QUAL case studies (n = 7), to include the original cases, as well as many more cases to create a bigger QUAN sample (n = 90)	Separate and multilevel: -From 26 middle schools, 334 teachers -Eleven principals from pool of high achieving middle schools	Identical and multilevel: -Medical student sample same throughout (n = 421) -SPIs same for QUAN and QUAL assessments
Hierarchical levels of sampling:	QUAL sample -For cases: industry size-major, senior, intermediate, junior (n = 7) -For subjects: manager level-senior and middle-level executives (n = 27) QUAN sample: -All eligible companies based on revenue	QUAN sample: -From high-performing (n = 21) and low-performing (n = 5) middle schools enrolled 334 teachers QUAL sample: -Enrolled 11 principals	Two levels: -QUAN and QUAL sample—all enrolled medical students. -SPIs same sample for QUAN and QUAL assessments
Qualitative sampling strategies:	For company cases, continuum sampling based on industry size and management roles within companies (n = 7). For subjects in cases, initially snowball sampling of managers (n = 19); emerging phenomenon sampling during analysis (18/19 plus nine new subjects)	Positive deviance sampling as "information rich cases" of principals of high-achieving middle schools and (n = 11) and maximum variation sampling to represent schools of varying size, socioeconomic (SES) status, geography (suburban, small town, and rural)	All students in trial provided qualitative data, but students were randomized to five different qualitative questions for reflective essays that provided the qualitative data.

Sampling Consideration	Business Example (Sharma & Vredenburg,1998)	Education Example (Harper, 2016)	Health Sciences Example (Kron et al., 2017)
Quantitative sampling strategies:	Population sampling: 110 companies—the total population of Canadian oil and gas companies of a minimum size, surveyed mid- and senior-level managers (n = 162)	Nonprobabilistic stratified sampling (based on SES and student achievement) of schools (n = 26), volunteer sampling for teachers (n = 334)	Population sampling: -421 medical students (210 for intervention, 211 for control) -All SPIs tasked with evaluating students
Mixed methods sampling strategies:	Exploratory sequential design sampling	Explanatory sequential design sampling where schools from the QUAN phase provided sample for the subsequent QUAL phase	Mixed methods trial with convergent sampling for trial and posttrial convergent assessments
Organization function level of sampling:	Three levels by firm activities: -Upstream (exploration, drilling, crude oil production) -Downstream (refining, marketing) -Integrated (both)	Two levels within 21 high-performing and five low-performing middle schools -Teachers -Principals -Sampling strategy required assistance of superintendents and principals to gain access	Two levels within three medical schools: -Second-year medicals students -SPIs assessing students
Geographic location and sampling:	National level (Canada)	Districts containing schools: from four relatively large Alabama metropolitan areas (Huntsville, Birmingham, Montgomery, and Mobile) and from rural areas and small towns across the state	Northern United States (n = 1) and Eastern United States (n = 2).

Workbox 9.1.2: Your Sampling Choices

Sampling Consideration	Relevance to Your Study
Target/study population(s):	
Sampling timing:	
Sampling relationships:	
Hierarchical levels of sampling:	
Qualitative sampling strategies:	
Quantitative sampling strategies:	
Mixed methods sampling strategies:	
Sampling and organization function:	
Geographic location and sampling:	

TARGET POPULATION

To get started, you should identify a population of individuals for inclusion in your research. Quantitative researchers and qualitative researchers think somewhat differently about samples relative to a population of people (Figure 9.1). First, quantitative researchers are thinking about many people. Moreover, quantitative researchers often talk about the **target population**, that is the *entire* group of individuals that serves as the source from which a smaller number of individuals, the sample, can be drawn. It can be thought of as the referent group that the sample represents. The **sampling frame** serves as a window and includes the individuals from the target population who are available for sampling. The **sample** represents the individuals drawn from the sampling frame chosen with the intent of representing the individuals of the entire population. By using **probability sampling, inferences** can be made, that is, conclusions drawn from the findings of the individuals in the sample to the target population.

Qualitative researchers are interested in knowing in great depth about a much smaller number of people. Rather than talking of the target population, qualitative researchers will tend to talk more about a **study population**, the individuals for whom the researcher is taking an interest. Rather than using a sampling frame, qualitative researchers choose a sample using **purposeful sampling**, that is, choosing participants with a specific rationale or intent. The number of individuals chosen may be as small as one. Generally, as the sample gets smaller, the expectation for deeper information about the case goes up. Based on a very in-depth exploration of the phenomenon as experienced by the study sample, the qualitative researcher then considers **the transferability**, or the extent the findings can extrapolate to others from the study population. These similar but different views are depicted in Figure 9.1.

FIGURE 9.1 ■ Sampling in Quantitative and Qualitative Research

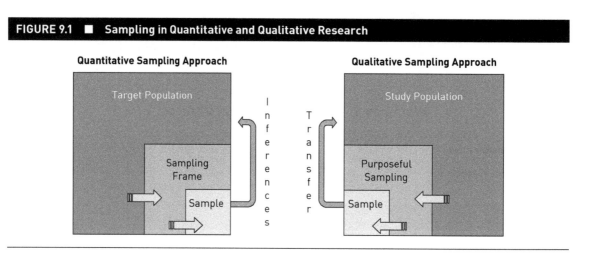

Activity: Identifying the Study Population(s)

Using the examples in Workbox Illustration 9.1.1 and Figure 9.1, fill in the target/study population or populations into Workbox 9.1.2 that you intend to utilize in your research. It may be populations of individuals or social institutions (e.g., small companies, school districts, hospital systems). The more details provided, the better.

SAMPLING TIMING

One of the first issues to consider with MMR sampling is the timing of the mixed methods data collection. **Sampling timing** refers to the temporal relationship between when the qualitative and the quantitative data are collected. Figure 9.2 shows three variations in the sampling timing that can occur in mixed methods projects, based on the timing of the qualitative data and quantitative data collection. In simultaneous timing, both the qualitative and the quantitative data are collected at essentially the same time. This pattern characterizes a convergent MMR design. With sequential QUAL to QUAN timing, the qualitative data are collected first, and the quantitative data are collected subsequently. This pattern characterizes an exploratory sequential MMR design. With sequential QUAN to QUAL timing, the quantitative data are collected first, and the qualitative data are collected subsequently. This pattern characterizes an explanatory sequential MMR design. In the business example where Sharma and Vredenburg

(1998) sought to explore linkages between environmental strategies and the development of capabilities, and understand the nature of any emergent capabilities and competitive outcomes in the oil and gas industry, the timing was *asynchronous*—qualitative case studies were followed by a quantitative survey. In the educational example where Harper (2016) sought to understand how principals could improve student achievement by improving school culture, the timing was asynchronous as the teacher sample for a survey was followed at a later time with qualitative individual interviews with principals. In the health sciences study, Kron et al. (2017) sought to examine the impact of the virtual human intervention to teach communication skills on medical students. The timing was *synchronous*. Medical students were enrolled at the beginning of the study, and while they were followed longitudinally, the different data collection procedures were conducted with the same sample regardless of the data collection points in the study. Standardized patient instructors differed across sites and were involved only during a single timeframe.

Activity: Identifying the Sampling Timing

Using the examples in Workbox Illustration 9.1.1 and Figure 9.2, fill in the sampling timing section of the Workbox 9.1.2. Pick from the three choices, synchronous, asynchronous–QUAL to QUAN, or asynchronous–QUAN to QUAL. If you are doing a multistage project, insert the information by phase or stage. Include as much detail as possible.

FIGURE 9.2 ■ **Sampling by the Timing Dimension in Mixed Methods Data Collection**

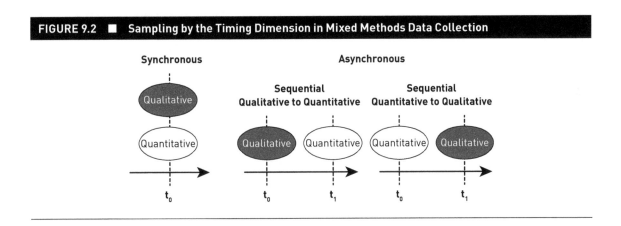

SAMPLING RELATIONSHIPS

The sampling relationship during mixed methods data collection constitutes the second factor for consideration. The **sampling relationship** is defined as how the sample or samples for the qualitative and quantitative data collection are related to each other and generally can have identical, nested, enlarged, separate, or multilevel hierarchical relationships (Figure 9.3). In an *identical* relationship, both qualitative and quantitative data are collected from an identical sample, the same individuals. In a *nested* relationship, the qualitative sample is identified from within the larger quantitative sample. This type of sampling will primarily occur in a convergent design or in an explanatory sequential mixed methods core design. The arrow for the nested relationship in Figure 9.3 indicates how the qualitative sample derives from the larger quantitative sample. In an *enlarged* relationship, an initial qualitative sample expands to include both the original qualitative participants as well as additional participants to create a larger quantitative sample. While relatively unusual, it occurs most commonly in an exploratory sequential design. The arrow for the enlarged relationship in Figure 9.3 indicates how the qualitative sample can be expanded and included in a larger quantitative sample. In a *separate* relationship, the qualitative data and quantitative data are collected from completely different samples. In a *multilevel hierarchical relationship*, different units or social levels from the hierarchy in an organization are included in the mixed methods project. Illustrations of various social units as might be relevant to a mixed methods study in business, education, and the health sciences are presented in Table 9.1. In the business example (Sharma & Vredenburg, 1998), the sample relationship was *enlarged* as the original companies from the seven QUAL case studies were apparently included, or at least eligible, in the bigger QUAN study (n = 90), although the authors were not explicit. In Harper's (2016) education study investigating how principals could improve student achievement by improving school culture, the sample was *separate* because teachers were sampled in the quantitative phase, and principals were sampled separately in the subsequent qualitative phase. Harper also conducted *multilevel* hierarchical sampling since the study included teachers and principals. In the health sciences study by Kron et al. (2017), looking at the impact of the virtual human intervention, the samples of medical students and SPIs were *identical*, and there was multilevel hierarchical sampling of students and teachers who were at different organizational levels.

FIGURE 9.3 ■ Sampling Relationship of Mixed Methods Data Collection

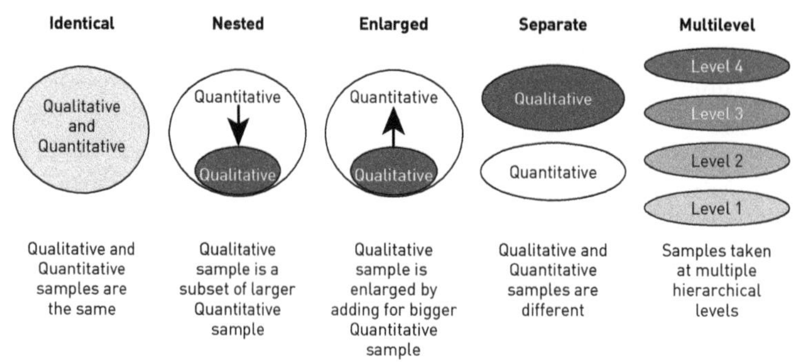

Identical	Nested	Enlarged	Separate	Multilevel
Qualitative and Quantitative samples are the same	Qualitative sample is a subset of larger Quantitative sample	Qualitative sample is enlarged by adding for bigger Quantitative sample	Qualitative and Quantitative samples are different	Samples taken at multiple hierarchical levels

TABLE 9.1 ■ Hierarchical Multilevel Sampling Levels Possible in Business, Education, and Health Sciences

Level	Business	Education	Health Care
1	Consumers	Students, parents	Patients/families
2	Staff-clerks, custodial	Staff-clerks, custodial	Staff, clerks, custodial
3	Workers	Teachers	Clinical workers
4	Mid-level managers	Principals	Mid-level administrators
5	Top-level managers, e.g., CEO, CMO, CFO	Superintendent	Top-level leaders, e.g., CEO, CMO, deans

Activity: Identifying Opportunities for Multilevel Sampling

Consider the potential for hierarchical multilevel sampling for your own project. If you will not be using hierarchical multilevel sampling, you can move to Part II below.

Part I: Using as a reference the hierarchical levels illustrated in Workbox Illustration 9.1.1, Table 9.1, and Figure 9.3, review the examples and draft as relevant to your study in Workbox 9.2. Write in each box the level and participant type you are targeting for your study. Use one row for each unique combination of hierarchical level and participant type. Having populated the first column, now populate the specific type of qualitative and quantitative data collection you envision you could, might, or will conduct, depending on the stage of your project. Use the last column to record any concerns, ideas, etc. For example, you might want to check with a colleague, advisor, a biostatistician, or a person of authority from qualitative research or quantitative research who could give you access. You might also record other questions it raises for you relative to compensation, stage of research, or other. It is your space to use to help you.

Part II: Having completed Workbox 9.2, go to Workbox 9.1.2 to provide a refined, edited version of your choices made in Workbox 9.2.

Workbox 9.2: Multilevel Hierarchical Sampling Example—Identifying the Sample Timing Relationship Using Business, Education and Health Sciences Examples

Study	Hierarchical Level and Participant Type	Sampling for Qualitative Data Collection	Sampling for Quantitative Data Collection	Comments
Business example (Sharma and Vredenburg, 1998)	Qualitative case studies: For companies, industry size For subjects, manager level For survey: All Canadian gas and oil companies with annual sales revenue in excess of $20 million	Industry sizes: major, senior, intermediate, junior (n = 7) Manager levels: senior, middle level, executives (n = 27), CEO, top management team member, environmental assessment manager, staff manager, line/operations manager	Canadian oil and gas companies (n = 90) from target population of N = 110	Companies participating in the survey apparently included the seven case study companies (authors not explicit).

Study	Hierarchical Level and Participant Type	Sampling for Qualitative Data Collection	Sampling for Quantitative Data Collection	Comments
Education example (Harper, 2016)	For survey: middle school teachers For QUAL interviews: middle school principals	Principals of high-performing middle schools (n = 11)	Teachers from high- (n = 21) and low- (n = 5) performing middle schools	The study required a variety of sampling strategies to recruit the survey sample.
Health sciences example (Kron et al., 2017)	For trial: medical students For clinical performance assessments: standardized patient instructors (SPIs)	All 2nd-year medical students transitioning to 3rd-year clinical rotations (n = 421); all SPIs who assess the students	Same students and SPIs	-In two sites, all students in the 2nd-year class -In one site, all students who did not opt out
Your study				

INCORPORATING TIMING AND SAMPLING RELATIONSHIPS INTO SPECIFIC MIXED METHODS RESEARCH DESIGNS

Having considered both the sampling timing and the sampling relationship of the qualitative and quantitative data collection, the next step involves incorporating these concepts into your specific mixed methods design. If you have not already committed to a mixed methods design, you should review Chapter 7 about core mixed methods designs and Chapter 8 about scaffolded mixed methods designs. As you will recall, the three core mixed methods designs are convergent, explanatory sequential, and exploratory sequential. Sampling always needs to be considered with the intent of the design. Workbox 9.3 is organized by the type of core mixed methods design, the sampling strategy for this type of design, sampling considerations, and a comment box.

Activity: Linking the Timing, Sampling Relationship, and Mixed Methods Design

Part I. Review Workbox 9.3. For the design you are planning to use, consider the different sampling strategies and options. In the final column, write in any comments (e.g., consider the relevance for your own project, jot down any questions or concerns). If you are implementing a multiphase or multistage research or evaluation project, you may choose to fill out several sections. In the comment box, you may want to add the particular phase/stage when it applies.

Part II. Having completed Workbox 9.3, succinctly complete the section on mixed methods sampling in Workbox 9.1.2.

Workbox 9.3: Sampling Strategies in Mixed Methods Research According to the Three Core Designs and Identification of Your Sampling Strategy

Type	Sampling Strategies	Sampling Considerations	Comments
Convergent design sampling	1. Use a quantitative sampling strategy to be able to generalize findings, demonstrate relationships, effect sizes, etc. 2. Use purposeful sampling strategy that will enhance interpretation of the quantitative findings, expand ideas tested, develop a theory, validate the findings, look for positive deviants, and look for contradictory cases.	1. Will you use the same individuals or different individuals for two approaches to data collection? 2. Will the qualitative sample size include the same individuals (identical) a subgroup (nested) of the larger quantitative sample or different (separate)? 3. Will you sample at a single social level or multiple social levels? 4. Will you sample for the quantitative and qualitative data and analysis to examine the same or different concepts?	
Explanatory sequential design sampling	1. Use a sampling strategy for the quantitative data collection to examine constructs of interest across a population; perhaps identify risk factors or develop a quantitative model. 2. Identify a qualitative sample to use based on the quantitative data analysis to interpret, illustrate, and illuminate what the quantitative research findings mean, and identify variations among subgroups; identify cases that are typical, intense, on a continuum, or outliers; validate a theory generated through quantitative modeling. Sampling may be driven by need to validate the quantitative findings, or help explain variance.	1. Will you use the same individuals (identical) or different individuals (separate) for two phases of data collection? 2. Will the qualitative sample size include the same individuals (identical) a subgroup (nested) of the larger quantitative sample or different individuals (separate)? 3. Will you sample at a single social level or multiple social levels (multilevel)? 4. Will you sample for the follow-up qualitative data and analysis using probability sampling or purposeful sampling to examine typical cases, intense cases, a continuum of cases, outliers, or positive deviants? Will you sample to create a theory? 5. Will you examine the same or different concepts? 6. During iterative data collection and analysis, do you need to employ additional or alternative sampling strategies? 7. During analysis, what type of analytical sampling should you consider?	
Exploratory sequential design sampling	1. Identify a qualitative sample to use based on the intent to develop a theory for subsequent testing in the quantitative phase, elucidate constructs and specific language used in real life to identify subpopulations for inclusion or exclusion, to test data collection instruments, to identify cases that are typical, intense, on a continuum or outliers; to culturally and/or linguistically adapt an existing instrument. 2. Use a sampling strategy for the quantitative data collection to examine constructs of interest across a population, clarify relationships and variables, identify intensity of relationships, and validate a qualitatively generated model.	1. Will you use the same individuals (identical) or different individuals (separate) for two phases of data collection? 2. Will the qualitative sample size include the same individuals (identical) as a subgroup (nested) of the larger quantitative sample or different individuals (separate)? 3. Will you sample at a single social level or multiple social levels (multilevel)? 4. Will you sample for the follow-up quantitative data collection and analysis using probability sampling or nonprobability sampling strategy? 5. Have the qualitative findings identified variations suggesting the need for stratified random sampling or a type of cluster sampling? 6. Will your sample help you examine all the concepts identified, a subgroup of those concepts, or an expanded group of concepts?	

QUANTITATIVE AND QUALITATIVE SAMPLING STRATEGIES TO INCORPORATE INTO YOUR MIXED METHODS DESIGN

With a clearer understanding of your sampling needs according to the type of mixed methods design you are using, you now need to clarify the specific type of quantitative and qualitative sampling strategies for you to use in your MMR or evaluation project. In the following, you will review some of the most recognized sampling strategies in quantitative research and qualitative research and fill out both Workbox 9.4 for the quantitative strand and Workbox 9.5 for the qualitative strand so as to identify the particular sampling strategies that might be useful in your project.

SAMPLING IN QUANTITATIVE RESEARCH

The language of sampling used in quantitative methodology involves several key terms (Johnson and Christensen, 2017). The **sample** represents participants of a group taken from a bigger population. The N is the population size while n represents the actual sample size. Researchers seek to **generalize** study results to a larger **population**. By using probability methods and certain measures, quantitative methodology has measures that can be used to control against **bias**, deviation in the interpreted value from the actual value.

Probability and Nonprobability Sampling

In quantitative research methodology, researchers often use probability sampling, which involves the use of a random selection approach to help ensure the sample chosen can be considered representative of the target population. Highly valued by quantitative researchers, probability sampling best enables one to make conclusions about the generalizability of study findings, that is, the extent that the findings from the participants in the study represent the population from which the subset was chosen. Random sampling moreover is a powerful tool for minimizing selection bias. Quantitative researchers also frequently employ *nonprobability sampling*. While characterized by what it "is not" in this terminology, a sample not chosen based on probability, it lacks a better term. While probability samples are particularly powerful, researchers often can make powerful conclusions using other strategies as well.

SAMPLING STRATEGIES FOR QUANTITATIVE DATA COLLECTION IN MIXED METHODS RESEARCH

Mixed methods sampling strategies are defined as an approach that draws upon the procedures in quantitative research for the selection of individuals for the quantitative sample and procedures common in qualitative research for selection of the qualitative sample. After collection of the data, analysis of the qualitative and quantitative data, if using a mixed methods approach, will reveal a merged or integrated understanding of the combined findings. The preferred approaches to sampling can be understood relative to the intent of the data collection. Hence, qualitative data collection in an early part of a mixed methods investigation or evaluation may be different during field observations and subsequent fieldwork, and later yet during the late analysis phase.

Activity: Identifying Sampling Strategies That Could Be Used for Quantitative Data Collection in Your Project

Workbox 9.4 illustrates sampling strategies commonly used in quantitative methodology. The table includes the type of sampling strategy, a brief definition, and a box for your completion. Use these boxes to make any comments to yourself. Is this a strategy you could use? If so why, or on the contrary, why not? You might want to make a note to learn more about the strategy. After going through the table, you may have only one strategy marked (especially if you have already completed your data collection), you may have several marked if a multistage **design**, or you may have none marked if undecided and still planning the design of your project.

Workbox 9.4: Sampling Strategies in Quantitative Research and Identification of Your Sampling Strategy

Type	Description	Relevance as Sampling Strategy in Your Project
1. Probability sampling	Select participants from the target population for study using some form of random selection	
a. Simple random/ equal probability sampling	Select participants using a probability sampling procedure such that every person or case in the target population has an equal *chance* of being selected for participation	
2. Systematic sampling	Select the sample for participation by determining a sampling interval k (size of the population divided by desired sample size N/n, which then equals k), selecting at random a starting point between 1 and k, and then selecting every kth person	
a. Panel sampling	Initially, a researcher selects participants using a random sampling approach and then follows the same group of individuals over time	
3. Stratified sampling	Select the sample by identifying mutually exclusive groups, dividing the population into these groups, and then randomly selecting a sample from each group	
a. Proportional stratified sampling	A subgroup of stratified sampling. Select the sample in proportions that are the same as the population proportions of the variable chosen for stratification	
b. Disproportional stratified sampling	A subgroup of stratified sampling. Select the sample in proportions to be of different size than the population proportions of the variable chosen for stratification	
c. Quota sampling	Set quotas of participants to be selected based on a project variable. Select participants randomly until quotas are filled, then select random participants to fill the individual quotas. Proportional and nonproportional quota sampling approaches are possible	
4. Cluster random sampling	Select randomly a sample based on clusters defined as a unit with multiple elements (e.g., retail outlets, schools, universities, clinics, hospitals), rather than individual elements (e.g., customers, sales representatives, and clerks; students, parents, and teachers; and nurses, physicians, administrators)	
a. One-stage cluster sampling	Select all the cases (e.g., customers, sales representatives, clerks) within a cluster selected at random from among the other clusters in the sample	
b. Two-stage cluster sampling	After a set of clusters is randomly selected, select a sample of cases at random from within the clusters	
Nonprobability sampling	A diverse group of procedures may be used. The individuals potentially eligible for being chosen to participate do not have an equal chance of being selected	
1. Population sampling	Select the entire population of eligible individuals for participation (this is not actually a sample, as all eligible individuals are offered enrollment)	
2. Voluntary sampling	Enroll only individuals who volunteer to participate when participation is announced	

SAMPLING IN QUALITATIVE RESEARCH

In stark contrast to sampling in quantitative research, qualitative researchers often use small samples that they study in great depth. Qualitative researchers sometimes examine only a single case in great depth. This contrasts with quantitative researchers who typically work with, or at least prefer, large sample sizes. In qualitative methodology, some key concepts merit discussion. **Information-rich cases** refer to cases that can illuminate the qualitative question being pursued by virtue of their nature and substance. While in quantitative methodology scientists endeavor to control bias, in qualitative methodology researchers seek to use *preconceptions*. For example, researchers can use their own ideas about a phenomenon of interest to start framing understanding about the phenomenon of interest. They will also intentionally use their preconceptions as a referent to look for contrary information or alternative interpretations than their own.

Purposeful Sampling Strategies in Qualitative Research

The preferred sampling strategy of researchers using qualitative methodology is called **purposeful sampling**. This entails the selection of participants with an explicit intent, rationale, or criterion in a qualitative study. Variations on the language of purposeful sampling also include intentional or criterion sampling. Purposeful sampling is one category of "nonprobability sampling" (language sometimes used by quantitative researchers; see Workbox 9.4.), though the downside of this language is that it defines the strategy by what it is not, rather than what it is. Also problematic in the eyes of many researchers is that nonprobability sampling also includes convenience sampling, an often-used term, but an approach generally spurned by quantitative and qualitative researchers alike.

Convenience Sampling

The term **convenience sampling**, also known as accidental sampling, grab sampling, haphazard sampling, or opportunity sampling, describes when researchers use in their research participants who were most readily available and easy to access. As both convenience and purposeful sampling are forms of nonprobability sampling, there may be an unfortunate, even if unintentional, tendency to implicate purposeful sampling as an inferior approach when, in fact, purposeful sampling strategies can be quite elaborate. Patton (2015), a leading qualitative research scholar, takes a clear stance that convenience sampling is to be avoided, and in the fourth edition of his book on qualitative research and evaluation, he removed convenience sampling from his master table of purposeful sampling strategies (pp. 266–272). Whenever possible, an intentional strategy should be used or properly identified as illustrated in Story From the Field 9.1. Also considered a dubious strategy, a variation on convenience sampling is quota convenience sampling, when the researcher determines the sample size for specific groups and then fills the sample size for each group using convenience sampling procedures.

STORY FROM THE FIELD 9.1
CONVENIENCE SAMPLING REFLECTIONS

I have two anecdotes to share about convenience sampling. First, I have often heard researchers, usually those who are very junior or trained only in a quantitative tradition, who mistakenly interpret convenience sampling as synonymous with qualitative research. Second, I have also encountered individuals during research consultations who state they intend to use convenience sampling in their research, or that they have already used it in their research. But when I question them closely, they have actually used one of the many variations of purposeful sampling. In short, I advise clarifying when you hear a coinvestigator or colleague use the language of convenience sampling. You would be wise to understand well the variations in qualitative purposeful sampling. If you or colleagues are planning a convenience sample, consider an alternative, accepted approach of purposeful sampling.

Additionally, check whether the actual strategy was actually a legitimate strategy and the colleague was just unaware of the language used to express how the qualitative sampling was conducted.

SAMPLING STRATEGIES FOR QUALITATIVE DATA COLLECTION IN MIXED METHODS RESEARCH

In his highly detailed articulation of purposeful sampling strategies used in qualitative research, Patton (2015) lays out 38 different options (pp. 266–271), and two mixed methods options (p. 272). These are presented with modification in Table 9.2. He divides the first 38 into seven major categories. In *significant single case strategies* (pp. 273–276), researchers choose one case to examine in great depth to provide a rich and deep understanding about a phenomenon of interest. In-depth examination can lead to breakthrough insights or may have specific features of great prominence. Within this category, Patton includes six categories. In *comparison-focused sampling* (pp. 277–282), the strategy involves sampling to create a group of cases that can provide in-depth information for data gathering and analysis with the intent of comparing and contrasting across the cases to illustrate similarities and differences, and Patton includes six strategies. In *group characteristics sampling,* the strategy is to select cases that will form an information-rich sample that can be used to illustrate group patterns—Patton identifies seven subcategories (pp. 283–287). In *theory-focused and concept sampling,* cases are selected to illuminate concepts and theories—Patton presents seven types (pp. 288–294). In *instrumental-use multiple case sampling,* researchers choose multiple case studies to illuminate changes in practices, programs, and policies that can be generalizable—Patton presents two types (pp. 295–297). In sequential and emergence-driven sampling strategies, cases are chosen during fieldwork as data collection proceeds when new leads or directions arise during data analysis—Patton identifies five (pp. 298–301). In the seventh qualitative purposeful sampling category, *analytically focused sampling,* cases are chosen to support and deepen qualitative analysis of patterns and themes—Patton (2015) identifies four categories (pp. 302–304). One of these, qualitative research synthesis, has emerged as a field unto itself (Jenson & Allen, 1994; Patton, 2015; Sandelowski, Docherty, & Emden, 1997). A critical point about the various sampling strategies described is that a qualitative researcher might use a combination of two, three, or more sampling strategies in the same line of inquiry. For example, in the qualitative strand of a mixed methods study developing a health care quality assessment tool, one research team used criterion sampling to identify four language groups, as well as maximum variation sampling to achieve diversity according to age, gender, and cultural background within each of the four language groups (Abdelrahim et al., 2017; Killawi et al., 2014).

Activity: Identifying Purposeful Sampling Strategies That Could Be Used for Qualitative Data Collection in Your Project

Workbox 9.5 illustrates purposeful sampling strategies commonly used in qualitative methodology. The table includes the type of sampling strategy, a brief definition, and a box for you to complete. As noted above, there are multiple types of strategies, some used at the onset of the research, some during fieldwork, and some during the analytical phase. Begin by reviewing the seven major categories. Then examine the subcategories for relevance. You likely will identify multiple strategies. Use these boxes to make any comments to yourself. Is this a strategy you could use? If so, why or why not? You might want to make a note to learn more about the strategy. After going through the table, you may have only one strategy marked (especially if you have already completed your data collection), or you may have several marked as you have a multistage project or you are still designing your project.

Workbox 9.5: Purposeful Sampling Strategies Used in Qualitative Research and Identification of Your Sampling Strategy

General Type	Description	Relevance as Sampling Strategy in Your Project
1. Single significant case	**A single in-depth case used to provide rich understanding**	
a. Index case sampling	Select the first case identified illustrating a phenomenon of interest	
b. Exemplar of phenomenon of interest sampling	Select a case that manifests major dimensions of a phenomenon of interest	
c. Self-study sampling	Select oneself to illustrate own experience with the phenomenon of interest	
d. High-impact case sampling	Select highly visible case powerful for illuminating a phenomenon of interest	

General Type	Description	Relevance as Sampling Strategy in Your Project
e. Teaching case sampling	Select a case powerful for educating others about a phenomenon of interest	
f. Critical case (or crucial case) sampling	Select a single case that embodies features for logical generalization and maximum application to other cases	
2. Comparison-focused sampling	**Select cases to compare and contrast, to illustrate similarities and differences**	
a. Outlier sampling	Select cases on tails of statistical distribution that have pronounced features of the phenomenon of interest	
b. Intensity sampling	Select cases that are information rich about the phenomenon of interest but are not extreme examples	
c. Positive-deviance comparison sampling	Select individuals or communities that have found solutions or done better for problems that otherwise endure	
d. Matched comparison sampling	Select cases to compare features that differ so as to understand what factors explain differences	
e. Criterion-based case selection (includes critical incident)	Choose cases based on a specific condition to implicitly or explicitly compare with cases without the condition	
f. Continuum or dosage sampling	Choose cases along a spectrum of interest to understand the nature of differences of manifestations of a phenomenon	
3. Group characteristics sampling	**Select cases to form an information-rich sample to illustrate group patterns**	
a. Maximum variation (heterogeneity) sampling	Purposefully choose a broad range of cases based on a dimension of interest to (1) document diversity and (2) identify patterns consistent across the sample	
b. Homogeneous sampling	Choose cases that are similar to study shared characteristics	
c. Typical cases sampling	Select several cases that are average to illustrate typicality and normality	
d. Key informant sampling	Choose subjects based on their knowledge or reputation for phenomenon of study	
e. Complete target population selecting	Select all individuals of a group comprised by their unique interest	
f. Quota sampling	Choose a predetermined number of cases to ensure certain categories of participants are included in a study regardless of their size and distribution	
g. Purposeful random sampling	Choose participants using a procedure such that each has an equal chance of selection	
h. Time-location selecting	Choose all individuals present during the same period and in the same setting	
4. Theory-focused and concept sampling	**Select cases for investigation that exemplify a concept or construct to inform theoretical ideas**	
a. Deductive theoretical sampling, operational construct sampling	Choose cases that manifest a theoretical construct of interest to amplify and verify understanding, variations, and implications of the theory	
b. Inductive grounded and emergent theory sampling	Choose participants initially based on emerging ideas, concept and theory, and subsequently to focus and hone the theory	

(Continued)

(Continued)

General Type	Description	Relevance as Sampling Strategy in Your Project
c. Realist sampling	Based on existing theory, choose subjects to test and refine the theory through examining what is known, what is emerging, and what can be grounded in empirical accounts	
d. Causal pathway case sampling	Pick cases to understand the underlying mechanisms leading to an outcome of interest	
e. Sensitizing concept exemplars sampling	Choose information-rich cases to illustrate sensitizing concepts, that is, terms, labels, phrases (empowerment, inclusivity) that are given meaning in a particular context	
f. Principles-focused sampling	Choose cases to illuminate the nature, implementation, outcomes, and implications of values or doctrine	
g. Complex, dynamic systems selection; ripple effect sampling	Choose cases to track, study, and document any complex and ever-changing phenomenon of interest	
5. Instrumental-use multiple case sampling	**Choose multiple cases to develop generalizable findings of a phenomenon to illuminate changes in practices, programs, and policies**	
a. Utilization-focused sampling	Choose specific cases of a problem/issue that can support rigorous identification of factors to inform decision making	
b. Systematic qualitative evaluation reviews	Choose completed evaluation studies to synthesize findings across the studies to identify what is effective	
6. Sequential and emergence-driven sampling strategies during fieldwork	**During fieldwork, choose cases that build on each other by following emerging leads and new directions**	
a. Snowball or chain sampling	Initially choose information-rich individuals, who then provide contacts of others to the researcher they feel could provide different/confirming information	
b. Respondent-driven sampling, network sampling, link-tracing sampling	Initially choose a few "seed" participants for study about a phenomenon who in-turn recruit (usually for pay) from their social network several other hard-to-reach participants	
c. Emergent phenomenon or emergent subgroup sampling	During an ongoing study, when unknown subgroups form or critical issues arise affecting some, but not others, select participants to examine the newly emerging phenomenon	
d. Opportunity sampling	During fieldwork, seize the occasion to choose individuals or events for study that could not have been planned for in advance	
e. Saturation or redundancy sampling	Choose participants during iterative data collection and analysis of fieldwork to select participants until nothing new is being learned	
7. Analytically focused sampling	**Choose cases to support and deepen the qualitative analysis of patterns and themes**	
a. Confirming and disconfirming case sampling	Choose additional cases during analysis to identify variations or exceptions to previously identified patterns	
b. Illuminations and elaboration sampling	Pick cases during analysis specifically to illuminate and deepen understanding of an emerging finding	
c. Qualitative research synthesis	Choose qualitative studies about a phenomenon using specific criteria (content and quality) to elucidate crosscutting findings	
d. Sampling politically important cases	Select politically important cases for inclusion or exclusion to attract attention to a study	

Source: Adapted with permission from Patton, M. Q. (2015). *Qualitative research and evaluation* (4th ed.). Thousand Oaks, CA: Sage.

SAMPLING OPPORTUNITIES ARISING FROM ORGANIZATIONAL ROLES AND FUNCTIONS

As you considered different quantitative and qualitative sampling strategies, you may have noted the need to consider more detailed questions about sampling with different organizational levels. Organizations connect in social networks within many levels. These different levels give mixed methods researchers opportunities to examine a phenomenon with these different organizational levels. The vast array of socially interconnected organizational levels also presents a challenge for thinking about sampling. Table 9.2 illustrates various levels of organizations that could be a target for sampling in an MMR and evaluation investigation. A given mixed methods project may be conducted within only one of these levels or it may be conducted in multiple levels.

TABLE 9.2 ■ Levels of Organizational Roles and Functions			
Level	Business	Education	Health Sciences
A	Retail in home	Home schooling	Home care
B	Brand-specific retail store	Early intervention	Nurse clinics
C	General retail stores	Nursery school	Free clinics
D	Retail outlets	Prekindergarten	Primary care clinics
F	Online sales	Online education	Specialty care clinics
G	Liquidation center	Middle school	Prehospital emergency care providers
H	Suppliers	High school	Emergency room
I	Distributors	Technical school	Hospital ward
J	Sales representatives	Two-year college	Intensive care unit
K	Business staff	College/university	Rehabilitation
L	Mid-level management	Graduate school	Nursing home
M	Upper management	Professional development/continuing education	Institutional palliative care

Activity: Identifying Organizational Role/Function-Based Sampling Levels That Could Apply in Your Mixed Methods Research or Evaluation Project

Part I. Using the organizational role/function-based sampling levels of Table 9.2 as a reference, fill out the Organizational Roles and Functions-Based Sampling row in Workbox 9.1.2, based on your study. Using Workbox Illustration 9.1.1 as a reference, populate the specific type of qualitative and quantitative data sampling you have already collected or envision, you could, might, or will conduct for your project. Use the last column to record any concerns, ideas, etc. For example, you record the rationale or questions to be answered before making a final decision. Again, it is your space to help advance your project.

SAMPLING OPPORTUNITIES BASED ON GEOGRAPHIC LOCATION

As you considered different quantitative and qualitative sampling strategies and organizational levels, additional questions may have arisen about the actual geographic location and where to sample. Table 9.3 provides six different types of locations that could be relevant in business, education, or health sciences projects. These different locations give mixed methods researchers opportunities for sampling in different locations. While a choice may not be required depending on the specific MMR or evaluation project that you are working on, this activity may nonetheless trigger you to think about the geographic locations you are choosing as part of your mixed methods sampling strategy. It may also lead you to ideas for sequel or future work from your current, active project.

Level	Business	Education	Health Sciences
Single location	Branch of an office, headquarters	Single school or school system	Single clinic or hospital system
Local	Multiple businesses within a single city	Multiple school systems or district in a single city	Multiple clinics or hospitals in a single city
Regional	Local franchises that have expanded to multiple cities, towns, or counties	Multiple school systems in regional communities or districts	Multiple clinics or hospitals in regionally linked communities or districts
State/Province	Locations at the state or provincial level	All schools in a state or province	Multiple clinics or hospitals at the state or provincial level
National	Nationally based companies	All schools across the country	Multiple clinics or hospitals across the country
International	Internationally based companies	Schools from multiple countries	Multiple clinics or hospitals from multiple countries

TABLE 9.3 ■ Geographic/Location Differences and Opportunities for Mixed Methods Sampling

Activity: Identifying Geographical/Location-Based Sampling Opportunities That Could Apply in Your Mixed Methods Research or Evaluation Project

Using Table 9.3 as a reference, complete the last row of Workbox 9.1.2 based on your study. Reference the examples from Workbox Illustration 9.1.1. Write in the geographic location(s) you are targeting for your study. If you are still in the brainstorm mode, you may choose several to aid your choosing. If you have already made these decisions, it will only be necessary to complete relevant sections.

Application Activities

1. **Peer Feedback**. If you are working on your project as part of a class or in a workshop, pair up with a peer mentor, and one of you spend about 5 minutes talking about Workbox 9.1.2. Take turns talking about your sampling choices and giving feedback. Focus on the mixed methods implications, especially the decisions that you struggled with the most. If you are working independently, share your output with a colleague or mentor.

2. **Peer Feedback Guidance**. As you listen to a partner, consider the overall picture and provide feedback. Do the sampling

timing and sampling relationships make sense? Does it link well with the proposed mixed methods design? Are there organizational levels or geographic locations that have been left out that should be included? Is there a good justification for the choices made?

3. **Group Debrief**. If you are in a classroom or large-group setting, take volunteers to present the areas of Workbox 9.1.2 that were most difficult. Reflect on how these same issues may play out in your own project.

Concluding Thoughts

Use this checklist to assess your progress in achieving the Chapter 9 objectives:

☐ I can explain major differences in the sampling intent and process for quantitative and qualitative approaches.

☐ I examined multiple quantitative sampling strategies.

☐ I recognize the broad range of qualitative sampling strategies available.

☐ I reviewed the impact of sampling choices on the conduct of mixed methods projects.

☐ I can extrapolate how sampling strategies are closely linked to mixed methods designs.

☐ I formulated a sampling strategy for my own mixed methods project.

☐ I reflected on my sampling strategy with a peer mentor or colleague.

Now that you have completed these objectives, Chapter 10 will help you develop integration strategies for data collection and analysis in your mixed methods project.

Key Resources

1. **FURTHER READING ON QUALITATIVE SAMPLING**

   - Creswell, J. W. (2016). *30 essential skills for the qualitative researcher*. Thousand Oaks, CA: Sage.

   - Miles, M. B., Huberman, A. M., & Saldaña, J. (2014). *Qualitative data analysis: A methods sourcebook* (3rd ed.). Thousand Oaks, CA: Sage.

   - Patton, M. Q. (2015). *Qualitative research and evaluation* (4th ed.). Thousand Oaks, CA: Sage.

2. **FURTHER READING ON QUANTITATIVE SAMPLING**

   - Johnson, R. B., & Christensen, L. (2017). *Educational research: Quantitative, qualitative, and mixed approaches* (6th ed.). Thousand Oaks, CA: Sage.

3. **FURTHER READING ON MIXED METHODS SAMPLING**

   - Creswell, J. W., & Plano Clark, V. L. (2018). *Designing and conducting mixed methods research* (3rd ed.). Thousand Oaks, CA: Sage.

   - Curry, L. A., & Nunez-Smith, M. (2015). *Mixed methods in health sciences research: A practical primer*. Thousand Oaks, CA: Sage.

   - Teddlie, C., & Tashakkori, A. (2009). *Foundations of mixed methods research: Integrating quantitative and qualitative approaches in the social and behavioral sciences*. Thousand Oaks, CA: Sage.

IDENTIFYING THE INTENT OF INTEGRATION AND ILLUSTRATING INTEGRATION FEATURES IN MIXED METHODS PROCEDURAL DIAGRAMS

Integration strategies formulated for data collection and analysis within mixed methods studies can be understood relative to the intent of data collection and the intent of the analysis. While you may (and should!) feel compelled to use integration in your data collection and analysis, the procedures may still seem to be a mystery. This chapter and its activities will help you distinguish among seven intents of integration during mixed methods projects, consider two intents of integration specific to sequential designs, learn six integration strategies for analysis, recognize three integration strategies for adjunctive data collection, choose integration strategies based on intent of the data collection and analysis, and incorporate integration planning into your mixed methods procedural diagram. As a key outcome, you will identify the intent of the integration procedures for your mixed methods and evaluation projects and situate the integration procedures in an expanded mixed methods procedural design figure.

LEARNING OBJECTIVES

To help you clarify and identify your integration strategies during data collection and analysis for your mixed methods research (MMR) or evaluation, this chapter will help you

- Distinguish among seven intents of integration during data collection used in MMR and evaluation projects

- Consider two intents of integration used in sequential mixed methods designs

- Learn six integration procedures used in the analysis of mixed methods projects

- Recognize three integration procedures for adjunctive data collection in mixed methods projects

- Choose integration strategies based on your intent during mixed methods data collection and analysis for your own project

- Incorporate integration planning during data collection and analysis into your mixed methods procedural figure

INTEGRATION DURING
DATA COLLECTION AND ANALYSIS

For the purposes of this chapter, **intent of integration** during mixed methods data collection and analysis refers to the specific purposes of linking qualitative and quantitative data as they are gathered and/or the findings are examined together for examination during mixed methods studies. An important challenge facing mixed methods researchers and evaluators is to clearly articulate mixed methods purposes for data collection and analysis during the study planning as this informs analysis procedures (Chapters 13–15). Clarity about integration procedures also identifies parameters for consideration when assessing research integrity (Chapter 16). **Integration intents during mixed methods data collection and analysis** include building, connecting, exploring, comparing, matching, expanding, diffracting, and constructing a case. Two integration procedures used in two-phase data collection and analysis specific to sequential designs are generating and testing hypotheses and developing and validating a model. Integration procedures for analysis in mixed methods designs include explaining, corroborating, enhancing, initiating, transferring, and generalizing. Integration procedures for adjunctive data collection include ascertaining (or documenting need), optimizing, and monitoring. Integration strategies are not necessarily exclusive of each other within a mixed methods project and can be formulated during the design phase for planning a mixed methods project or *post facto* to describe the integration procedures used.

Activity: Identifying Integration Strategies During Data Collection for Mixed Methods Research and Evaluation Designs

Review Workbox 10.1 and consider the mixed methods integration procedures during data collection. As you review explanations of the various strategies in Workbox 10.1, check those that may have application in your own work. This will help you complete the specific procedural diagrams later in the chapter based on your choices.

Workbox 10.1: Integration Procedures for Data Collection in Mixed Methods Designs

Integration Type	Description
☐ Building	Using the data collection and analysis of one form of data to inform the data collection approach of the other type of data collection and analysis
☐ Connecting	Using results from one type of data collection to inform selection of subjects for the other type of data collection
☐ Exploring	Using initial qualitative data collection and analysis to discover relevant information or to study a concept prior to conducting the quantitative strand
☐ Comparing	Collecting both qualitative and quantitative data about a phenomenon of interest with the intent of examining how the two types of data relate to each other
☐ Matching	With forethought about specific potential for comparison, collecting both qualitative and quantitative data about a phenomenon of interest to examine how the two types of data relate to each other
☐ Expanding	Using both qualitative and quantitative data collection to elucidate a broader yet overlapping view of a phenomenon
☐ Diffracting	With forethought about specific potential for examining different facets of a phenomenon, conducting qualitative and quantitative data collection to examine different "cuts" or aspects of a phenomenon of interest
☐ Constructing a case	Collecting qualitative and quantitative data to develop a robust understanding about a specific example under investigation

INTEGRATING DATA COLLECTION STRATEGIES INTO MIXED METHODS STUDIES

The data collection strategies for integration in mixed methods studies illustrated in Workbox 10.1 are described in further detail in the following.

a. **Building** refers to the intent of using the data collection and analysis of one form of data to inform the data collection approach of the other type of data collection and analysis (Fetters, Curry, & Creswell, 2013). Building represents one aspect of *development* as presented by Greene, Caracelli, and Graham (1989). This procedure occurs commonly in both types of sequential designs (Fetters et al., 2013). In an exploratory sequential design starting with qualitative data collection, the themes can become scales, codes can become variables, and quotes can become items in a survey (Figure 10.1). In an explanatory sequential design, survey findings can inform the constructs for examination in subsequent qualitative interview questions (Figure 10.2).

FIGURE 10.1 ■ Building as an Integration Strategy During Data Collection for an Exploratory Sequential Design

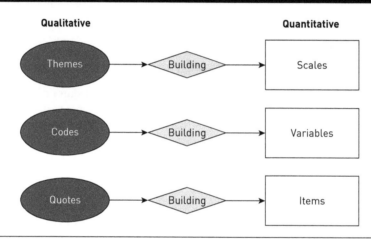

Acknowledgment: Adapted with permission of Timothy C. Guetterman, who developed the original version of this diagram.

FIGURE 10.2 ■ Building as an Integration Strategy During Data Collection for an Explanatory Sequential Design

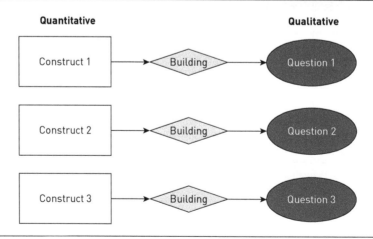

b. **Connecting** describes the intent of using results from one type of data collection to inform selection of subjects for the other type of data collection (Fetters et al., 2013). This concept falls under the broader meaning of *development* as presented by Greene et al. (1989). This occurs most commonly in an explanatory sequential design when based on initial quantitative data collection from a large population; a mixed methods researcher/evaluator can use demographic characteristics or some other findings obtained from the collected quantitative data to select participants for the qualitative data collection (Figure 10.3). That is, quantitative results are used to decide who to *sample* for follow-up interviews, focus groups, etc. Typically, subjects from one strand of data collection will be involved in the subsequent strand of data collection.

FIGURE 10.3 ■ Connecting as an Integration Strategy for Identifying Participants From the Quantitative Data Collection for the Qualitative Data Collection

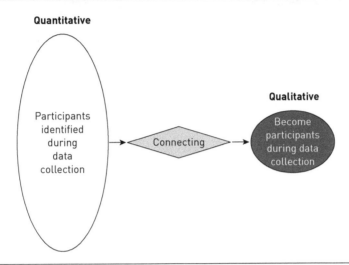

c. **Exploring** denotes the intent of using initial qualitative data collection and analysis to discover relevant information or to study a concept *prior* to conducting a quantitative follow-up study used to confirm or generalize initial qualitative findings (Figure 10.4). This is the overarching intent of an exploratory sequential MMR design (Creswell & Plano Clark, 2018).

FIGURE 10.4 ■ Exploring as an Integration Strategy for Identifying the Unknown for Subsequent Measurement

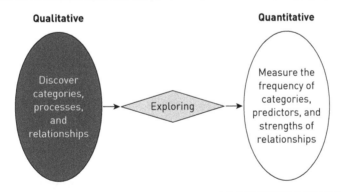

d. **Comparing** describes the intent of collecting both qualitative and quantitative data about a phenomenon of interest, and then examining how the two types of data relate to each other (Figure 10.5). Comparing is the most encompassing of additional merging strategies, namely, matching, expanding, and diffracting. To the extent possible, at the design level, the well-prepared mixed methods investigator will have more than just a vague plan that the data will be compared. Matching, expanding, and diffracting are three intents that illustrate how advanced planning can facilitate clarity in data collection procedures. Some authors may use the word *triangulate* to convey the intent of comparing (Greene et al., 1989). But using *triangulation* in mixed methods studies may be problematic because the term has become almost synonymous with the field of qualitative research, while *integration* has become the term most synonymous with the field of

MMR. In addition, the original meaning of triangulation from navigation derived from using multiple angles to identify an exact location. The suggestion that combining information together leads to an "exact understanding is incompatible with postmodernist views about the social construction of reality (Denzin, 2010; Fetters & Molina-Azorin, 2017a; Janesick, 1994; Richardson, 1994).

FIGURE 10.5 ■ Comparing as an Integration Strategy During Data Collection

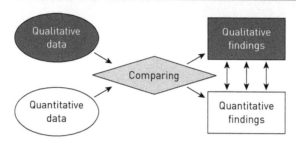

e. **Matching** conveys the intent of collecting both qualitative and quantitative data about the *same* domains, constructs, or ideas. It differs from comparing, a generic approach, through forethought about what data will be collected using both methods to ensure that information across both types of findings will be related closely (Figure 10.6). For example, in an actual convergent mixed methods study, the researchers collected information about quality of life and activities of daily living of cancer patients using standardized instruments, while also interviewing individuals about their quality of life and activities of daily living (Moseholm, Rydahl-Hansen, Lindhardt, & Fetters, 2017).

FIGURE 10.6 ■ Matching as an Integration Strategy During Data Collection

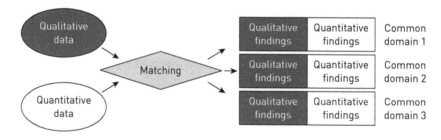

f. **Expanding** refers to the intent of extending the breadth and range of inquiry by using different methods in an MMR or evaluation project (Greene et al., 1989). Greene et al. (1989) describe the rationale of expansion as increasing the scope of inquiry through selection of methods as needed for mixed methods inquiry. In a convergent mixed methods design, a researcher will seek to collect qualitative and quantitative data about a central phenomenon, as well as additionally related data that extends beyond the central phenomenon (Figure 10.7).

FIGURE 10.7 ■ Expanding as an Integration Strategy During Data Collection

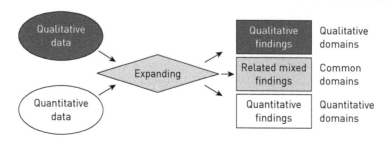

g. **Diffracting** describes the intent of seeking different cuts or slices of data with qualitative and quantitative data collection, respectively as illustrated in Figure 10.8 (Uprichard & Dawney, 2016). It differs from other strategies by specifically planning with forethought, and then collecting data to examine different "cuts" or aspects of a phenomenon. This strategy conveys a more specific focus than the more general strategy of *expansion*, as articulated by Greene et al. (1989). The analogy of the white light going into a prism—the researcher going into the field—and coming out on the opposite side in seven different colors—at the end of data collection with different aspects and data. Referring back to the analogy, the quantitative data may address the "red, orange, and yellow" cuts of data, while the qualitative data address the "green, blue, indigo, and violet" cuts of data. In a convergent mixed methods design, a researcher using diffraction may collect qualitative data about experiences of one group, while quantitative data may be collected from a larger group to examine other aspects of a phenomenon. The two methods are used to examine *different* aspects of the same phenomenon with *different* philosophical assumptions and *different* kinds of data collection and analysis procedures (Uprichard & Dawney, 2016).

FIGURE 10.8 ■ Diffracting as an Integration Strategy During Data Collection

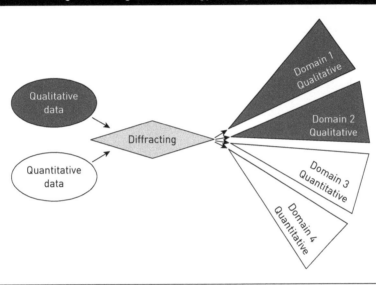

h. **Constructing a case** describes the intent of collecting qualitative and quantitative data to develop a robust understanding about a specific example under investigation (Creswell & Plano Clark, 2018). The intent is to obtain the qualitative and quantitative data necessary to answer the research or evaluation question about a case (Figure 10.9). Constructing a case can occur with both types of sequential designs, as well as with convergent designs. Case studies can be one component or the overarching component of a mixed methods study (Guetterman & Fetters, 2018). Constructing-a-case procedures are possible with any core or advanced/complex/scaffolded design. For example, Wakai, Simasek, Nakagawa, Saijo, and Fetters (2018) constructed a mixed methods case study using a scaffolded intervention design and quality improvement process.

FIGURE 10.9 ■ Constructing a Case as an Integration Strategy During Data Collection

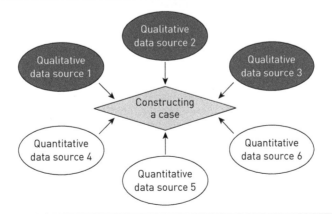

INTEGRATION PROCEDURES IN TWO-PHASE DATA COLLECTION AND ANALYSIS USED IN SEQUENTIAL DESIGNS

Mixed methods researchers use two important two-phase data collection and analysis integration procedures in sequential designs: generating and testing hypotheses, and developing and validating a model/theory (Workbox 10.2).

Workbox 10.2: Integration Procedures in Two-Phase Data Collection and Analysis Used in Sequential Designs

Integration Type	Informs Data	First Phase Role	Second Phase Role	Comment
☐ **Generating and testing hypotheses**	Collection and analysis	Creating hypotheses	Testing the hypotheses	Often qualitatively developed hypotheses to test quantitatively
☐ **Developing and validating a model**	Collection and analysis	Developing a model/theory	Validating the model/theory	Either sequence can occur—qualitatively developed model tested quantitatively, or quantitatively developed model tested quantitatively

Activity: Identifying Two-Phase Data Collection and Analysis Integration Strategies for Use in Sequential Mixed Methods Research and Evaluation Designs

Review Workbox 10.2 and consider the potential use of the mixed methods integration procedures for your exploratory sequential (QUAL to QUAN) mixed methods design, or for your explanatory sequential (QUAN to QUAL) mixed methods design. As you review the explanation of the various strategies, in Workbox 10.2 you can check the relevance of these special strategies that may have application in your own work. Identifying the potential relevance will help you complete the specific procedural diagrams later in the chapter. The two-phase data collection and analysis integration procedures in sequential designs are described in more detail below.

a. **Generating and testing hypotheses** describes the intent of developing postulations based on one type of data that can then be tested with the other type of data. This intent of integration can occur in both types of sequential designs and over two phases. Generating occurs during the first phase of the data collection and analysis, and testing of developed hypotheses occurs in the second phase of data collection and analysis. In an exploratory sequential design, initial qualitative data collection may inform hypotheses that can be explored empirically in the subsequent quantitative phase. In an explanatory sequential design with initial quantitative analysis, correlations or relationships identified can be examined qualitatively for confirmation, disconfirmation, or expansion.

b. **Developing and validating a model** refers to the intent of creating a theoretical or conceptual framework with one form of data collection and analysis, and then testing its validity with the other form of data collection and analysis (Kelle, 2015). This intent of integration also can occur in both types of sequential designs and in convergent designs. In an explanatory sequential design, analysis of quantitative data may result in a model that is then examined through the collection and analysis of qualitative data. For example, Crooks, Schuurman, Cinnamon, Castleden, and Johnston (2011) refined a location analysis model in human geography using qualitative interviews. Conversely, the relationships identified through a model based on qualitative data could then be tested and validated quantitatively. Haase, Becker, Nill, Shultz, and Gentry (2016) conducted a qualitative study to examine male breadwinning ideology and developed a model to advance the theoretical analysis of the phenomenon that they then examined experimentally using vignette studies.

INTEGRATION PROCEDURES FOR MIXED DATA ANALYSIS

The mixed data analysis strategies for integration in mixed methods designs are found in Workbox 10.3 and include explaining, corroborating, enhancing, initiating, transferring, and generalizing.

Workbox 10.3: Integration Procedures for Analysis in Mixed Methods Designs

Integration Type	Description
☐ **Explaining**	Qualitative data used to explain previously obtained quantitative findings
☐ **Corroborating**	Finding information from one data form to support the other
☐ **Enhancing**	Using information from the two types of data for increasing interpretability and meaningfulness
☐ **Initiating**	Seeking discovery of paradox and contradiction by recasting questions or findings from one method with the other method
☐ **Transferring**	Considering the relevance of qualitative findings from the study participants to a larger population, phenomenon of interest, context, or theory
☐ **Generalizing**	Extrapolating quantitative findings from the study population to a target population, usually in larger studies

Activity: Identifying Integration Strategies for Mixed Data Analysis

Review Workbox 10.3 and consider the potential use of integration procedures during mixed data analysis for your MMR or evaluation project. As you review the explanations of the various strategies, in Workbox 10.3, you can check relevant boxes for choices that may have application in your own work. Identifying the potential relevance will help you complete the specific procedural diagrams later in the chapter. For the purposes of this chapter, these are presented as intents, but after data collection and analysis is complete, these may also represent the outcomes of the integrated analysis. The mixed data analysis strategies for integration introduced in Workbox 10.3 are presented in greater detail below.

1. **Explaining** describes the intent of describing or explicating initial quantitative findings with subsequent qualitative data collection and analysis. This is the overarching integration intent of an explanatory sequential mixed methods design (Creswell & Plano Clark, 2018). After completing the mixed data analysis, researchers may report the findings were explained, example qualitative data explain previous quantitative findings.

2. **Corroborating** portrays the intent to use one type of data to verify the findings of the other form of data (Greene et al., 1989). It differs from matching, as matching occurs during the data-planning process, whereas corroboration can be sought and confirmed or disconfirmed during the analysis after the data are collected. In a convergent design, a researcher may corroborate findings from the quantitative analysis with findings from qualitative investigation. Alternatively, in a mixed methods evaluation, the evaluator may corroborate qualitative findings with quantitative findings. Some researchers refer to this as *triangulating*, though I believe *corroborating* does provide a more specific inference. After completing the mixed data analysis, researchers may report that one type of finding corroborated the other.

3. **Enhancing** designates the intent of using information from both the qualitative and quantitative data to increase interpretability and meaningfulness. Enhancing is a strategy that derives from the condition of complementarity, as articulated by Greene et al. (1989). As a noun, *complementarity* reflects a state, while *enhancing* describes the intent of the analysis. Ostensibly, one could use complementing, but Greene

et al. (1989) operationalized complementarity to have multiple meanings (e.g., elaboration, enhancement, illustration and clarification of results, and as a rationale for increasing interpretability, meaningfulness, and validity of constructs and inquiry results). After completing the mixed data analysis, researchers may report that one type of findings enhanced understanding of the other.

4. **Initiating** depicts the intent of searching for paradox and contradiction. Initiating is a strategy that derives from the term *initiation* described by Greene et al. (1989). The term has been recast here as a gerund to indicate an active process. The initiating strategy involves recasting questions based on findings, or recasting findings from one method with findings of the other method. After completing a preliminary mixed data analysis, researchers may report they initiated further analysis of the data or even further data collection and analysis.

5. **Transferring** conveys the intent to consider the relevance of the findings from the study participants to a larger population, phenomenon of interest, context, or theory. The highly renowned qualitative research methodologists Lincoln and Guba (2000) developed the concept of transferability. Transferability is roughly analogous to generalizability relative to external validity in quantitative research. While generalizability is framed from the perspective of inferential statistics, transferability is based on a qualitative assessment of how the study population holds related features and commonality with other settings, contexts, participants, or theoretical contexts (Kelle, 2015). In the second phase of an explanatory sequential mixed methods design, how a sample is chosen to draw conclusions about the implications of the qualitative findings for the full study requires careful thought. In the case of convergent designs, the researcher may need to consider simultaneously how to plan for transferability for the qualitative findings from a smaller number of individuals when the sample is embedded, separate, or multilevel. If there also is a larger sample, then generalizability may be a consideration as well. After completing the mixed data analysis, researchers may report how the qualitative findings transfer to a larger group or population.

6. **Generalizing** indicates the intent of extending findings and conclusions drawn from an initial qualitative phase, through the use of a subsequent quantitative phase conducted with a representative population of individuals where findings are assessed by using inferential statistics (Creswell & Plano Clark, 2018). This represents a common intent in exploratory sequential mixed methods designs where a phenomenon of interest is initially explored qualitatively, and then subsequent data collection is conducted with the intent of developing a broader understanding of qualitative findings among a wider population. After completing the mixed data analysis, researchers may report how the quantitative findings generalize to the target population.

INTEGRATION PROCEDURES FOR ADJUNCTIVE DATA COLLECTION IN MIXED METHODS STUDIES

Mixed methods researchers have used and identified additional strategies that can be critical for conducting rigorous mixed methods studies, even though the data collection strategy may serve primarily as an adjunctive approach (Workbox 10.4). Three strategies for discussion here include ascertaining the need, optimizing, and monitoring. These integration procedures are most common in longitudinal studies, and particularly in intervention studies.

Workbox 10.4: Integration Procedures for Adjunctive Data Collection in Mixed Methods Studies

Integration Type	Convergent, Sequential, or Both	Description
☐ **Ascertaining (documenting) need**	Usually sequential	Justifying the need for further research using either form of data
☐ **Optimizing**	Usually sequential	Adjusting data collection procedures using either form of data in preparation for primary data collection
☐ **Monitoring**	Both	Checking fidelity to study protocols and procedures using either form of data

Activity: Identifying Adjunctive Strategies for Use in Your Mixed Methods Research and Evaluation Studies

Review Workbox 10.4 and consider the potential use of the adjunctive mixed methods integration procedures for your mixed methods design. These strategies may apply in sequential and convergent studies. As you review the explanation of the various strategies, in Workbox 10.4, you can check relevant boxes for choices that may have application in your own work. Identifying the potential relevance will help you complete the specific procedural diagrams later in the chapter.

1. **Ascertaining the need** refers to the intent of collecting qualitative or mixed methods data prior to conducting the main component of an MMR or evaluation study to document the need or confirm that an investigation or evaluation is actually indicated (Creswell, Fetters, Plano Clark, & Morales, 2009). Many community-based mixed methods studies and mixed methods evaluation studies use this integration strategy. While not necessarily the main focus of an investigation, the consequence of not conducting an assessment in advance can be quite large. In one example, investigators conducted an intervention based on the assumption of need without clearly understanding the perspective of the population for whom a trial was designed (Catallo, Jack, Ciliska, & MacMillan, 2013). After data collection, researchers may report they ascertained the need.

2. **Optimizing** describes the intent of using qualitative or mixed methods data collection and analysis early in an MMR or evaluation study to ensure that study instruments or interventions have been developed appropriately for the study intent. Optimizing can include planned activities such as recruiting participants or study sites, understanding the participants, context, and environment to ensure these factors are optimized for the investigation (Creswell et al., 2009). Occurrences may be found in any of the core designs (Chapter 7) and, by extension, scaffolded designs (Chapter 8). After data collection, researchers may report they optimized their data collection tools, strategies, etc.

3. **Monitoring** signifies the intent to use qualitative or mixed methods data collection and analysis to watch for events during a mixed methods study or evaluation. This strategy can include examining the impact on participants including unexpected experiences (good or bad), documenting unexpected or expected events or incidents that could have an impact on the study, identifying resources that could facilitate or deter conduct of the study, checking for fidelity to the study procedures, and identifying potentially mediating or moderating factors that occur during the study that could have an impact on study outcomes, or could illuminate information that could be germane to interpreting the study results (Creswell et al., 2009). After data collection, researchers may report how they monitored aspects during the study.

ADDING THE INTENT OF INTEGRATION INTO MIXED METHODS PROCEDURAL DIAGRAMS

In the planning of your procedural diagram, you will want to consider the level of detail as this may vary depending on your purpose. For example, you may prefer more detail in a version prepared for a grant or publication and less detail in a version for an oral presentation. Addition of the intents of integration can add significant clarity to a mixed methods proposal, especially when under development for a mixed methods dissertation or funding application. At this time, include as much detail as possible, as it will be easier to remove detail than add it later. The exercises will help you logically develop your figure. If your data collection or analysis procedures are complete, using past tense of the data collection and analysis strategies may be effective.

Procedural Diagram Activities

The Workbox Illustrations and Workboxes that follow cover all three core designs. As the scaffolded designs (Chapter 8) can be constructed with the core designs (Chapter 7), you should use the core design figures if you have a scaffolded design. Your task is to consider Workbox Illustration 10.5.1 for an explanatory sequential mixed methods design, Workbox Illustration 10.6.1 for an exploratory sequential design, and Workbox Illustration 10.7.1 for a convergent design. These Workboxes are modified versions of the procedural diagram workboxes from Chapter 7. Workboxes 10.5.2, 10.6.2, and 10.7.2 have been modified to create space specifically designed for you to add integration strategies during the data collection phase. The

Workboxes build upon previous design figures, by showing integration. The sequential design figures will not be complete without consideration of integration after both phases, that is, the quantitative then qualitative in explanatory sequential designs, and the qualitative then quantitative in the exploratory sequential designs. Often times, the final integration step has just been referred to as "merging," which conflates the strategies of integration as part of data collection and integration during mixed methods analysis procedures that occur after completing data collection.

DATA COLLECTION AND ANALYSIS INTEGRATION STRATEGIES FOR EXPLANATORY SEQUENTIAL MIXED METHODS RESEARCH DESIGNS

Workbox Illustration 10.5.1 provides the integration procedures for an explanatory sequential mixed methods design utilized by Harper (2016). He sought to understand how principals can improve student achievement by improving school culture. Harper assessed this relationship in 26 of Alabama's 218 middle schools through use of a survey (Harper, 2016). As illustrated by the integration diamond in Workbox Illustration 10.5.1, he used integration procedures of *connecting* to identify a sample for subsequent interviews and *building* to develop the content for the interviews. Based on statistical modeling, he found academic optimism was a significant predictor of academic achievement, so he then *explored* qualitatively how three dimensions of academic optimism, namely, faculty trust, collective efficacy, and academic emphasis, were related to student achievement through interviews with 11 principals of high-achieving middle schools. As illustrated by the second integration diamond in Workbox Illustration 10.5.1, for the analysis Harper used the integration procedures of *expanding* and *corroborating* (Harper, 2016).

Workbox Illustration 10.5.1: Data Integration and Analysis Strategies in an Explanatory Sequential Mixed Methods Research Design from Education

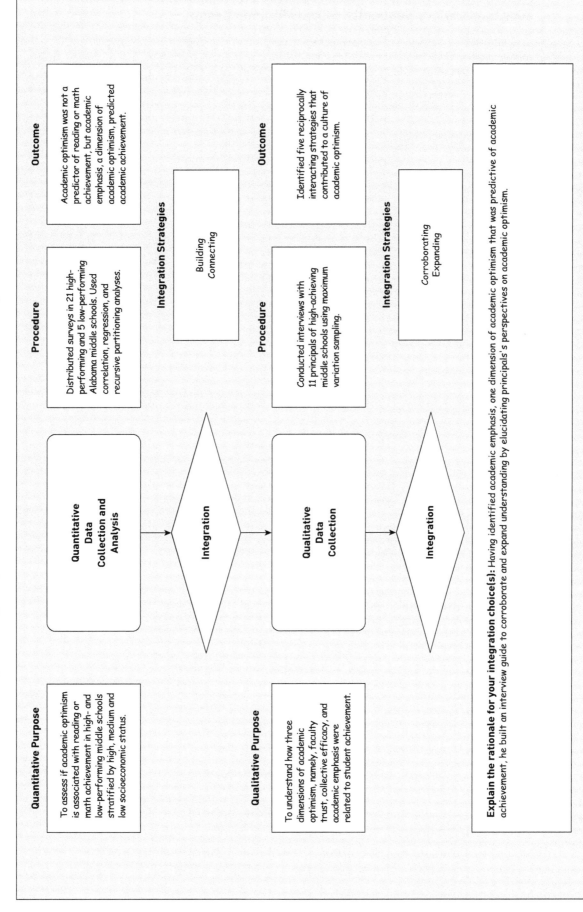

Quantitative Purpose

To assess if academic optimism is associated with reading or math achievement in high- and low-performing middle schools stratified by high, medium and low socioeconomic status.

Procedure

Distributed surveys in 21 high-performing and 5 low-performing Alabama middle schools. Used correlation, regression, and recursive partitioning analyses.

Outcome

Academic optimism was not a predictor of reading or math achievement, but academic emphasis, a dimension of academic optimism, predicted academic achievement.

Quantitative Data Collection and Analysis

Integration

Integration Strategies

Building
Connecting

Qualitative Purpose

To understand how three dimensions of academic optimism, namely, faculty trust, collective efficacy, and academic emphasis were related to student achievement.

Procedure

Conducted interviews with 11 principals of high-achieving middle schools using maximum variation sampling.

Outcome

Identified five reciprocally interacting strategies that contributed to a culture of academic optimism.

Qualitative Data Collection

Integration

Integration Strategies

Corroborating
Expanding

Explain the rationale for your integration choice(s): Having identified academic emphasis, one dimension of academic optimism that was predictive of academic achievement, he built an interview guide to corroborate and expand understanding by elucidating principals's perspectives on academic optimism.

Source: Harper (2016, p.210) with adaptations by the *Mixed Methods Research Workbook* author.

133

Activity: Identifying Common Integration Strategies Associated With Your Explanatory Sequential Mixed Methods Design

Workbox 10.5.2 provides a template for explanatory sequential mixed methods designs. An efficient strategy for completing the Workbox involves writing your quantitative purpose, procedures, and outcomes. Then complete the qualitative purpose, procedures, and outcomes. Using Workboxes 10.1–10.4 and the full definitions, decide what integration strategies you have after the quantitative phase. Fill in the integration strategies planned after the subsequent qualitative phase in the diamond figure.

Workbox 10.5.2: Your Data Collection and Analysis Integration Strategies for an Explanatory Sequential Mixed Methods Research Design

Quantitative Purpose

Procedure

Outcome

Quantitative Data Collection and Analysis

Integration

Integration Strategies

Qualitative Purpose

Procedure

Outcome

Qualitative Data Collection

Integration

Integration Strategies

Explain the rationale for your integration choice(s):

DATA COLLECTION AND ANALYSIS INTEGRATION STRATEGIES FOR EXPLORATORY SEQUENTIAL MIXED METHODS RESEARCH DESIGNS

Workbox Illustration 10.6.1 provides the integration procedures for an exploratory sequential mixed methods design utilized by Sharma and Vredenburg (1998). They conducted extensive qualitative data collection. This included initially 19 in-depth interviews with senior and middle management executives to *construct case studies* of seven firms in the Canadian oil and gas industry. They then longitudinally interviewed 27 executives between two to five times over 1.5 years. They used the interview findings and literature to *build* a survey. During this phase they *generated hypotheses* for testing in the subsequent phase (see the first integration diamond, Workbox Illustration 10.6.1). The authors then distributed a survey and received 99 completed instruments (response rate 90%) that allowed them to measure environmental strategies of the Canadian oil and gas industry. They then *tested the hypotheses* from the first phase. In their analysis, they further *compared* their mixed findings (see the second integration diamond, Workbox Illustration 10.6.1) to *corroborate* and *expand* their findings (Sharma & Vredenburg, 1998).

Workbox Illustration 10.6.1: Integration Strategies for an Exploratory Sequential Mixed Methods Research Design from Business

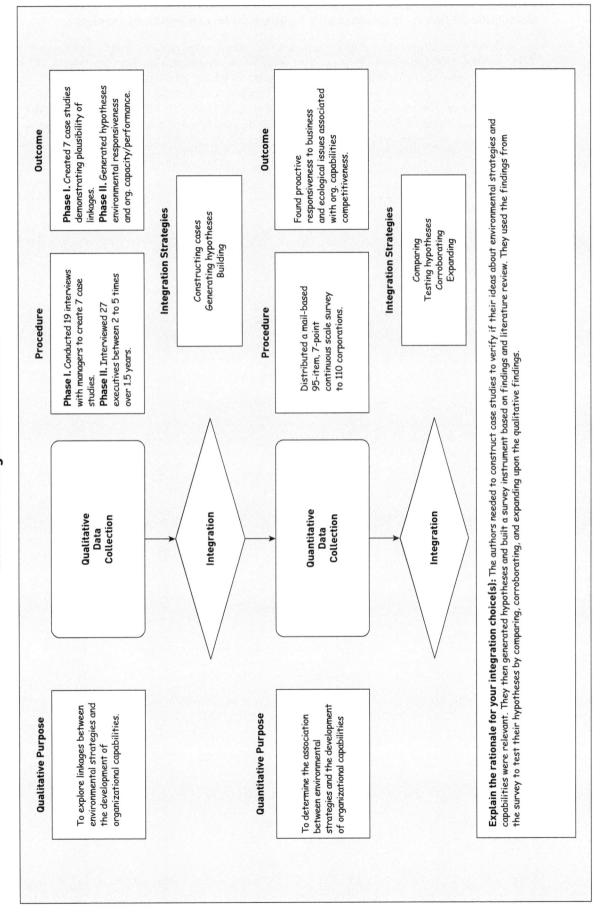

Qualitative Purpose

To explore linkages between environmental strategies and the development of organizational capabilities.

Quantitative Purpose

To determine the association between environmental strategies and the development of organizational capabilities

Procedure

Phase I. Conducted 19 interviews with managers to create 7 case studies.
Phase II. Interviewed 27 executives between 2 to 5 times over 1.5 years.

Procedure

Distributed a mail-based 95-item, 7-point continuous scale survey to 110 corporations.

Outcome

Phase I. Created 7 case studies demonstrating plausibility of linkages.
Phase II. Generated hypotheses environmental responsiveness and org. capacity/performance.

Outcome

Found proactive responsiveness to business and ecological issues associated with org. capabilities competitiveness.

Integration Strategies

Constructing cases
Generating hypotheses
Building

Integration Strategies

Comparing
Testing hypotheses
Corroborating
Expanding

Qualitative Data Collection

Integration

Quantitative Data Collection

Integration

Explain the rationale for your integration choice(s): The authors needed to construct case studies to verify if their ideas about environmental strategies and capabilities were relevant. They then generated hypotheses and built a survey instrument based on findings and literature review. They used the findings from the survey to test their hypotheses by comparing, corroborating, and expanding upon the qualitative findings.

Source: Sharma and Vredenburg (1998). Procedural diagram created by the *Mixed Methods Research Workbook* author.

Activity: Identifying Common Integration Strategies Associated With Your Exploratory Sequential Mixed Methods Design

Workbox 10.6.2 provides a template for exploratory sequential mixed methods designs. First complete the qualitative purpose, procedures, and outcomes. Then complete the quantitative purpose, procedures, and outcomes. Using Workboxes 10.1–10.4 and the full definitions, decide what integration strategies you have after the qualitative phase. Fill in the integration strategies planned after the subsequent quantitative phase. Then explain the rationale for your choice and the next steps you could take in a subsequent study. This will be particularly valuable for multistage designs, as well as for future planning of steps after the current research or evaluation is completed.

Workbox 10.6.2: Your Data Collection Integration Strategies for Exploratory Sequential Mixed Methods Research Design

Qualitative Purpose

Qualitative Data Collection

Integration

Procedure

Outcome

Integration Strategies

Quantitative Purpose

Quantitative Data Collection

Integration

Procedure

Outcome

Integration Strategies

Explain the rationale for your integration choice(s):

DATA COLLECTION AND ANALYSIS INTEGRATION STRATEGIES FOR CONVERGENT MIXED METHODS RESEARCH DESIGNS

Workbox Illustration 10.7.1 provides the integration procedures for a convergent mixed methods design utilized by Shultz et al. (2015), who were evaluating the benefit of a standardized training session for Japanese doctors during an international training elective while in the United States. In addition to the underlying convergent design, there was an overlaid mixed methods case study design based on their framing of the case for investigation. As illustrated by the integration diamond in the figure, for their integration procedures, they *compared* qualitative and quantitative data and used their findings to *construct a case* (Shultz et al., 2015).

Workbox Illustration 10.7.1: Integration Strategies for Convergent Mixed Methods Research Design from Medical Education

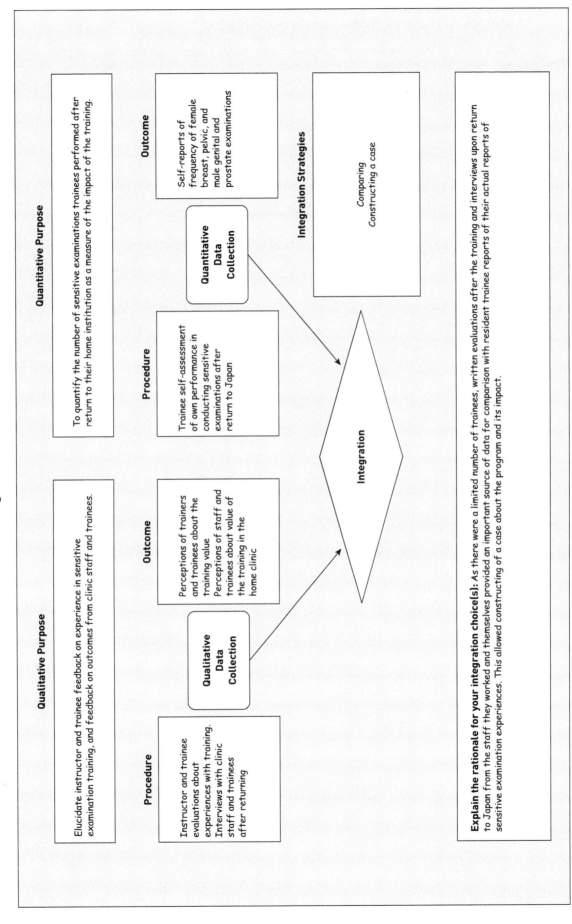

Qualitative Purpose

Elucidate instructor and trainee feedback on experience in sensitive examination training, and feedback on outcomes from clinic staff and trainees.

Quantitative Purpose

To quantify the number of sensitive examinations trainees performed after return to their home institution as a measure of the impact of the training.

Procedure

Instructor and trainee evaluations about experiences with training. Interviews with clinic staff and trainees after returning

Procedure

Trainee self-assessment of own performance in conducting sensitive examinations after return to Japan

Outcome

Perceptions of trainers and trainees about the training value
Perceptions of staff and trainees about value of the training in the home clinic

Outcome

Self-reports of frequency of female breast, pelvic, and male genital and prostate examinations

Qualitative Data Collection

Quantitative Data Collection

Integration

Integration Strategies

Comparing
Constructing a case

Explain the rationale for your integration choice(s): As there were a limited number of trainees, written evaluations after the training and interviews upon return to Japan from the staff they worked and themselves provided an important source of data for comparison with resident trainee reports of their actual reports of sensitive examination experiences. This allowed constructing of a case about the program and its impact.

Source: Shultz et al. (2015) Procedural diagram created by the Mixed Methods Research Workbook author.

Activity: Identifying Common Integration Strategies Associated With a Convergent Design

Workbox 10.7.2 provides a template for convergent mixed methods designs. First complete the qualitative purpose, procedures, and outcomes. Then complete the quantitative purpose, procedures, and outcomes. Using Workboxes 10.1–10.4 and the full definitions, decide what integration strategies you have for the two integration levels, then fill in the intent of integration. Explain the rationale for your choice and the next steps you could take in a subsequent study. This will be particularly valuable for multistage designs, as well as for future planning of steps after the current research or evaluation is completed.

Workbox 10.7.2: Your Data Collection Integration Strategies for a Convergent Mixed Methods Research Design

Qualitative Purpose

Quantitative Purpose

Procedure

Outcome

Procedure

Outcome

Qualitative Data Collection

Quantitative Data Collection

Integration

Integration Strategies

Explain the rationale for your integration choice(s):

Application Activities

1. **Peer Feedback.** If you are working on your project as part of a class or in a workshop, please pair up with a peer mentor, and one of you spend about 5–10 minutes talking about your integration strategies. You should focus on the integration selections made. After quickly reviewing your overall procedures with your partner, turn to the integration diamonds that were most challenging. Check with your partner if the chosen integration strategies make sense? Are there additional integration strategies to add? Do each of the integration strategies listed involve an interfacing of the qualitative and quantitative data to your mixed methods design? Take turns talking about your projects and giving feedback.

2. **Peer Feedback Guidance.** Continue honing your critiquing skills. Your goal is to help your partner refine the integration strategies. Are the integration strategies appropriate? Inclusive? Are their strategies missing? Do all the strategies listed relate to both the qualitative and quantitative data collection and the study design?

3. **Group Debrief.** If there is time, have someone present their procedural diagram with the integration strategies to the class or workshop participants.

Concluding Thoughts

Use this checklist to assess your progress in achieving the Chapter 10 objectives:

☐ I can distinguish seven intents of integration during data collection in MMR and evaluation projects.

☐ I considered two intents of integration used in sequential mixed methods designs.

☐ I learned six integration procedures used in the analysis of mixed methods projects.

☐ I examined three integration procedures for adjunctive data collection in mixed methods projects.

☐ I chose integration strategies based on my intent during mixed methods data collection and analysis for my mixed methods project.

☐ I incorporated specific integration planning during data collection and analysis into my mixed methods procedural figure.

☐ I reviewed my Chapter 10 integration approaches with a peer or colleague to refine the planning for integration in my data collection and analysis.

Now that you have completed these objectives, Chapter 11 will help you develop an implementation matrix for your MMR or evaluation project.

Key Resources

FURTHER READING ON INTEGRATION DURING DATA COLLECTION

- Creamer, E. G. (2018). *An introduction to fully integrated mixed methods research.* Thousand Oaks, CA: Sage.
- Creswell, J. W., & Plano Clark, V. L. (2018). *Designing and conducting mixed methods research* (3rd ed.). Thousand Oaks, CA: Sage.
- Fetters, M. D., Curry, L. A., & Creswell, J. W. (2013). Achieving integration in mixed methods designs-principles and practices. *Health Services Research, 48,* 2134–2156. doi:10.1111/1475-6773.12117
- Fetters, M. D., & Molina-Azorin, J. F. (2017). The journal of mixed methods research starts a new decade: The mixed methods research integration trilogy and its dimensions. *Journal of Mixed Methods Research, 11,* 291–307. doi:10.1177/1558689817714066

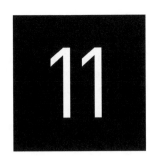

CREATING AN IMPLEMENTATION MATRIX FOR A MIXED METHODS STUDY

Mixed methods projects are complicated, as they feature multiple forms of data collection and analysis and often occur in multiple phases. You may be facing difficulty portraying your different mixed methods project steps and how they relate to study questions or aims, data collection, and expected outcomes. An implementation matrix is an illustration succinctly summarizing project aims, procedures, analysis plans, and expected outcomes. This chapter and its activities will help you understand the value and multiple applications of an implementation matrix, examine variations other researchers have incorporated into their implementation matrices, consider the potential relevance to your mixed methods project, and develop an implementation matrix for your project. As a key outcome, you will develop a mixed methods implementation matrix specific to your project.

LEARNING OBJECTIVES

To effectively convey the details of your mixed methods plan in a single matrix or table, this chapter will help you

- Recognize the value of an implementation matrix for writing a mixed methods research (MMR) proposal, conveying to others your research procedures during the review process, guiding conduct of your project, and representing your project during publication
- Explore different variations for constructing an implementation matrix and consider them as potential models for your own projects
- Develop an implementation matrix for your own project

WHAT IS AN IMPLEMENTATION MATRIX?

An **implementation matrix** is a table that illustrates an overview of your mixed methods research plan in a concise way. The elements of the simplest implementation matrix will include project aims or phases, procedures that will be used, and expected products or outcomes. For example, Figure 11.1 is an implementation matrix used in a grant called the *Medical Marvels Interactive Translational Research Experience* that was funded by the National Library of Medicine of the National Institutes of

Health (NIH). The purpose of the grant was to build in collaboration with a public science center an exhibit that would engage individuals to take a greater interest in research participation. As illustrated, Figure 11.1 features three columns: the phases, procedures, and products. Through the rest of chapter, you will learn more about using and building an implementation matrix, but first you have to understand how an implementation matrix differs from a figure.

FIGURE 11.1 ■ An Implementation Matrix With Three Basic Features

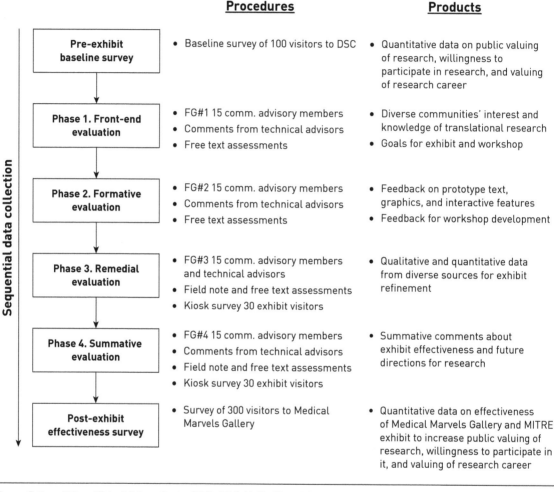

Procedures

Products

Sequential data collection

Pre-exhibit baseline survey
- Baseline survey of 100 visitors to DSC
- Quantitative data on public valuing of research, willingness to participate in research, and valuing of research career

Phase 1. Front-end evaluation
- FG#1 15 comm. advisory members
- Comments from technical advisors
- Free text assessments
- Diverse communities' interest and knowledge of translational research
- Goals for exhibit and workshop

Phase 2. Formative evaluation
- FG#2 15 comm. advisory members
- Comments from technical advisors
- Free text assessments
- Feedback on prototype text, graphics, and interactive features
- Feedback for workshop development

Phase 3. Remedial evaluation
- FG#3 15 comm. advisory members and technical advisors
- Field note and free text assessments
- Kiosk survey 30 exhibit visitors
- Qualitative and quantitative data from diverse sources for exhibit refinement

Phase 4. Summative evaluation
- FG#4 15 comm. advisory members
- Comments from technical advisors
- Field note and free text assessments
- Kiosk survey 30 exhibit visitors
- Summative comments about exhibit effectiveness and future directions for research

Post-exhibit effectiveness survey
- Survey of 300 visitors to Medical Marvels Gallery
- Quantitative data on effectiveness of Medical Marvels Gallery and MITRE exhibit to increase public valuing of research, willingness to participate in it, and valuing of research career

Source: Fetters, M.D. and Detroit Science Center. (2008–2011). *Medical Marvels Interactive Translational Research Experience*. National Library of Medicine/NIH, R03 LM010052-02.

FIGURE 11.2 ■ Perspectives on the Procedural Diagram, Implementation Matrix, and the Narrative for Comprehending Details of a Mixed Methods Research Project

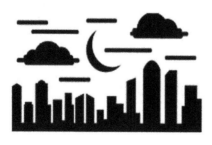

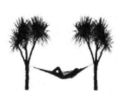

"Bird's Eye View"
Procedural Diagram

"Forest View"
Implementation Matrix

"Ground View"
Research Narrative

Differences Between a Procedural Diagram and Implementation Matrix

An implementation matrix somewhat resembles a procedural diagram (see Chapters 7 and 8). However, the procedural diagram is more concise and dynamic with arrows to show relationships and other features visually to suggest flow or movement. A procedural diagram and an implementation matrix serve different purposes. The procedural diagram provides a "bird's-eye" perspective, that is, the study "topography" can be understood from a big picture perspective, but with fewer details (Figure 11.2). In contrast, an implementation matrix provides a "forest-level" perspective, that is, details on how the proposed methods would be implemented in the field. The "research narrative" as a written project proposal or ultimately a publication, then becomes a "ground-level" perspective of the project. If you have not yet developed an MMR procedural diagram, review Chapters 7 and 8 as having a procedural diagram can help to develop an implementation matrix.

HOW CAN AN IMPLEMENTATION MATRIX BE USED?

MMR projects are complex. A mixed methods implementation matrix can be used multiple times in the course of a research project. This spans from conception to dissemination. For example, an implementation matrix can be used for (1) writing an MMR proposal; (2) conveying the complex mixed methods procedures to those reviewing your proposal; (3) conducting the actual procedures of the project after the grant is funded; and (4) publishing and writing reports about your research methodology. Below, I provide more details and examples of each.

If a picture is worth a thousand words, then an implementation matrix may be worth $100,000 or more.

1. Writing a Mixed Methods Research Proposal

When developing your MMR proposal, using an implementation matrix can be very helpful for developing the details of how you will conduct your project. If writing a dissertation or thesis proposal, you may find working with multiple advisors to be much easier if you begin with a one-page document detailing your plans. If you have to make changes, it is easy to make a change in the matrix and share with your advisor(s) and other mentors. It can be miserable and overwhelming to get feedback from advisors or a mentor when you have sunk your heart into a multiple page draft only to get a rash of red ink that looks like the chicken pox. By printing or sharing an electronic version of your implementation matrix, mentors/advisors/supervisors can all write/edit on the same draft.

Over many years of writing and working on research proposals, my approach to grant writing has evolved. Rather than writing the text or outline, I begin by working on a detailed implementation matrix and then writing the narrative section of the grant by explaining the content of the matrix. During the actual writing of the grant narrative, or while creating a budget, plans change for any number of reasons, including revisions to the scientific plan, feasibility issues due to budget constraints, etc. The matrix fundamentally serves as the working outline or overview of the project, so it can be used as the repository for adding or changing things. As many mixed methods researchers work on teams, starting with a one-page document as an implementation matrix can literally and figuratively get the entire team "on the same page." If you use the implementation matrix as the definitive document for your procedures, when changes are made as you write the text, the implementation matrix can be used as a reference for editing the text

STORY FROM THE FIELD 11.1

USEFULNESS OF AN IMPLEMENTATION MATRIX FOR WRITING THE METHODS OF A MIXED METHODS GRANT APPLICATION: EXAMPLE FROM THE ADAPT-IT PROJECT

I was invited to participate in a grant developing an innovative approach to the conduct of clinical trials using adaptive clinical trial designs for neurological emergencies (Meurer et al., 2012). In the initial conference call, I learned the grant deadline was 3 weeks away, and my task was to create the evaluation plan in two pages. We began by developing an implementation matrix over an hour-and-a-half conference call to develop the evaluation aims, the potential data collection procedures, the number of potential participants, and evaluation outcomes. On a second call

1 week later, we discussed the matrix to ensure agreement about the aims, procedures, and outcomes. Using the finalized implementation matrix as a guide, I developed the evaluation section. After feedback by the team members on the initial draft, this section was ready to go. The submitted project was successfully funded under the U01 mechanism to the National Institutes of Health. This experience illustrates the value of an implementation matrix for *figuratively and literally getting all project members on the same page* for the evaluation procedures.

narrative. This may be particularly important if you are developing a proposal requiring team science (i.e., collaborative research) with investigators of many backgrounds. Story From the Field 11.1 illustrates a pivotal experience that reinforced the value of first writing the implementation matrix to guide the MMR project depicted in Figure 11.3.

2. Conveying Mixed Methods Research Procedures to Others Reviewing Your Project

If you are submitting any kind of a proposal, for example, proposal for funding, doctoral student proposal, etc., you must be clear about what you are planning. Grant reviewers for national grants are highly successful but

FIGURE 11.3 ■ Implementation Matrix That Contributed to Successful Funding of an Adaptive Clinical Trial Development Process Evaluation

Purpose	Approach	Data Collection	Expected Outcome
To understand the concerns and strategies of personnel participating in FTF meetings, both prior to initiation of design activities (pre-FTF-1) and after completion of substantial design activities (pre-FTF-4)	• VAS ratings of ACT features • Pre-meeting MFGIs with three expert panels: 1. NETT clinical leadership 2. NETT statistical leadership 3. Statisticians experienced in ACT design	• Seven VAS ratings per person on general ACT features (14* persons for two FTF meetings • N = six MFGIs (three MFGIs prior to FTF-1 and three MFGIs prior to FTF-4)	• Quantitative assessments of seven general ACT features to be examined pre-/post-FTF meetings • Identify variations in views of experts regarding potential value, barriers, risks, and advantages of ACTs • Establish baseline views on ACTs to delineate how those views change after participating in design processes
To understand interactions that occur during FTF meetings with respect to ACT development	• Unstructured observations and audio recordings during four FTF meetings to assess participants' nonverbal reactions	• 32 hours direct observation (5 hours per four FTF meetings)	• Process evaluation regarding constructive and unconstructive approaches to resolution of disagreements during the development of ACTs
To determine participants' assessments of each proposed ACT's strengths, weaknesses, and probability of success using both quantitative and qualitative measures	• Administer VAS-based assessments after the discussion of each proposed trial in all four FTF meetings • Written, short-answer, qualitative assessments at each FTF meeting by all participants	• Six VAS ratings per person on each trial (14* persons and two trials per meeting for four meetings) • N = 72 (18R per FTF meeting) per four trials	• Quantitative assessments of six ACT features per trial that will be compared with funding success • Assessment by all participating members regarding the design and meeting processes • Examination of degree that qualitative assessments support or conflict with VAS results
To identify the views of stakeholders external to the project	• Stakeholder interviews including NIH and FDA personnel, patient advocates, and peer reviewers	• N = 12 semi-structured telephone interviews of key informants in Years 1 and 2	• Stakeholders' knowledge and views regarding potential value, barriers, risks, and advantages of ACTs
To elicit assessments of participants on the ACT design process	• Summative evaluations, using individual interviews at end of 2 years	• N = 12 evaluations conducted in early Year 3	• Global assessments of the clinical trials design development process
To evaluate grant reviewer responses to submissions that include ACTs	• Summary statement ("pink sheets") document analysis of four trials submitted for funding	• N = 4 documents of around six pages each in Year 3	• Grant reviewers' knowledge and views regarding potential value, barriers, risks, and advantages of ACTs

*While 18 people will participate in each FTF meeting during a day, only 14 are anticipated to participate in the discussion of each individual trial.

Acronyms: FTF, face-to-face; ACTs, adaptive clinical trials; VAS, visual analog scale; MFGI, mini-focus group interviews; NIH, National Institutes of Health; FDA, Food and Drug Administration.

Note: A substantively revised version of this figure appears in Wisdom and Fetters (2015, p. 324).

Source: Barsan, W. (2010–14). *Accelerating Drug and Device Evaluation through Innovative Clinical Trial Design-Adaptive Design Trial.* National Institutes of Health Common Fund, 1U01NS073476.

often overextended individuals. For grant reviews, they have the responsibility of evaluating grant proposals for scientific merit and making recommendations for funding. Faculty members reviewing dissertation proposals are chronically stretched for time. These time-pressed individuals need to quickly grasp your complex MMR plans. The implementation matrix provides concise, but sufficiently detailed summary of the information needed to grasp a project's overall process and outcomes.

The implementation matrix provides an anchor to help reviewers know where to find information in the narrative based on your systematic writing about the methods. Story From the Field 11.2 provides an experience from the field from when I served on a study section for NIH Fogarty grants. An author of a grant did not provide any kind of table or implementation matrix for a complex study. There were inconsistencies and contradictions in the grant. If the grant author had used an implementation matrix, the study procedures and proposed outcomes could have been clearer. There is no good grant rejection, though rejection based on reviewer skepticism about your science is preferable to rejection from reviewer frustration with *not* understanding your mixed methods plan.

STORY FROM THE FIELD 11.2
OBSERVATIONS ON A SOURCE OF CONFUSION DURING A GRANT REVIEW SECTION

When sitting on my first National Institutes of Health grant review committee to evaluate and rank grant proposals, I observed that study section members have to quickly decide which grants they will and will not review. The first step is to "triage" grants, that is, to reject those considered to have too many flaws to be considered for full review. In this study section, a grant was confusing because the authors had written inconsistently about their study procedures and the number of subjects they intended to recruit. The confusion contributed to rejection of the grant. An implementation matrix, had it been used, could have ensured consistency. An implementation matrix will not ensure funding through peer review, but at minimum you will be able to ensure that your proposal is evaluated based on what you propose to do rather than misunderstandings.

The value of having an implementation matrix has also become clear through my own experience on grant submissions. In one of my early grant proposals that was funded, the grant reviewers, who typically only comment about problems, praised the implementation matrix in the proposal. See Story From the Field 11.3 for an example with a successfully funded mixed methods Small Business Technology Transfer project from the National Institutes of Health.

STORY FROM THE FIELD 11.3
FEEDBACK ON AN IMPLEMENTATION MATRIX FROM A FUNDED PROJECT

For federal grant submissions, most reviewers don't give many positive comments, as their job is to critique and tell you what's wrong with your proposal, or what they feel you should do differently. After using an implementation matrix in several projects, we noticed that reviewers were commenting about how useful the matrix was for understanding the overall project. We were so surprised by positive comments that we included a few quotations in a book chapter on how to acquire funding for mixed methods. For example, one reviewer stated, "[The figures] were quite helpful and the case illustration was very effective in showing the difference between what you propose and what is available" (Wisdom & Fetters, 2015, p. 327).

3. Conducting a Mixed Methods Research Project

The complexity of mixed methods projects occurs not only during the design phase but also during implementation. Through the course of conducting multiple MMR projects, we discovered the utility of the implementation matrix as a quick reference for guiding the conduct of the project. Despite the best-developed and clearest design plans, many projects require adjustments as the project proceeds. As illustrated in Story From the Field 11.4, one such mixed methods investigation was a project I conducted in collaboration with colleagues in Qatar. In the course of the project, we frequently referred back to the project's implementation matrix to discuss team progress and next steps.

STORY FROM THE FIELD 11.4
USING AN IMPLEMENTATION MATRIX DURING PROJECT IMPLEMENTATION

One of the most complex, challenging, and interesting projects I have worked on has been the Qatar Consumer Assessment of Health Plan Survey project I conducted with colleagues in Qatar, major grant that was funded by the Qatar National Research Fund. This project involved primary data collection in the four languages of Arabic, English, Hindi, and Urdu (Hammoud et al., 2012). We had multiple team members involved in the cultural adaptation of a health care quality instrument and then testing of the instrument. As illustrated by the implementation matrix from the proposal, the grant involved five specific aims (Figure 11.4). The primary data collection occurred in Qatar. While I made several trips to Qatar during the study, I was based in the United States and collaborated with my co-principal investigator and the Qatar-based team remotely. On multiple occasions, we referred to the implementation matrix to assess our grant progress, to organize data collection, and to consider next steps.

The implementation matrix as submitted in a grant to the Qatar National Research Fund and used as a reference during the project can be seen in Figure 11.4. We conducted this challenging project in four languages, Arabic, English, Hindi, and Urdu. This implementation matrix features three columns, the Steps, Procedures, and Products. With each progressive step, the matrix includes concise information about the approach, the procedures used, and what products are to be delivered. In this matrix, the "Steps" also corresponds to the five specific aims of the study. The "Procedures" column illustrates what was done. For example, in Step 1, the research team translated an existing instrument and used translation dilemmas to culturally adapt it. In the last column, "Products," the two bullets summarize the primary outcome of Step 1 and how the results would build to the work of Step 2. Sequentially, subsequent steps all built upon the preceding step. This depiction sends a clear message that each step provides findings that build to the subsequent step. A caveat of this approach is to avoid writing steps/aims dependent upon a specific or positive outcome for addressing the subsequent step/aim. If there is a significant chance of not having a positive outcome, the science of the procedures may be considered flawed by reviewers.

Under the procedures, the matrix includes terms such as the *translation procedures, qualitative assessments, validity assessments using qualitative interviews,* and *survey.* The key third column lists the expected product. The term here could also be *outcome* depending on your own preference, local academic culture, or preference of your funding agency. The key product of Step 1 was to be the identification of phrases and concepts that were difficult to translate, so-called translation dilemmas. Step 2 then depicts how translation dilemmas would be used to gain feedback from patients coming for ambulatory care visits. Hence, each step has procedures and products. The implementation matrix shows how Step 2 would lead to Step 3 procedures and outcomes, and Step 4 procedures and outcomes would lead to Step 5. Under Step 5, the final product would be the culmination of the research proposal.

4. Writing and Publishing Your Mixed Methods Research and Evaluation Project

As a fourth reason, an implementation matrix can be used for disseminating information about your research at a scientific meeting or in dissertations, theses, book chapters, or other publications.

Using an implementation matrix to present your research. An implementation matrix is a highly effective way to present research. For an oral presentation, I usually encourage mentees to use a horizontally designed implementation matrix to explain their mixed methods studies. The dimensions of slides are more conducive to the "landscape" format that tends to be horizontal, or widened. A portrait style or landscape implementation matrix (see example in Wisdom & Fetters, 2015, p. 324) can be used effectively in a poster presentation.

Using an implementation matrix when writing a mixed methods paper for publication. An implementation matrix can be used for disseminating the results of your MMR through publication. Depending upon your need and purpose, you may need to choose between the detailed implementation matrix or a less detailed procedural figure for submission in a publication. In original research publications a concise figure may be preferable. For a methodology publication where the readership is interested in methodological detail, the more comprehensive implementation matrix may be preferred. In the *Journal of Mixed Methods Research*, authors are encouraged to include a figure or illustration such as an implementation matrix to consolidate the methodological details. Readers of methodological articles want to understand what you did in detail, why you were doing it, how much you did, how many people you worked with, what your analytic procedures were, and what your outcomes were. An implementation matrix places this critical information in one readily accessible place.

FIGURE 11.4 ■ Implementation Matrix Guiding Project Execution in a Cross-Cultural Project Assessing Health Care Quality

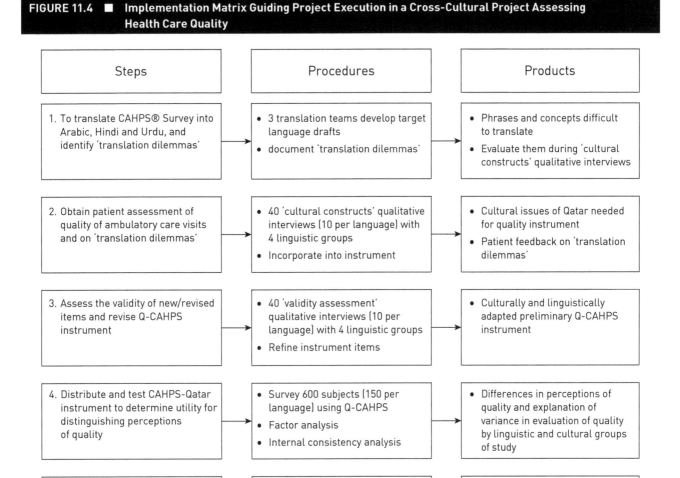

Steps	Procedures	Products
1. To translate CAHPS® Survey into Arabic, Hindi and Urdu, and identify 'translation dilemmas'	• 3 translation teams develop target language drafts • document 'translation dilemmas'	• Phrases and concepts difficult to translate • Evaluate them during 'cultural constructs' qualitative interviews
2. Obtain patient assessment of quality of ambulatory care visits and on 'translation dilemmas'	• 40 'cultural constructs' qualitative interviews (10 per language) with 4 linguistic groups • Incorporate into instrument	• Cultural issues of Qatar needed for quality instrument • Patient feedback on 'translation dilemmas'
3. Assess the validity of new/revised items and revise Q-CAHPS instrument	• 40 'validity assessment' qualitative interviews (10 per language) with 4 linguistic groups • Refine instrument items	• Culturally and linguistically adapted preliminary Q-CAHPS instrument
4. Distribute and test CAHPS-Qatar instrument to determine utility for distinguishing perceptions of quality	• Survey 600 subjects (150 per language) using Q-CAHPS • Factor analysis • Internal consistency analysis	• Differences in perceptions of quality and explanation of variance in evaluation of quality by linguistic and cultural groups of study
5. To organize results on use and interpreting linguistic and cultural influences on health care quality for use by others	• ANOVA and regression analysis to examine intergroup variation • Integrate qualitative and quantitative data into guide	• Final Q-CAHPS in 4 languages • Q-CAHPS user guide that describes use and interpretation of cultural and linguistic groups

Source: Fetters, M.D. and Khidir, A. (2009–12). *Providing Culturally Appropriate Health Care Services in Qatar: Development of a Multilingual "Patient Cultural Assessment of Quality" Instrument.* Qatar Foundation, NPRP08-530-3-116.

DEVELOPING AN IMPLEMENTATION MATRIX[1]

For the main activity of this chapter, you will be developing an implementation matrix. You can build on the examples in Figures 11.1, 11.3, or 11.4 by adding the analysis for each step. Workbox Illustration 11.1.1 displays an implementation matrix for a sequential mixed methods design. This features Harper's (2016) educational leadership research investigating how principals can improve student achievement by improving school culture. Workbox Illustration 11.1.2 displays an implementation matrix for a multiphase design with sequential and convergent components. In the example, Simões, Dibb, and Fisk (2005) from the world of business sought to develop an interdisciplinary measure of corporate identity management.

Implementation Matrix of an Explanatory Sequential Mixed Methods Design

Harper conducted an explanatory sequential mixed methods design (he referred to it as a sequential QUAN to QUAL mixed methods design). In Workbox Illustration 11.1.1, there are four headers, Phases, Procedures, Analysis, and Products. Compared to Figure 11.4, the example has two differences in the columns. Rather than using the language of steps, this implementation matrix uses the language of phases. For Phase I and Phase II, the implementation

---

[1] *A note on flexibility:* Remember, templates provide a starting point for building your implementation matrix. But bear in mind, adaptations and deviations to the headers to reflect your field, the particular end product of greatest interest to you, the grant mechanism, and even artistic inclination are all valid reasons to change the matrix structure!

Workbox Illustration 11.1.1: An Implementation Matrix Illustrating Mixed Methods Procedures for a Project From Education

Title: Investigating How Principals Can Improve Student Achievement by Improving School Culture: An Implementation Matrix of an Explanatory Sequential Mixed Methods Design

PHASES	PROCEDURES	ANALYSIS	PRODUCTS
1. Quantitative Phase **Questions:** (a) What is the relationship between academic optimism in Alabama middle schools and student achievement in math and reading? (b) What is the relationship between the three dimensions of academic optimism (faculty trust, collective efficacy, and academic emphasis) and student achievement in math and reading?	• Two hundred and eighteen Alabama schools stratified into high and low categories of student achievement based on proficiency in reading and math • Schools stratified into high-, medium-, and low-SES status based on free and reduced program for lunch • Teachers from 26 participating schools completed School Academic Optimism Scale to measure the degree of academic optimism in each school.	• Correlation, regression, and recursive partitioning analyses to examine how academic optimism predicted reading or math achievement when controlling for SES	• Identified how different dimensions of academic optimism predict student achievement • Regression identified academic efficacy (one of the dimensions of academic optimism) as a significant predictor of student achievement • Identified a representative sample of principals from high-achieving schools who were selected for follow-up interviews in Phase 2
2. Qualitative Phase **Question:** What strategies do principals use to create a culture of academic optimism to foster high student achievement in Alabama middle schools? **Subquestions:** (a) What strategies might account for the unusually strong association of academic emphasis with levels of academic achievement? (b) What strategies do principals use to develop faculty trust? (c) What strategies do principals use to develop collective efficacy?	• Used purposive, maximum variation sampling to identify 11 principals of high-achieving middle schools	• Used inductive coding to identify three a priori themes and categories, faculty trust, collective efficacy, and academic emphasis • Leadership style emerged as the fourth theme during inductive analysis of principal interviews. • Used NVivo 10 for computer-aided analysis	• Identification of strategies for developing academic optimism that fosters high student achievement in high- and low-SES middle schools. 1) Faculty trust grows out of normative social interactions in which the principal is caring, consistent, and collaborative. 2) Collective efficacy is nurtured by support from the principal for teachers. 3) Academic emphasis emerges from goals, extra student help, and celebrating achievement 4) Leadership style influences how principals impact the three dimensions of academic optimism.

Acronyms: SES, socioeconomic status

Source: Harper (2016). Implementation matrix created by the *Mixed Methods Research Workbook* author.

matrix features the quantitative research questions of Phase I and the qualitative research questions of Phase II. It features a column called Analysis to show the analysis procedures used in both Phase I and Phase II.

Phases. The phases refer to the stages of the study, but according to your field or your professors', colleagues', or own preferences, the first column can also be labeled with Aims, Steps, Questions, Hypotheses, or Tasks (the latter may be preferred in engineering proposals). (Note that Figure 11.2 used steps.) If writing a grant, and there are instructions for the writing of the proposal, follow the specific language used/advised. Be aware, different fields have different conventions. The template provides an organizing structure, and it can be edited as appropriate. Harper had two phases, an initial quantitative Phase I that addressed two research questions, and a subsequent qualitative Phase II that involved asking a primary question and three subquestions.

Procedures. Moving across the top of the implementation matrix, the next header is the Procedures section. The purpose of this section is to write the essential information needed to understand what data collection procedure is used, and how many participants will be included in each procedure. In continuation of the Phase I row, the procedures section depicting Harper's work illustrates how there was a pool of 218 Alabama schools, how he stratified them, and how he ultimately surveyed teachers from 26 schools about academic optimism. In the qualitative Phase II, Harper conducted qualitative interviews with 11 principals from high-performing schools.

Analysis. Moving further across to the right into the third column, the statistical procedures conducted and the information sought are succinctly summarized. In Phase I, Harper's statistical analysis sought to delineate how academic optimism predicted reading or math achievement when controlling for socioeconomic status. In Phase II, for the qualitative analysis he used three *a priori* themes and a fourth emergent theme to code the data. He used computer software to support his analysis.

Products. The products column depicts the results produced through the analysis of the particular phase. For example, in Harper's study, he identified in Phase I how different dimensions of academic optimism predicted student achievement, the best predictor of student achievement, and a sample for follow-up questions he could use in Phase II, an integration procedure known as connecting. In Phase II, he identified four strategies used by principals to encourage academic optimism.

Implementation Matrix for a Convergent Mixed Methods Design

Creating an implementation matrix for a convergent mixed methods design can be challenging because the qualitative and quantitative data collection and analysis often occur at roughly the same time. A choice must be made whether to have the qualitative and quantitative data collection listed in the same row or in separate rows. A rationale for using the same row is when there is intramethod data collection, that is, qualitative and quantitative data collection using the same procedure. Another rationale for using a single row occurs when the sample for both the qualitative and quantitative data collection are the same. A rationale for two rows is the use of different data collection procedures for the qualitative and quantitative data. Even though decisions about how to structure a convergent mixed methods design may pose challenges, the structure of the implementation matrix can be adjusted according to the needs of any project.

Implementation Matrix of a Multiphase Mixed Methods Study With Convergent Phases

Workbox Illustration 11.1.2 portrays a multiphase mixed methods study. In this research, Simões et al. (2005) conducted a three-phase mixed methods design and the aims align with each phase. For each of the three phases and aims, they employed multiple forms of data collection within the phase. This implementation matrix thus illustrates multiple data collection procedures depicted within each row.

Phases. An implementation matrix can show extensive detail, even for specific aims using multiple forms of data collection within a phase. This depiction of the Simões et al. (2005) study illustrates this through three aims. In the first phase, they aimed to "understand corporate identity" by using a qualitative approach. In the second phase, they sought to develop and test an instrument for which they used an exploratory sequential mixed methods survey design. In the third phase, they aimed to validate, interpret, and develop the findings using a mixed methods convergent design.

Procedures. The Procedures section depicts the data collection approach(es), including the number of participants planned for inclusion in the study. Using a simultaneous data collection strategy (e.g., the quantitative and qualitative data are collected using the same methodology) requires listing only one procedure (e.g., survey with 100 people). If using different data collection procedures, these should be listed separately. For example, if conducting a battery of structured surveys and focus groups, these would be inserted separately. In the Simões et al. (2005) study, Phase I utilized qualitative data collection from three sources of information, namely, published documents, tourism materials, and interviews with 18 experts. In Phase II, they developed an initial pool of items for a survey, then progressively used interviews, piloting, and psychometrics testing of their new instrument. In Phase III, the investigators simultaneously collected qualitative and quantitative data through 10 interviews with managers and a mail survey to 110 additional managers.

Analysis. Depicting the analysis in an implementation matrix when each phase has multiple data collection procedures proves most challenging for aligning the analysis procedures with the previous data collection procedures. For example, in the Simões et al. (2005) study, for the Phase I analysis, the authors focused on developing formation for three scales: (1) product and service identity, brand development, and communication; (2) hotel industry context; and (3) how corporate identity or corporate brand is developed/managed at the hotel unit level. In Phase II, their analysis involved multiple steps for developing and validating their survey. In Phase III, their analysis centered on the validation, interpretation, and development of the findings.

Products. Depending on the aim of the phase, the products column may have varying degrees of complexity. In the Simões et al. (2005) study, the modest product of Phase I comprised a pool of information potentially relevant to corporate identity management. In contrast, the two key products of Phase II were a functional instrument and compelling information on the psychometric properties of the newly developed instrument. The Phase III product was the resulting instrument and potential applications of the instrument.

Workbox Illustration 11.1.2: An Implementation Matrix for Multiphase Design With Sequential and Convergent Components From Business

Title: Development of an Interdisciplinary Measure of Corporate Identity Management: An Implementation Matrix for a Multiphase Design			
PHASES AND AIMS	**PROCEDURES**	**ANALYSIS**	**PRODUCTS**
First aim: To gain an in-depth understanding of corporate identity management (CIM)	• Collected published documents, in-depth interviews (n = 18 experts), and material from tourism and hotel industry events	• Analyzed for (1) product and service identity, brand development, and communication; (2) hotel industry context; (3) how corporate identity or corporate brand is developed/managed at hotel unit level; (4) CIM scale development and initial refinement	• Information appropriate for inclusion in the Phase II scale development phase
Second aim: To develop and test a CIM survey questionnaire	• Based on Aim 1 results and literature review, developed pool of 70 Likert scale items • Three interview rounds • Five academic experts reduced to 44 items • Ten hotel/sales marketing experts; reduced to 31 items • 24 stake holders • Pilot testing with 14 hotel managers • Questionnaires from 533 hotel general managers	• Item reduction • Interrater reliability assessment • Interobserver reliability • Descriptive statistics of hotels, participants, and demographics • Exploratory factor analysis • Confirmatory stage analysis • Convergent and discriminant validity check • Internal consistency assessment	• Well-developed CIM survey with three subscales: Cohesiveness Communications Visual identity • Compelling statistics on the psychometric properties of the newly developed instrument
Third aim: To validate, interpret, and develop the findings of the CIM	• Part I: Interviews with 10 hotel managers, cognitive interviews about CIM scale • Part II: Mail survey to 110 managers to assess CIM scale, representativeness of their hotel, and overall evaluation of the measure	• Merged findings from interviews and surveys to finalize instrument	• Refined CIM survey deemed useful for identifying CIM activities needing attention Diagnosing CIM activity Monitoring/ assessing CIM programs/activities

Source: Simões, C., Dibb, S., & Fisk, R. P. (2005). Implementation matrix created by the *Mixed Methods Research Workbook* author.

CREATING A MIXED METHODS IMPLEMENTATION MATRIX

Having reviewed multiple rationales for an implementation matrix and examined several examples (Figures 11.1, 11.3, or 11.4), you can now focus on your creating an implementation matrix for your own project based on the two Workbox Illustrations 11.1.1 and 11.1.2.

Activity: Developing Your Implementation Matrix

The Implementation Matrix Template (Workbox 11.1.3) is generic and can be used for any mixed methods design. For the purpose of the Mixed Methods Workbook, the template has five headers. In structuring your own implementation matrix, you are not locked into the headers provided. You may opt to change them depending on your needs and rhetoric of your field. A final column called Comments has been added, as invariably questions come up, and this column provides the necessary space for recording for these thoughts. This can be used to record any concerns, questions, ideas, hesitations, etc. If you do not need all the rows, ignore them. Or if you have more than five aims, you can expand the number of rows. You have options of using the hard copy in the workbook or creating an electronic version on your computer.

Workbox 11.1.3: Creating Your Implementation Matrix

PHASES / AIMS / RESEARCH QUESTIONS	PROCEDURES	ANALYSIS	PRODUCTS	COMMENT
1				
2				
3				
4				
5				

If you have already conceptualized the details of your aims, procedures, analysis, and outcomes, you can populate all these areas straight away. This may work if you have already developed the narrative of your proposal and you seek to add an implementation matrix to facilitate ease of understanding of your procedures. If you are like many people however, you may be using your implementation matrix to help develop or expand your mixed methods design procedures. It will be particularly helpful if you have completed an MMR design figure from Chapters 7 and 8. With this information in hand, you can begin completing an Implementation Matrix Template. Workbox 11.2 provides a checklist for completing a Mixed Methods Implementation Matrix.

Workbox 11.2: Checklist for Completing a Mixed Methods Implementation Matrix

Check off the steps as you complete them as you develop an implementation matrix:

☐ Assemble the documents you have already created

☐ Add a title for your implementation matrix

☐ Insert your phases, specific aims, research questions, and/or hypotheses

(Continued)

(Continued)

☐   Complete the easiest components of the implementation matrix template

☐   Record any concerns in the comments header

☐   Populate the missing areas

☐   Clarify and update your choices

☐   Update the narrative

☐   Edit the implementation matrix to optimal size

☐   Edit for aesthetic appearance

STEPS FOR CREATING AN IMPLEMENTATION MATRIX

The following 10 steps will assist you in building an implementation matrix.

1. *Assemble the documents you have already created.* Find and have accessible all the related documents related to the study so that you will have these at your fingertips and will be able to efficiently fill in the table. If you have been using worksheets in the book, they will already be accessible. Put a sticky note on the relevant pages, and maybe jot a note about the content. If you have been creating electronic versions on your computer, know where they all are and that they are easy to open. If you plan to work on the paper version in the workbook, you may want to use a pencil or a pen with erasable ink.

2. *Add a title for your implementation matrix.* When creating a title, I advise putting the content topic first, and then adding afterwards that this illustration is an implementation matrix. Most consumers of your research will probably be most interested in your topic area. By having reference to the methods second, you show that the methods have a supportive role for examining the topic area. You may want to reference the title you created in Chapter 1 and refined in Chapter 5.

3. *Insert your phases, specific aims, research questions, and hypotheses.* You should now add in the Phases Column your study aims, questions, and hypotheses. You may be able to use or adapt the MMR questions/hypotheses you developed in Chapter 6.

4. *Complete the easiest components of the implementation matrix template.* You will find it most efficient to complete the information you already have committed to use. In workshops, I often find people have identified the methods that they want to use (e.g., interviews, surveys, document analysis, observations, secondary dataset). Add this information first. The more difficult information requires estimating how many of each type of data will be collected. A common mistake for researchers less familiar with qualitative methodology is to overestimate the number of participants.

5. *Record any concerns in the Comments header.* The Comments header is there to help remind you to clarify your choice of a particular point. For example, it could be about any difficulties, uncertainties, and feasibility questions. Maybe you record you have a certain colleague who you want to review a particular aim. You might need to do a power analysis to determine your sample size. You might want some colleagues' opinions about feasibility issues. Perhaps you want to check with the IRB about possible ethical complications. It is your space to use as needed, and it is *optional!*

6. *Populate the missing areas.* Gradually add in the more difficult cells or questions based on your further reading or consultation with others.

7. *Clarify and update your choices.* Iteratively add and update your choices. Check with others to determine if you have included sufficient detail for the reader of the implementation matrix to understand your qualitative, quantitative, and mixed methods integration procedures.

8. *Update the narrative.* If you are working on the narrative of a research proposal or paper, develop the habit of updating the implementation matrix first, and then update all related locations in the text. Keeping the implementation matrix as the repository for the most up-to-date thinking and text helps avoid conflicting information in the text.

9. *Edit to optimal size.* As you add more and more information to the implementation matrix, you may find that one section takes up an inordinate amount of space. For example, the procedures section may seem very long. You will find yourself editing and re-editing to shorten it. If using an electronic table in a word-processing program, you will want to resize the column width using the table function.

10. *Edit for aesthetic appearance.* As a final step, edit the implementation matrix to be aesthetically appealing. The matrix will receive a lot of interest, and by having it appeal to the eye, it is much easier to engage the reviewer. Do you have consistent capitalization and punctuation? Have you used bullets effectively? Are all sections within a single column similarly formatted? Busy reviewers will likely use the matrix to quickly grasp the overall picture of your study; hone in on areas they may be particularly interested in learning more about. For example, if you are conducting interviews, they may want to use the matrix to find for what point in the study you are using them, and then flip to that section. In this way, the matrix is somewhat like an expanded index.

ADDITIONAL ELEMENTS THAT CAN BE ADDED TO AN IMPLEMENTATION MATRIX

There are a number of variations that can be added to an implementation matrix. These may be more or less relevant, depending on your circumstances and are thus treated as optional. While you could envision adding all these columns, it does add further complexity. So, there must be a balance in weighing how many columns to actually add. There is probably space to add such discussion to one or two of these in the comments section, but all will become prohibitive. When a large number of columns are added, it may be necessary to switch the orientation from a vertical "portrait" to a horizontal "landscape" view. Additions discussed here are theory, point of integration, and validity threat.

Theory. A variation in the mixed methods implementation matrix is the addition of a second column titled Theory. This iteration was introduced by Justine Wu who is conducting a mixed methods grant, a career development award, on increasing access to contraception for women with disabilities (Wu et al., 2018). For each phase, she wanted to emphasize how the specific aim tied to reproductive justice theory. If you are working in an area where theory has specific relevance in different ways for each phase, this can be worthwhile. If the theory is more general, and the language would be repetitive, then the additional column and text may take up space unnecessarily.

Point of integration. Another iteration attributable to Wu is the addition of a final column titled Point of Integration (Wu et al., 2018). I like this header for settings or contexts that are focused on the methodology. Hence, in a mixed methods course where the focus is on learning and incorporating integration, this can be very helpful. For a lay publication or a grant review panel, the reviewers may be more interested in the research in service of the content under investigation. In such cases, the point of integration column may have less utility.

Validity threats. In presenting an implementation matrix about a project to an NIH project officer, Wu suggested adding a final column on validity threats (Wu et al., 2018). Study sections increasingly expect grant authors to present these threats in their proposals. As to whether to include your assessment in the matrix or in the narrative will be up to you. If you choose to add it, you should succinctly state the validity threat and justify your choice. I prefer not to highlight limitations in such attention-getting space, but it is a choice.

Application Activities

1. **Peer Feedback.** If working as part of a class or in a workshop, pair up with a peer mentor, and each of you spend about 5–10 minutes talking about your implementation matrix sheet. If available, also bring or refer to Chapter 5 to assess how your qualitative, quantitative, and mixed methods questions can be answered by implementing the procedures in your implementation matrix. In addition, bring or refer to your mixed methods design from Chapters 7 or 8. The presenter in each pair should switch roles. If there is time, have someone present a well-developed sequential and convergent implementation matrix to the class or workshop participants.

2. **Presenter Guidance.** You should *focus on the overall logic and flow of your study implementation plans.* After quickly reviewing your overall procedures with your partner, turn to the areas you were least comfortable with. Ask your partner to help identify resources for answering your question. As you talk about it, make a candid assessment to yourself as

to where you need to focus energy to improve your matrix and consult with others who can answer your questions. Consider how you might streamline your implementation matrix. Be respectful of time and save time to critique your partner's work!

3. **Feedback Guidance.** As you listen to your partner, hone your critiquing skills. Help your partner refine the implementation matrix. What gaps are there in the matrix? Are there clear data collection procedures, numbers of

participants, etc.? Has your partner articulated important outcomes? Are the outcomes achievable with the proposed methods and sample size? For any sequential components, does the subsequent aim/question meaningfully build on the previous aim/question?

4. **Group Debrief.** If you are in a classroom or large-group setting, take volunteers to present their implementation matrices. Reflect on the format consider revisions to your own implementation matrix.

Concluding Thoughts

Use this checklist to assess your progress in achieving the Chapter 11 objectives:

☐ I learned the purpose and value of an implementation matrix.

☐ I explored variations for constructing an implementation matrix and considered them as potential models for my own project.

☐ I developed an implementation matrix for my own project.

☐ I reviewed my Chapter 11 implementation matrix with a peer or colleague to refine my mixed methods procedures.

Now that you have completed these objectives, Chapter 12 will help you consider the ethical conduct of research with human subjects and to develop a research protocol for your MMR or evaluation project.

Key Resources

FURTHER READING ABOUT MATRICES, GRIDS, AND TABLES TO GUIDE MIXED METHODS RESEARCH AND EVALUATION PROJECTS

- Patton M. Q. (2015). *Qualitative research and evaluation methods* (4th ed.). Thousand Oaks, CA: Sage.

- Wisdom, J. P., & Fetters, M. D. (2015). Funding for mixed methods research: Sources and strategies. In S. Hesse-Biber & R. B. Johnson (eds.), *The Oxford handbook of multimethod and mixed methods research inquiry* (pp. 314–332). New York, NY: Oxford University Press.

12

ENSURING ETHICAL CONDUCT OF RESEARCH WITH HUMAN SUBJECTS AND DEVELOPING A MIXED METHODS RESEARCH PROTOCOL

This chapter addresses the unique challenges mixed methods researchers encounter in the ethical conduct of human subjects research that must be considered and submitted for approval by human subjects review committees. The regulatory requirements and complexities can feel overwhelming and tedious even if you are an experienced researcher. This chapter and its activities will help you review the importance of compliance with human subjects research regulations, understand the grounds for possible exemption, recognize unique ethical considerations that can arise in mixed methods projects, contrast the regulatory language of human subjects and participants, review elements of a research protocol, consider the applications of a research protocol, and create a tailored research protocol for submission in a human subjects research application. As a key outcome, you will complete a mixed methods protocol that can be used in a human subjects approval application.

LEARNING OBJECTIVES

This chapter aims to guide you how to navigate the human subjects review process and how to develop a research protocol so you will be able to

- Comply with human subjects research regulations

- Determine whether your mixed methods study is exempt from human subjects regulations

- Recognize unique ethical considerations that can arise relative to conduct of a mixed methods research (MMR) or evaluation project and how to address those issues in a protocol

- Compare the regulatory language of *human subjects* and *participants*, that is, language describing individuals who engage in mixed methods studies

- Review the elements that constitute an MMR or evaluation protocol

- Consider applications of a research protocol

- Recognize how elements of a research protocol may vary depending on your purpose

- Create a human subjects research application

WHY IS COMPLIANCE WITH HUMAN SUBJECTS RESEARCH REGULATIONS IMPORTANT?

All investigators involved in the conduct of research involving human subjects need to have an adequate understanding of the ethical principles of research and compliance requirements. Prior to establishment of these principles, a number of egregious violations of human subjects have been documented in both the medical and social sciences (McNeill, 1993; Rothman, 1991). Major national funding organizations of research such as the National Institutes of Health (NIH) in the United States (NIH, 2012), the National Science Foundation in the United States, the National Health Service through the Health Research Authority in England (National Health Service, 2017), and the Canadian Institutes of Health Research in Canada (Canadian Institutes of Health Research, 2015), all require investigators to be trained and certified to be adequately knowledgeable of ethical principles for the conduct of human subjects research. Moreover, most major international journals require confirmation that approval was obtained for research involving human subjects.

In most cases, key personnel, including the investigator and key support staff involved in any aspect of recruitment, enrollment and consent procedures, data collection, and analysis, will be required to demonstrate training in the ethical conduct of research. For example, my host institution has a series of online courses that provide training required by university, state, and federal regulations for the responsible conduct of research. Thousands of institutions worldwide rely on the Collaborative Institutional Training Initiative (CITI) to provide training in human subjects and ethical conduct. While not a requirement, the NIH Office of Extramural Research offers a free tutorial on the ethical conduct of research that can be used for education in the protection of human subjects, including a Spanish language version (NIH, 2016).

DOES THE STUDY QUALIFY AS EXEMPT FROM REGULATORY OVERSIGHT?

Many business, education, social science, and health sciences researchers engage in research that human subjects research committees exempt from oversight. For example, in the United States, the Office of Human Research Protections of the Department of Health and Human Services has a regulatory policy to guide researchers engaged in health and human services-related research. The criteria from the regulations that determine if a study is considered exempt are provided in Table 12.1. For example, the MPathic-VR study was deemed "exempt" at my host institution based on criterion (1) under the Office of Research Protections Policy. (Kron et al., 2017)

Importantly, even if you believe your research is exempted from regulations on the conduct of research with human subjects, you will most likely still need to submit your application to your institutional ethics review committee for approval as an exempt study. This will be particularly important if you wish to publish your study as official approval may be required by the publication venue. Criteria for what is considered regulated and what is exempt research will vary from country to country. You should identify in your own environment whether your research is regulated or not regulated and secure approval accordingly. Furthermore, you should understand what exempt research means at your institution as interpretations of requirements vary considerably.

TABLE 12.1 ■ **Criteria for Determining if Research Is Exempt From Regulation Under the U.S. Department of Health and Human Services, Office for Human Research Protections Policy for Protection of Human Research Subjects (2009)**

(1) Research conducted in established or commonly accepted educational settings, involving normal educational practices, such as (i) research on regular and special education instructional strategies, or (ii) research on the effectiveness of or the comparison among instructional techniques, curricula, or classroom management methods

(2) Research involving the use of educational tests (cognitive, diagnostic, aptitude, achievement), survey procedures, interview procedures, or observation of public behavior, unless:

(i) information obtained is recorded in such a manner that human subjects can be identified, directly or through identifiers linked to the subjects; and (ii) any disclosure of the human subjects' responses outside the research could reasonably place the subjects at risk of criminal or civil liability or be damaging to the subjects' financial standing, employability, or reputation.

(3) Research involving the use of educational tests (cognitive, diagnostic, aptitude, achievement), survey procedures, interview procedures, or observation of public behavior that is not exempt under paragraph (b)(2) of this section, if

  (i) the human subjects are elected or appointed public officials or candidates for public office; or (ii) federal statute(s) require(s) without exception that the confidentiality of the personally identifiable information will be maintained throughout the research and thereafter.

(4) Research involving the collection or study of existing data, documents, records, pathological specimens, or diagnostic specimens, if these sources are publicly available, or if the information is recorded by the investigator in such a manner that subjects cannot be identified, directly or through identifiers linked to the subjects.

(5) Research and demonstration projects conducted by or subject to the approval of department or agency heads, and designed to study, evaluate, or otherwise examine:

  (i) Public benefit or service programs

  (ii) Procedures for obtaining benefits or services under those programs

  (iii) Possible changes in or alternatives to those programs or procedures

  (iv) Possible changes in methods or levels of payment for benefits or services under those programs

(6) Taste and food quality evaluation and consumer acceptance studies, (i) if wholesome foods without additives are consumed or (ii) if a food is consumed that contains a food ingredient at or below the level and for the use found to be safe, or agricultural chemical or environmental contaminant at or below the level found to be safe, by the Food and Drug Administration or approved by the Environmental Protection Agency or the Food Safety and Inspection Service of the U.S. Department of Agriculture.

WHY DOES HUMAN SUBJECTS PROTECTION IN MIXED METHODS RESEARCH MATTER?

The Office of Behavioral and Social Sciences Research (OBSSR) at the NIH in the United States was established in 1993 in response to the evolving understanding in the 1980s that health outcomes are influenced by behavioral, social, and biological factors (NIH Office of Behavioral and Social Sciences Research, n.d.). As illustrated in the Office of Behavioral and Social Science Mixed Methods Research Best Practices documents, the first (Creswell, Klassen, Plano Clark, & Smith, 2011) and second editions (NIH Office of Social and Behavioral Research, 2018), identify unique issues that arise in the conduct of MMR conducted directly with human subjects. First, mixed methods researchers need to be aware of the ethical issues that may arise through the conduct of both qualitative and quantitative research procedures. For example, in quantitative research studies, investigators may manipulate conditions, and in qualitative research studies, the collection of detailed personal information through stories, observations, and audio/visual recordings could be used to identify the subject. How you protect subjects as a researcher is a key issue (Creswell et al., 2011; NIH Office of Social and Behavioral Research, 2018).

Before embarking on MMR study, the investigator should fully consider whether the additional burden on subjects from mixed methods data collection justifies the added value that conducting a mixed methods project will produce. In other words, is the benefit of collecting both types of data, and the associated burden on the subject, justified relative to the incremental burden encompassed by a mixed methods study? Second, when conducting advocacy and participatory studies such as a transformative design, the investigator needs to carefully choose community members who can represent the targeted population. Following below is a discussion of potential risks and benefits to subjects participating in MMR investigations. While no claim is made relative to the comprehensiveness of the list, the discussion is focused on the particulars of engagement in MMR studies.

WHAT ARE POTENTIAL RISKS TO HUMAN SUBJECTS RAISED BY PARTICIPATION IN A MIXED METHODS RESEARCH STUDY?

Relatively little has been written about ethical considerations specific to MMR. Here, I review and add to ideas raised in Mixed Methods Research Best Practices Guidelines from the Office of Behavioral and Social

Sciences Research (Creswell et al., 2011; NIH Office of Social and Behavioral Research, 2018). First, relative to the issue of informed consent, a subject participating in both qualitative and quantitative data collection will need to understand more complex procedures than if just one form of data collection is used. This may render obtaining a subject's informed consent more complicated, challenging, and burdensome. Second, subjects who are requested to provide information during both qualitative and quantitative data collection procedures may have a greater burden than if only one data collection procedure was used. Third, MMR may require the collection of identifying information that may not have been collected otherwise. For example, when using a survey to collect quantitative data, there may not be a need to collect personal information, while in a mixed methods study, such as one using an explanatory sequential mixed methods design, the researcher may need to collect identifying information to follow up with subjects during the qualitative phase. Fourth, mixed methods researchers who want to have follow-up contact with subjects will require more time from subjects than if they had not participated in the mixed methods study. Fifth, mixed methods researchers who are engaged in a participatory or transformative mixed methods study need to consider the risks to individuals who advocate on behalf of others.

DISCUSSION OF THE LANGUAGE OF HUMAN SUBJECTS VERSUS HUMAN PARTICIPANTS

The term *human subjects* has become the regulatory language of research. Many **institutional ethics review boards** refer to participants in research as human subjects. If required, you will of course need to use such language. As possible, I avoid this language, which has an unnecessarily negative connotation of a human being as an "object" of research. For example, as a verb, *subject* means to "cause or force to undergo." With the era of informed consent, and other safeguards, I believe the term *participant* is preferable as it captures the nuance of voluntary for the subject. However, in many historical discussions about the ethical treatment of humans in research, humans were indeed "subjects" and not "participants." Further debate about this rhetoric extends beyond the purpose of this chapter. In the interest of consistency with the regulatory language, in this chapter, I have predominantly used the term *human subjects*. Suffice it to say, you may find or be required to use the terms *human subjects* or *participants* in your own institution.

Activity: Identifying Potential Risks to Subjects in Mixed Methods Research

Workbox Illustration 12.1.1 provides an example of potential risks identified in the application for the MPathic-VR Mixed Methods Virtual Human Communications Education Trial. You can use this as a reference for on your own protocol if you are uncertain how or what to write about your own mixed methods project in Workbox 12.1.2.

Workbox Illustration 12.1.1: Potential Risks of Being a Subject in the MPathic-VR Mixed Methods Medical Education Study

Minimal risk is expected. Breach of confidentiality is possible, though very unlikely, and in the unlikely event it occurred, potential harm seems minimal. The potential risks arising from use of the educational system are no more significant than for students participating in normal educational practices.

Sources: Kron et al. (2017) and Fetters, M.D. and Kron, F.W. (2012–15). Modeling Professional Attitudes and Teaching Humanistic Communication in Virtual Reality (MPathic-VRII). National Center for Advancing Translational Science/NIH 9R44TR000360-04.

Based on your current proposal, write the potential risks to subjects who would participate in your mixed methods project in Workbox 12.1.2 You should consider each of the potential factors listed above, but remember there may be additional potential risks that fall outside of those listed.

Workbox 12.1.2: Potential Risks of Being a Human Subject in Your Mixed Methods Research Project

WHAT ARE POTENTIAL BENEFITS OF PARTICIPATION IN A MIXED METHODS RESEARCH STUDY?

The potential benefits of being in an MMR study that are unique to MMR are more limited, and perhaps more nuanced, than the potential risks. First, there may be a more substantive benefit to subjects who provide both qualitative and quantitative information for a study. Study subjects who choose to participate in a mixed methods study may find it personally meaningful to be able to share more comprehensively their own situation or story. Providing both qualitative and quantitative information may provide a greater level of satisfaction for such subjects. Second, if a subject engages in a participatory or transformative mixed methods study, the subject may find it rewarding to represent a community of interest and bring a voice to those without a voice in the context of an advocacy-focused MMR design (e.g., transformative, community-based participatory, or action research).

Activity: Identifying Potential Benefits Unique to Human Subjects Participating in Mixed Methods Research

Workbox Illustration 12.2.1 provides an example of potential benefits identified in the application for the MPathic-VR Mixed Methods Virtual Human Communications Education Trial. You can reference this example as your work on your own protocol in Workbox 12.2.2.

Workbox Illustration 12.2.1: Potential Benefits of Being a Subject in the MPathic-VR Mixed Methods Medical Education Study

Subjects will learn information that can be expected to be useful to them during their medical training. Many subjects find the opportunity to provide an opinion during research studies and helping advance science to be rewarding.

Sources: Kron et al. (2017) and Fetters, M.D. and Kron, F.W. (2012–15). Modeling Professional Attitudes and Teaching Humanistic Communication in Virtual Reality (MPathic-VRII). National Center for Advancing Translational Science/NIH 9R44TR000360-04.

Based on your current proposal, write the potential benefits to subjects who would participate in your mixed methods project in Workbox 12.2.2. You should consider each of the potential factors listed above, but remember there may be additional potential benefits that fall outside of those listed.

Workbox 12.2.2: Potential Benefits of Being a Subject in Your Mixed Methods Study

Identifying Ethical Issues Raised by Your Mixed Methods Research Study

A final issue, also raised in the Best Practices Reports (Creswell et al., 2011; NIH Office of Social and Behavioral Research, 2018) considers the need to educate human subjects review boards about the features and qualities of MMR. While MMR has seen exponential growth in use, it may be less familiar to human subjects review committee members. First, it can be helpful to add some general language in your human subjects research application that your study is a mixed methods study and that a mixed methods involves the collection, analysis, and integration of qualitative and quantitative data.

In creating an application for human subjects research approval, the applicant will be wise to minimize jargon and define any mixed methods – specific language. For example, when indicating that the project will involve an exploratory sequential mixed methods design, it is easy to explain that information initially collected qualitatively will be linked to the development of subsequent data collection through a survey. This approach helps a reviewer unfamiliar with MMR to eliminate the need to look up information about MMR (and possibly delay your approval). It also provides succinct education about mixed methods procedures.

Articulating potential ethical issues unique to a mixed methods study, including those presented in this chapter and any others you may identify, and specifically the procedures you're taking to minimize risks and burdens on subjects will help mitigate follow-up questions from your human subjects committee. This may help educate committee members unfamiliar with MMR as well. For example, consider the extra burden on a participant in a convergent mixed methods study that involves multiple questionnaires, interviews, and observations. Multiple data collection procedures can be a burden to potential subjects. Thus, an investigator might note that compensation will be increased concomitant to the burden and that data collection will be spread out to avoid fatiguing the subjects. Alternatively, if conducting a participatory project, for example, a community-based participatory research project, or transformative project, you may want to emphasize the benefits to participants of being in your mixed methods project for giving them a voice in a process of policy change and advocacy.

WHAT IS A MIXED METHODS RESEARCH PROTOCOL?

For the purposes of this MMR workbook, an MMR protocol is a document in a table format that contains all the essential components necessary for conducting an MMR study (e.g., the background, rationale, goals and objectives, design, methodology, statistical and text/media analysis, and implementation). There are many different ways that a **research protocol** can be defined and designed, and some organizations, host academic institutions, or funding agencies may even specify elements to be included. Despite the variations, there remains considerable overlap in suggested content. For example, the World Health Organization lists a relatively limited number of sections as illustrated in Table 12.1 and has more of a clinical focus than social sciences focus (World Health

Organization, n.d.). You may work in an institution that does not have a specific research protocol format, and you are free to develop one according to your own needs. Over time, you may even develop your own list of key elements to include based on the specific type of MMR you conduct. If you are conducting a thesis or dissertation, I strongly suggest checking with your institution and program for requirements. You might also seek consultation from your advisor or chair.

Table 12.1: Research Protocol Components Recommended by the World Health Organization

Part I

- Project summary (300 words or less)
- General information
  - Protocol title, protocol identifying number, and date
  - Name and address of sponsor/funder
  - Name, title, and contact information of investigators
  - Name and contact information of technical/laboratories involved
- Rationale and background information
- References
- Study design
- Methodology
- Safety considerations
- Follow-up
- Quality assurance
- Expected outcomes of study
- Dissemination of results and publication policy
- Duration of the project
- Problems anticipated
- Project management
- Ethics
- Informed consent forms

Part 2

- Budget
- Other support for the project
- Collaboration with other scientists or research institutions
- Links to other projects
- Curriculum vitae of investigators
- Other research activities of the investigators
- Financing and insurance

WHY HAVE A MIXED METHODS RESEARCH PROTOCOL?

An MMR protocol can be helpful in several ways. First, a research protocol has a series of key elements that should be addressed in your research, and the process of completing the research protocol may help you consider and plan for implementation. Second, a research protocol, somewhat like an implementation matrix (Chapter 11), can help ensure all mixed methods team members fully understand and agree with the proposed mixed methods project implementation procedures. Third, a research protocol can be used, and may be required, for communicating with funding agencies, collaborators, mentors, and institutional representatives. Fourth, you can use a research protocol to bring together all of the decisions and documents that you will need in preparation for your human subjects approval application. See Story From the Field 12.1 regarding the early "preprotocol" years of my research career, when I was still unfamiliar with the utility of a research protocol. Fifth, a research protocol can be helpful when you are preparing for data collection to ensure that all aspects of the project are ready for deployment.

STORY FROM THE FIELD 12.1
THE IMPORTANCE OF A RESEARCH PROTOCOL

When I first embarked on my own research projects back in the day of paper submissions, I started my first human subjects application. There were pages of instructions, and I started from the beginning and went to the end. I spent a lot of time combing through the project materials, and coming up with answers and resources that were not included in my application, such as the informed consent document, recruitment flyer, etc. The whole process was very inefficient, as I would make two steps forward in filling out the application, then take one step back as I needed to clarify issues relevant to the requirements of the submission or actually create documents for the submission. While human subjects applications are now mostly online, the need for optimally organizing the materials needed for the submission in advance has not gone away. This experience prompted me to begin projects and advise mentees submitting projects for the first time to develop their research protocol first. I am certain I have saved numerous mentees precious time!

Activity: Writing a Mixed Methods Research Protocol

Workbox Illustration 12.3.1 provides an example of how the research protocol was used from the MPathic-VR mixed methods medical education study (Kron et al., 2017). You can use this as a reference as you work on your own protocol if you are uncertain about what to write. In Workbox 12.3.2, you may choose to write directly in the workbook as a first draft, or you can create the research protocol using a word-processing program. Note that this research protocol template was developed to be comprehensive and is based on multiple experiences submitting to institutional review boards for approval. The order is not strict. The format is designed to be helpful to you and the institutional ethics committee that reviews your proposal.

Workbox Illustration 12.3.1: Mixed Methods Research Protocol MPathic-VR Mixed Methods Medical Education Study

Project title	Modeling Professional Attitudes and Teaching Humanistic Communication in VR (MPathic-VR) PHASE II
Date	2012_8_20
Funding source	National Center for Advancing Translational Sciences (NCATS)
Project numbers	NCATS: Project ID 2 R44 CA141987-02A1 UM IRB: HUM00067336
Project period	09/01/2012-06/31/2015

Summary/abstract	The investigators previously developed and tested an MPathic-VR prototype using an educational system with virtual humans to teach communication skills. In Phase II, the investigators will enhance the educational breadth and technical sophistication of the system. The team will rigorously evaluate the effectiveness of the program in a single-blinded mixed methods randomized controlled trial at Eastern Virginia Medical School (EVMS), the University of Michigan (UM) Medical School, and the University of Virginia (UVa) Medical School.
Project members	Co-principal Investigator: Dr. Frederick Kron, fkron@email.edu[b] Co-principal Investigator: Dr. Michael Fetters, mfetters@email.edu[b]
Philosophical stance	Pragmatism
Overarching objectives	To examine whether MPathic-VR Virtual Human Communications Education System is effective for teaching advanced communication skills, and if so, why.
Specific aims/ questions/hypotheses	The investigators will test these hypotheses: (1) students randomized to learn with MPathic-VR will improve their communication performance after engaging in a communication scenario, receiving feedback on their performance, and applying the feedback in a second run-through; and (2) knowledge acquired through MPathic-VR will be resilient (i.e., students will incorporate learned materials into their manner of communication) and the performance of MPathic-VR-trained students assessed in a subsequent advanced communication objective structured clinical exam (OSCE) will be scored higher than students trained with a conventional computer-based learning (CBL). The investigators will ask the mixed methods research question, how do qualitative findings from students' reflective comments and quantitative responses to an attitudinal survey compare for the MPathic-VR and the CBL experiences?
Background	Medical educators face great difficulty teaching verbal and nonverbal communication skills. While standardized patient instructors (SPIs) have also been used to evaluate these competencies, they are time-consuming, costly, and perform inconsistently over multiple encounters. A novel approach that is effective, and an understanding as to why, is needed to improve the education of medical students in communication skills.
Design/methodology	Demonstrate the effectiveness of the MPathic-VR communications education program in a single-blinded, mixed methods, randomized controlled trial at three medical schools. Framed by an ethnographic approach, investigators will research students' experiences when taking the modules.
Setting	EVMS, UM, and UVa Medical Schools
Population	The entire medical school classes for the targeted 2nd-year medical students in the 2014–2015 year at EVMS, UM, and UVa.
Sampling	All students who participate from the three medical schools will represent the population for both the quantitative and qualitative data collection.
Recruitment	An announcement in advance of training will be made to medical students.
Intervention	Exposure to the MPathic-VR module versus a state-of-the-art CBL module.
QUAN data collection procedures	(1) Scoring on the modules from first and second time on each of two scenarios, (2) postintervention attitudinal survey about clarity, purpose, utility, and likelihood to recommend the experience, (3) scores on a posttrial OSCE to score performance in a realistic scenario
QUAL data collection procedures	Qualitative reflective essays collected postintervention from all students in the intervention and control groups
Project forms/ instruments	**Quantitative:** (1) Scoring rubric of the MPathic-VR system, (2) 12-item attitudinal survey with 7-point Likert-type scale choices, and (3) OSCE assessment with four domains: openness/defensiveness, collaborative/competitive, nonverbal communication, and presence. **Qualitative:** Reflective essay about how the module could be improved, three most important things learned, how interacting with the system influences views about patient-family-health professional interactions, and how interacting with the system influences thinking about nonverbal communication. **Other:** Notification of training procedures, instructions for taking the modules. **Informed Consent:** Not applicable, exempt.
Number of subjects	Approximately 480 second-year medical students eligible across the three sites

(Continued)

(Continued)

Inclusion criteria	Male or female, minimum age of 18, who has been apprised about use of student data through school's research in medical education process
Exclusion criteria	(1) Subject drops out of the medical school; (2) subject opts out; and (3) EVMS, UM, or UVa faculty request for a student to not participate.
Compensation	None
Expected benefits to society	Data from the study will help with the design of an educational system that utilizes virtual humans and virtual patients to teach medical students communication skills, professionalism, and patient-centered skills, for patients and families facing a diagnosis of cancer. The point of creating the MPathic-VR educational system is to improve current medical school curriculum in these areas. Knowing whether the MPathic-VR educational system works will benefit medical educators who want to use the program to improve student communication behavior.
Risks to public/ community	None
Informed consent type	Exempt: The lead investigator at each site obtained approval with exemption status from the respective Institutional Review Board.
Foreseeable benefits to subjects	From the activity, subjects will learn information that can be expected to be useful during their medical training. Many subjects find the opportunity to provide an opinion during research studies and help develop an educational tool rewarding.
Foreseeable risks to subjects	Minimal risk: Breach of confidentiality is possible, though very unlikely and in the unlikely event it occurred, potential harm seems minimal. The potential risks arising from use of the educational system are no more significant than for students participating in normal educational practices.
Why risk/benefit ratio is favorable?	Students should learn valuable information from both the MPathic-VR intervention and CBL control with minimal or no risk of harm.
Communicate results back to subjects	Deferred
Data analysis procedures	Quantitative: Descriptive statistics will be calculated for all demographic items. For the first hypothesis regarding improvement during the MPathic-VR simulation, we will compare scores for each run-through of the intercultural and inter professional scenarios with a repeated measures analysis of variance (ANOVA) to assess learning derived from the additional practice with the system. For the second hypothesis comparing the MPathic-VR arm, and the control arm, we will conduct both a multivariate analysis of variance (MANOVA) and univariate ANOVAs on the four OSCE rating scale domains with module (intervention or control) as the independent variable. For the last hypothesis regarding student attitudes toward MPathic-VR and CBL learning, we will compare the mean scores for each module aggregated across rating items with an independent t-test. All analyses will be evaluated with an alpha level of 0.05, unless stated otherwise.
	Qualitative: All qualitative data will be entered into a single file. MAXQDA software will facilitate the analysis. Two investigators will read through the text files and develop codes. The analytic approach will reduce the data into overarching themes. After reading through the entire qualitative database, segments of text will be identified and assigned a code, based on an emerging coding scheme. This will lead to an initial codebook. Analysts will review and discuss each code to calibrate coding and achieve intercoder agreement, and then refine and clarify the codes. After coding all text, they will organize related codes into the primary themes. As a validation strategy, a third researcher will review the coded data. The analytics will focus on students' experiences, while they were taking the MPathic-VR and the CBL modules.
	Mixed methods: After completing the qualitative and quantitative analyses, the qualitative findings from learners' reflections on their experiences will be linked with the quantitative results of the attitudinal scale. The purpose is to compare the two sources of data to gain a more complete understanding of learners' experiences. The analysis and interpretation will be represented in a visual joint display.
What will happen to data after study ends?	Qualitative and quantitative: When the primary and secondary analyses are complete, the data will be destroyed.

Expected outcomes	1. We anticipate students exposed to the MPathic-VR virtual human communications teaching modules will improve between the first run-through and the second run-through.
	2. We expect that students using the MPathic-VR (the intervention cohort) will score higher on the communication skills OSCE than the control and provide compelling evidence that MPathic-VR provides added value to educational approaches designed to help students learn critical communication skills.
	3. We expect that students will find the interactivity of the MPathic-VR module as an advantage over a standard computer-based learning module.
	4. Cumulatively, we anticipate a mixed methods trial will provide support for using virtual humans for teaching medical students doctor–patient, and through further research, doctor–family and doctor–nurse communication skills.
Implications	The study will provide evidence supporting the use of virtual human simulation for training communication skills. It is anticipated the study findings will demonstrate both improved communication performance with MPathic-VR training and successful transfer of communication skills acquired from MPathic-VR to a different, clinically realistic communication scenario. Mixed methods evaluation of students' training experience will favor MPathic-VR over traditional CBL due to the interactive approach. These will offer educators an effective and engaging means of training advanced communication skills.

[a] This is a truncated version of the original protocol used to illustrate the features of an MMR protocol from the MPathic-VR medical education trial (Kron et al., 2017).

[b] Alias email addresses used for illustrative purposes only.

Sources: Kron et al. (2017) and Fetters, M.D. and Kron, F.W. *Modeling Professional Attitudes and Teaching Humanistic Communication in Virtual Reality (MPathic-VRII)*.National Center for Advancing Translational Science/NIH 9R44TR000360-04.

As seen based on the length of the protocol, there are many issues to consider when preparing to submit your application for human subjects approval and implement your research. While the list seems daunting, most sections are self-explanatory and do not require long answers. Rather, your goal is to be succinct, yet thorough and complete. If you have this document created prior to starting your Institutional Review Board (IRB) application, you will be able to efficiently complete the process. There may be some categories that seem irrelevant to your situation or institution. These you can skip or leave out.

You may also find that the ordering in this template of qualitative, quantitative, and mixed methods (where relevant), as listed under project forms/instruments, number of subjects, inclusion criteria, exclusion criteria, incentive, foreseeable risks, data analysis procedures, and management of primary data after completion of the study, will not necessarily make sense for your study. For example, if you are conducting an explanatory sequential mixed methods design collecting quantitative data first, and qualitative data second, you may want to change the order to reflect your design and circumstances. As a rule, it makes most sense to list in the same chronological order as the data are collected. You may also find that your colleagues/institution/funding agency have additional requirements, which you should add. The explanations below will help guide you for any sections that seem unclear.

Workbox 12.3.2: Writing Your Mixed Methods Research Protocol*

Project title	
Date	
Funding source	
Project number	
Project period	
Summary/abstract	

(Continued)

(Continued)

Project members	
Philosophical stance	
Overarching objective(s)	
Specific aims/questions/hypotheses	
Background	
Design/methodology	
Setting(s)	
Population	
Sampling	Qualitative: Quantitative:
Recruitment	
Intervention	
QUAL data collection procedures	
QUAN data collection procedures	
Project forms/instruments	Qualitative: Quantitative: Informed Consent:
Number of subjects	Qualitative: Quantitative:
Inclusion criteria	Qualitative: Quantitative:
Exclusion criteria	Qualitative: Quantitative:
Compensation	Qualitative: Quantitative:
Expected benefits to society	
Risk to public/community	
Informed consent type	
Foreseeable benefits to subject	
Foreseeable risks to subject	Qualitative: Quantitative:
Why risk/benefit ratio is favorable?	
Communicate results back to subjects	
Data analysis procedures	Qualitative: Quantitative: Mixed Methods:
What will happen to the data after study ends?	Qualitative: Quantitative:
Expected outcomes	
Implications	

*Add or delete items as needed to personalize as your own template.

HOW TO FILL IN THE RESEARCH PROTOCOL?

The format in the blank research protocol in Workbox Illustration 12.3.1 varies slightly from the example in Workbox 12.3.2. This is intentional, as the purpose is to illustrate how the protocol can vary, and why, as will be explained below.

Project Title. Populate this section with the title of your project. If your title is long, you may want to consider also creating a shorter title that can be used on running headers in documents.

Date. Insert the date. Many researchers like using a format of YYYY_MM_DD in all research documents, especially in titles of saved documents. In contrast to spelled out dates, or alternative wording, this format always lists your documents in chronological order.

Funding Source. List the name and address of the funding agency. If you have more than one source, you can add both, and if you have no source, you can either state "none" or delete the line.

Project Number. You can list a number assigned by a funding agency, or specific IRB number, or both. As there were two project numbers associated with the MPathic-VR Mixed Methods Virtual Human Communications Education Trial, both the grant number and IRB number are listed.

Project Period. Insert the dates of the project. Ideally, you will be consistent in your presentation of dates (see note under "Date" above).

Summary/Abstract. In approximately 250 words or less, provide the study abstract. While you may be tempted to have a longer abstract, keeping it short is better, particularly because many online sources, where you might want to use the abstract in the future, have word count or space limits. If you can convey the main points in less than 250 words, that is acceptable.

Project Members. List your project members. Ideally, you will include at least their email contact information. You will find in the future that it is very helpful to have this information in an accessible place.

Philosophical Stance. For many researchers in the health sciences, this section may be considered optional, although in the social sciences, this information is often considered paramount. Would you believe that medical researchers and social scientists have a different culture (see Chapter 6)? if you are not certain what to write here and feel the quantitative and qualitative strands of your project follow different philosophical frameworks, you can list both.

Overarching Objective. Insert your primary objective that you hope to accomplish through your mixed methods study. Rigorous mixed methods studies will, at minimum, allude to the qualitative and the quantitative contributions that will be made by the research. You will note in the Workbox 12.3.2 objective that the word *effectiveness* refers to the trial's quantitative assessment, and the *why* suggests a component of qualitative assessment.

Specific Aims/Questions/Hypotheses. Record you MMR study aims, questions, and/or hypotheses. As illustrated in Chapter 2, you may use aims or hypotheses for your quantitative strand, research questions for the qualitative strand, and a mixed methods aim that foreshadows the kind of **metainferences** you anticipate being able to make when the study is complete. In the MPathic-VR Mixed Methods Virtual Human Communications Education Trial, we used hypotheses and an MMR question.

Background. Compose three to five sentences that reflect the main reasons the study is important. Depending on the length of what you have written in your background section in Chapter 4, you may be able to use that text here. This section in your research protocol should include at least one sentence about how your topic is important from a sociological or public health perspective and then language about why qualitative and quantitative data collection are indicated.

Design/Methodology. Describe the specific MMR design you will use. You may refer back to Chapter 7 for your core design or Chapter 8 for the design proposed in your project. Remember many others will not necessarily have the level of expertise that you have acquired relative to design names, so this is a good place to be certain to explain what you are doing by describing the methodology you plan to use, preferably in lay terms. Generally speaking, it is not necessary to duplicate many of the elements that are also part of the methodology (e.g., setting, population) that follow, but it is not wrong to include them here. It just creates unnecessary redundancy.

Setting(s). Describe the specific setting or settings where your project will take place. With a mixed methods study, it is possible that the setting will be the same for both strands or different for the two strands. If the setting is the same, you do not need to list qualitative and quantitative separately. As in Workbox Illustration 12.3.1, the setting did not change for the qualitative and quantitative data collection.

Population. Like the setting, the population for the qualitative and quantitative might be the same target population, or it may not be the same.

Sampling. The sampling framework may approximately align with the target population if everyone will be recruited to join. More often than not, researchers do not have the same targeted population as the sample. Particularly, in mixed methods projects, the sample for qualitative data collection and quantitative data collection will differ. Commonly, the qualitative sample will be smaller than the quantitative sample. In your protocol, you should explicitly state who will serve as your qualitative sample and who will serve as your quantitative sample. You may want to consult your notes from Chapter 9 about sampling and sampling relationship to complete this section.

Recruitment. Describe how you will recruit subjects into your study. You will need to explicate your procedures for both the qualitative and quantitative strands.

Intervention. If you are conducting a study with an intervention, here is where you will want to provide information about what kind of intervention you will be conducting.

QUAL data collection procedures. Record how you will collect your qualitative data, e.g., type of interview, observations, document reviews, etc. You may want to refer back to Chapter 5 on data sources if you need a reminder. As illustrated in Workbox 12.3.2, the order with QUAN data collection procedures was switched in the protocol, as the QUAN data collection occurred first.

QUAN data collection procedures. Record how you will collect your quantitative data (e.g., survey structured interview, structured observations, document reviews). If you are using numbers from an existing dataset, you may want to describe the procedures for procuring the dataset and cleaning it for your own research purposes. Refer back to Chapter 5 on data sources if you need a reminder. As illustrated in Workbox 12.3.2, the order with QUAL data collection procedures was switched to second in the protocol, as the QUAL data collection occurred after QUAN data collection.

Project Forms/Instruments. While this seems simple, a deceivingly large amount of effort is needed to complete this section, especially if you include the materials as part of your application. This is one of the most useful sections of the research protocol. It will be the first time you have considered comprehensively all documents you need to proceed with your study. To be comprehensive, think about the documents you will need in the order you will collect the data. Hence, this will include recruitment flyers, recruitment text (if doing a phone or online survey), radio announcements, or any other text that will be used during recruitment. If you need a protocol for collecting field observations, consider the 3Cs approach and template (Fetters and Rubinstein, forthcoming). Next, consider what specific documents will be needed for the recruitment and enrollment. Usually, this starts with the informed consent script and forms. It may also include a summary sheet you will provide to subjects. The next steps will be the data collection, so you will list your data collection instruments, including your surveys, interview guides, and observation protocols. I recommend all projects develop a field notes protocol for submission with their projects, to be certain that any study events that can affect the study can be recorded. If you are conducting audiovisual data collection (e.g., video recording interactions or behaviors), you will need to describe this as well. Ultimately, you may have a very large number of documents. In Workbox 12.3.2, a subcategory of other has been added for additional necessary documents.

Number of Subjects. You will need to project the number of subjects that you will recruit for both your qualitative and quantitative data collection. This requirement often annoys researchers who have primarily worked in a qualitative tradition, as they will tell you they cannot know in advance, as they will continue data collection until reaching the point of saturation, that is, the point when no substantively new information is generated about the phenomenon of one's qualitative inquiry. Despite the qualitative tradition and qualitative researchers' frustration, IRBs require a number. I advise listing the maximum number of subjects that you anticipate enrolling for the qualitative strand. IRBs may become alarmed if you recruit *more* subjects than you anticipated. The reason is that many proposals coming to a medical IRB are trials, and the IRB has a duty to ensure that not too many individuals are enrolled to meet the purposes of the trial. Hence, from a compliance perspective, it is easiest if you overestimate the number of subjects you plan to enroll in the qualitative strand.

Inclusion Criteria. For both the qualitative and quantitative strands of your study, you should list the criteria for including subjects in your research. As noted in Workbox 12.3.2, these were the same for the qualitative and quantitative data collection in the example, and subcategorization of the two parts was not needed. Your inclusion criteria section should reflect your design and any differences between the two strands.

Exclusion Criteria. For both the qualitative and quantitative strands of your study, you should record the criteria of excluding subjects from participation in your research. Note that you do not need to list as an exclusion criterion "a subject who does not meet inclusion criteria." As noted in Workbox 12.3.2, these were the same for the qualitative and quantitative data collection in the example. Hence, subcategorization of the two parts was not needed.

Compensation. Record the amount of the payment or remuneration, if any, that will be offered to your subjects. If conducting a convergent design with identical sampling for the qualitative and quantitative data collection, you may not need to list separately. Compensation may only occur for one strand of the mixed methods study (e.g., the qualitative strand), because collection of qualitative data does require a longer period of time for participation.

Expected Benefits to Society. Please write what potential benefit your study is likely to be delivered to society. This could include benefits such as developing a technology to improve a current practice, demonstrating the effectiveness of an intervention, or gaining knowledge that will drive a field forward.

Risks to the Public or Community. Like the previous item, this may require some thought. Researchers engaged in marginalized communities, with specific findings about serious social problems (e.g., drug or alcohol use, sexual behaviors) could result in stigmatization. The comprehensive nature of mixed methods inquiry might mistakenly produce a result that further marginalizes and stigmatizes a population.

Foreseeable Risks to the Subject. Will you engage subjects or record their information in any way that could put them at risk? For example, would participation by someone engaged in a risky behavior (e.g., illegal drug use) be at risk for being recognized based on specific qualitative information collected, voice, photo, stories disclosed?

Similarly, if there is too much detail collected quantitatively, especially in a smaller sample (e.g., with a convergent design), then this could also be identifying information.

Why Is Risk-to-Benefit Ratio Favorable? This section requires a candid assessment on the part of the investigator, as to whether there is a favorable risk-to-benefit ratio, and can include perspectives of society and individuals. The compelling nature of mixed methods data collection can arguably help provide a comprehensive and robust assessment of a researched topic.

Communicate Results Back to Subjects. If you have plans to communicate study findings back to subjects, then you should describe those procedures. For example, you might intend to send a summary of the mixed data findings individually through a letter or phone call. It might also be possible you would communicate the findings back through a public forum.

Data Analysis Procedures. Record what specific analytical procedures will be followed for the qualitative, quantitative, and mixed methods components of the study. For the mixed methods analysis, you may want to reference your activities from Chapters 13, 14, and 15, that address mixed methods analysis procedures. As shown in Workbox 12.3.2, the order of quantitative, qualitative, and mixed methods is consistent with the chronology of data collection and analysis in the study.

What Will Happen to the Data After Completion of the Study? Once study data have been collected, you will need to describe whether there are plans to destroy the original data source, especially any materials that have identifying information. This tends to be particularly risky with qualitative data. With the quantitative data, this may only involve discarding survey instruments (shredding, use of service, etc.) after data have been entered into study software.

Expected Outcomes. Record the information that is likely to be obtained upon completion of the study.

Implications. Record what the implications of the study findings are likely to be. For example, how do you anticipate your mixed methods study would significantly alter or enhance current approaches and procedures?

Application Activities

1. **Peer Feedback.** If working on your research protocol as part of a class or in a workshop, pair up with a peer mentor, and one of you spend about 5 minutes talking about your topic. Take turns talking about your protocol and giving feedback. The helpful parts to discuss are those that you struggled with the most. In particular, focus on the mixed methods components of your protocol, as these areas are often most challenging and the elements that a partner in a mixed methods course will likely have the greatest interest. If you are working independently, share your protocol with a colleague or mentor.

2. **Peer Feedback Guidance.** As you listen to your partner, focus on learning and honing the valuable skills of critiquing. Your goal is to help your partner refine the research protocol. Help him or her focus on the mixed methods tasks of the protocol. Try and avoid showmanship of what you know, but focus on sections or areas where your partner needs feedback the most. Are there any sections that don't make sense or seem infeasible?

3. **Group Debrief.** If you are in a classroom or large group setting, take volunteers to present the areas of the research protocol that were most difficult. Reflect on how these same questions may play out in your own project.

Concluding Thoughts

Use this checklist to assess your progress in achieving the Chapter 12 objectives:

☐ I understand the need for complying with human subjects research regulations.

☐ I determined whether my mixed methods study is exempt from human subject regulations.

☐ I recognize unique ethical considerations that can arise relative to conduct of an MMR project, and how to address those issues in my protocol.

☐ I can distinguish between the regulatory language of *human subjects* and *participants*, language describing individuals who engage in mixed methods studies.

☐ I reviewed the elements that constitute a research protocol.

☐ I recognize multiple potential uses of a research protocol.

☐ I considered the elements of a research protocol and how the elements may vary depending on my purpose.

☐ I created a research protocol for my mixed methods project.

☐ I reviewed my research protocol with a peer or colleague to refine it.

☐ I submitted my research human subjects research application using the research protocol.

Now that you have completed these objectives, Chapter 13 will alert you to fundamental steps of analysis for your MMR or evaluation project.

Key Resources

1. **FURTHER READING ON ELEMENTS OF A RESEARCH PROTOCOL**

   - Recommended format for research protocol. (2019). World Health Organization. Retrieved from http://www.who.int/rpc/research_ethics/format_rp/en/.

2. **FURTHER READING ON ETHICAL ISSUES UNIQUE TO MIXED METHODS RESEARCH**

   - NIH Office of Behavioral and Social Sciences. (2018). Best practices for mixed methods research in the health sciences (2nd ed.). Bethesda, MD: National Institutes of Health. Retrieved May 10, 2019, from https://obssr.od.nih.gov/wp-content/uploads/2018/01/Best-Practices-for-Mixed-Methods-Research-in-the-Health-Sciences-2018-01-25.pdf.

3. **FURTHER READING ON U.S. REGULATIONS RELATIVE TO CONDUCT OF HUMAN SUBJECTS RESEARCH**

   - U.S. Department of Health & Human Services. (2009). Title 45 public welfare. Part 46: Protection of human subjects. *Code of federal regulations*. Retrieved from https://www.hhs.gov/ohrp/regulations-and-policy/regulations#.

4. **FURTHER READING FOR AN OUTLINE TO DEVELOP A RESEARCH PROTOCOL**

   - Maxwell, J. A. (2013). *Qualitative research design: An interactive approach* (3rd ed.). Thousand Oaks, CA: Sage.

13

PERFORMING FUNDAMENTAL STEPS OF MIXED METHODS DATA ANALYSIS

Mixed methods data analysis involves a series of fundamental steps that have parallels in qualitative and quantitative approaches. Given the complexity of mixed methods projects, it may seem that mixed data analysis is a black box. This chapter and its activities will help you (1) conduct a data collection inventory, considering gaps in the data, and taking steps to address inconsistencies; (2) consider the mixed methods data relative to the specific hypotheses and questions; (3) identify patterns in the data; (4) use organizational structure to summarize findings; (5) check for inconsistencies, anomalies, or conflicting findings; (6) organize the findings for dissemination; and (7) use writing procedures to articulate the mixed methods findings for a sophisticated interpretation. Mixed methods data analysis involves a series of fundamental steps that have parallels in qualitative and quantitative approaches. As a key outcome, you will develop a mixed methods data analysis plan.

LEARNING OBJECTIVES

To help you create a mixed methods research (MMR) or evaluation analysis plan, this chapter illustrates key steps so you can

- Apply seven fundamental mixed methods data analysis steps in your MMR or evaluation project

- Assemble the mixed data, conduct a data collection inventory, consider gaps in the data sources, take steps to address deficiencies, and consider data reduction

- Evaluate the mixed data relative to the specific hypotheses and questions using an independent or interactive data analysis approach, and identify any new mixed methods questions given emerging findings

- Describe patterns found by identifying linkages about related constructs and merging the findings

- Recognize how researchers merge qualitative and quantitative findings using a narrative approach

- Assess for "fit" of the qualitative and quantitative data together for convergence, complementarity, expansion, and/or divergence

- Refine or reconstruct the mixed findings using tables, graphs, or figures

- Compose a written interpretation of the findings using a logical organizational structure, either a separate, "contiguous" structure or "weaving" structure, with qualitative and quantitative findings presented together

WHY FIND COMMONALITY BETWEEN YOUR QUALITATIVE AND QUANTITATIVE DATA?

While modern MMR has been evolving since its conceptualization in the late 1980s (Bryman, 1988; Greene, Caracelli, & Graham, 1989), merging or integration of the data has long captured the interest of MMR methodologists. Well into the early 2000s, effective integration in mixed methods studies lagged behind other aspects of mixed methods developments (Bryman, 2006, 2007). Contemporary scholars emphasize the importance of integration as a distinguishing feature of the methodology (Bazeley, 2018; Creamer, 2018; Creswell & Plano Clark, 2018; Fetters & Molina-Azorin, 2017c).

Bazeley and Kemp (2012) introduced a key idea for conceptualizing integrated analysis. They have described a critical distinction to be whether the analysis involves a "process of change in the structure of the data that initiates possibilities for further exploration of the data" (Bazeley & Kemp, 2012). For the purposes of this workbook, data analysis not involving a change in the structure of data will be considered fundamental mixed methods analysis procedures. Chapter 14 addresses the special case of a joint display, which does not necessarily but may change the structure of the data. Integrated analysis strategies that involve changes in the structure of the data are covered under advanced mixed methods analysis procedures (Chapter 15). This chapter focuses on strategies that do not involve a change in the structure of the data.

Here, **mixed methods data analysis** refers to the process of examining both the qualitative and quantitative findings to identify linkages across the two types of findings that comprise constructs with commonality, and making new interpretations or drawing metainferences for a more enhanced, detailed, or holistic understanding. Completing the readings and activities of this chapter will help guide the mixed methods data analysis of your MMR and evaluation projects.

SEVEN FUNDAMENTAL STEPS IN MIXED METHODS DATA ANALYSIS

In my experience conducting many workshops and individual research project consultations, junior and senior researchers alike often are uncertain about how to integrate data collected during mixed methods projects. To demystify this process, Table 13.1 illustrates how the primary qualitative data analysis, quantitative data analysis, and mixed methods data analysis have parallel steps, namely, (1) entering data, cleaning the database, and resolving inconsistencies; (2) framing the analysis in accordance with the study purpose; (3) conducting a preliminary, descriptive analysis; 4) using an organizational structure to summarize initial findings; (5) checking for inconsistencies; (6) organizing findings for dissemination; and (7) interpreting the findings and writing up results. As shown in Chapters 14 and 15, many studies conduct additional analysis using advanced techniques (Bazeley, 2018; Curry & Nunez-Smith, 2015).

TABLE 13.1 ■ Comparison of Primary Steps in Qualitative, Quantitative, and Mixed Methods Data Analysis			
Major Steps	**Qualitative Data**	**Quantitative Data**	**Mixed Data**
Step 1. Enter, clean, and address gaps or deficiencies in the data	Organize, transcribe (as relevant), review, clean audio-recorded data, review other textual or visual qualitative data for accuracy, and assess the dataset for completeness	Inventory all different data sources, review for erroneous data values, and implement strategies to rectify ambiguous, missing, or conflicting data	Assemble the data, conduct a data collection inventory, consider gaps in the qualitative and quantitative data sources, and take steps to address deficits
Step 2. Frame the analysis in accordance with the study purpose	Frame by descriptive purpose, theory testing or development, or evaluation purpose, and collect additional data to achieve saturation	Confirm independent or dependent outcomes relative to hypotheses or research questions, and create new variables by combining existing variables	Consider the mixed data relative to the specific hypotheses and questions, and identify any new mixed methods questions given emerging findings

Major Steps	Qualitative Data	Quantitative Data	Mixed Data
Step 3. Discern patterns in the data	Segment and code iteratively, as data are collected to construct and refine a coding scheme and develop qualitative themes	Conduct descriptive statistics by evaluating relevant summary measures, such as means, medians, tabulations, etc.	Identify commonalities between the two types of data using spiralled analysis, following a thread, or back-and-forth exchanges and merging related findings
Step 4. Use an organizational structuring to summarize initial findings	Develop a table of themes and/or develop a model or theory and identify illustrative quotes	Arrange findings in a series of tables according to major findings of scales or items and organize the findings within the tables for ease of understanding	Organize the linked qualitative and quantitative findings using a narrative approach, or by using one or more joint display(s) (Chapter 14)
Step 5. Check for inconsistencies, anomalies, or conflicting findings	Check the overall cohesiveness and completeness of the findings and the consistency of quotes with the interpretations	Examine overall trends and look for consistencies and discrepancies between related findings and resolve any unexpected findings	Look at the "fit" of the qualitative and quantitative data together for convergence, complementarity, expansion, and/or divergence
Step 6. Organize the findings for dissemination	Develop theme-based tables, figures, or graphics	Reconfigure tables, figures, graphs, heat maps, and other visualizations of data	Refine or reconstruct the mixed findings using tables, graphs, and figures
Step 7. Interpret the findings in writing up the results	Develop a study narrative based on the theme or resulting model or theory using illustrative examples and quotes	Report the findings based on identified trends seen in the observed patterns for each table and sequentially explain the findings for each	Compose an interpretation of the findings using a logical organizational structure, either a separate, "contiguous" structure or "weaving" structure with qualitative and quantitative findings presented together

As there are volumes of books and resources on conducting quantitative and qualitative analyses (Creswell, 2016; Miles, Huberman, & Saldaña, 2014; Patton, 2015), details about these approaches are beyond the scope of this chapter, and only sufficient detail to illuminate the comparable steps in a mixed methods study will be addressed. Moreover, there are many software programs for supporting statistical analysis, qualitative analysis, and increasingly mixed methods analysis (Guetterman, Creswell, & Kuckartz, 2015). Many mixed methods researchers routinely use software to support integrated mixed methods analysis, but deciding whether to use software can be made in conjunction with other research or evaluation team members or dissertation committee members. The primary steps in analysis as described below remain relevant, regardless of whether you will or will not use software support.

STEP 1. ENTER, CLEAN, AND ADDRESS GAPS OR DEFICIENCIES IN THE DATA BASED ON A DATA COLLECTION INVENTORY

The first step of MMR data analysis involves conducting an inventory of all different data sources, reviewing for erroneous data values, and implementing a strategy for handling ambiguous, missing, or conflicting data. A **data collection inventory** describes assembling a comprehensive list of the data collection elements from the qualitative and quantitative strands. After inventory, the researcher may wish to eliminate unrelated material that are not related to the study purpose, a process called data reduction (Johnson & Christensen, 2017).

In workshops and consultations, many individuals with questions about their MMR data analysis have never stopped to take an inventory of the sources available or consider their "mixed data collection portfolio." While a parallel step, conducting a data collection inventory goes beyond the initial "data cleaning" steps that occur in the qualitative and quantitative data analysis processes. Taking a data collection inventory requires a higher level of analysis that goes beyond traditional "data cleaning" typically associated with quantitative datasets (e.g., addressing missing data, double data entry, etc.) and qualitative data analysis (e.g., careful review of transcriptions for omissions, "beautification," i.e., inappropriately creating full sentences, correcting grammar). Conducting a mixed methods data collection inventory allows for "cleaning up" by organizing the contents of the data in a single place. Further, it provides an opportunity to look for gaps in either type of data, the possibility for additional qualitative data collection, or the building of quantitative variables from existing variables that may have a better fit with the qualitative themes. Through data reduction, it identifies data that may be useful primarily in a qualitative paper (due to the lack of related quantitative data), or useful in a quantitative paper (due to the lack of related qualitative data). Additionally, there may be data collected that were unexpected about other topics outside the scope of the study's aim.

Considering Your Methodological Dimension of Analysis

The methodological dimension of the analysis refers to "how the quantitative and qualitative strands are weighted relative to merging analytics" (Moseholm & Fetters, 2017) and involves qualitatively driven, quantitatively driven, and equivalently driven mixed methods studies (Johnson, 2015; Johnson, Onwuegbuzie, & Turner, 2007; Moseholm & Fetters, 2017). In brief, these approaches may associate with philosophical stances (Chapter 4), qualitatively driven constructivist-oriented, quantitatively driven as more postpositivistically driven, and equivalently driven where neither predominates and there is equal status. This has implications for the structure of your mixed methods data collection inventory. If your stance is quantitatively driven, structure your data collection inventory with the quantitative column first. If your stance is qualitatively driven, structure your data collection inventory with the qualitative content column first. If your stance is equivalently driven, choose a structure based on the specifics of your project.

A Mixed Methods Data Collection Inventory

Workbox Illustration 13.1.1 provides an example of a Mixed Methods Data Collection Inventory from the MPathic-VR mixed methods trial, a medical education study examining effectiveness in a mixed methods intervention of a virtual human to teach communication skills (Kron et al., 2017). The column "Quantitative Sources" contains the questions asked using a Likert scale rating completed immediately after student randomization to the virtual human simulation intervention, or computer-based learning module control. Moreover, it contains the items used by the standardized surgical assistant in the posttrial objective structured clinical examination (OSCE). The column "Qualitative Sources" contains qualitative questions used to stimulate reflective essays written by the medical students immediately after exposure to the intervention or control. The choice of how detailed or general to be with the content listed is study dependent and a personal choice. The data collection inventory table may initially resemble data sources (see Chapter 6) with subsequent versions becoming more detailed. As patterns of related information come together more clearly, updates to the data collection inventory sheet may be helpful.

Workbox Illustration 13.1.1: Data Collection Inventory of the MPathic-VR Mixed Methods Medical Education Study

Quantitative Sources	Qualitative Sources
Attitudinal Survey Items 1 Purpose of the training was clear. 2 Content was appropriate for my level of training. 3 Training was engaging. 4 Training was effective for learning verbal communication skills. 5 Training was effective for learning nonverbal communication skills. 6 Training was effective for learning how to handle emotionally charged situations. 7 Training will help me improve my clinical skills. 8 Based on training, my communication skills improved. 9 Visual media were effective for learning the material. 10 Interaction felt realistic. 11 Quality of feedback on my performance was high. 12 Overall, it was an excellent training experience. 13 I would recommend it to others at my level of training. 14 I want to take similar educational exercises in future.	Reflective Essay Questions (students were randomized to different questions) Question 1. In 75-500 words, reflect on how you think this learning experience in advanced communication skills could be improved. Use specific examples in your response. Question 2. In 75-500 words, reflect on the three most important things you learned from this interaction. Use specific examples in your response. Question 3. In 75-500 words, please reflect on how interacting with the system has influenced your views about human interactions (e.g., interprofessional, patient-provider, family-provider, patient-family). Use specific examples in your response. Question 4. In 75-500 words, please reflect on how interacting with the system has influenced your understanding about nonverbal communication. Use specific examples in your response.

Quantitative Sources	Qualitative Sources
Scores on Objective Structured Clinical Examination 1. Introduces self 2. Rephrases the surgical assistants, concern to check for mutual understanding 3. Asks clarifying questions to better understand situation 4. Admits own lack of knowledge 5. Names emotions/acknowledges feelings (empathy) 6. Makes statement to reframe situation in a positive light 7. Provides statement of support/collaboration 8. Provides statement of respect (acknowledgment) 9. Verbalizes an apology 11. Openness/defensiveness 13. Collaborative/competitive 15. Nonverbal communication 17. Presence	Proctors' Freehand Notes Recorded During the Trial Site 1. Notes Site 2. Notes Site 3. Notes Video Recordings From the Intervention Arm During the Trial Video recordings of students taken while interacting with the virtual human patient. Evaluator Comments of the Objective Structured Clinical Examination 10. "Verbalizes apology" comments 12. "Openness/defensiveness" comments 14. "Collaborative/competitive" comments 16. "Nonverbal communication" comments 18. "Presence" comments

Sources: Kron et al. (2017) and Fetters, M.D. and Kron, F.W. (2012–15). *Modeling Professional Attitudes and Teaching Humanistic Communication in Virtual Reality (MPathic-VRII).* National Center for Advancing Translational Science/NIH 9R44TR000360-04.

Activity: Conducting a Mixed Methods Data Collection Inventory

Using Workbox Illustration 13.1.1 as an example, complete Workbox 13.1.2 and create a mixed methods data collection inventory sheet for your project. Based on your mixed methods design, you may switch the order to qualitative content and quantitative items. If you have completed a data sources table (see Chapter 6), use this as a reference to help populate the columns. From your files, locate the best summaries of the instrument(s) used to collect the quantitative data. In addition, find the most up-to-date version of your qualitative data collection instruments or description of your sources. If there are unrelated sources, for example, process measures or other types of feedback, you may choose to leave these out, though at this stage, erring on the side of inclusiveness may be better. If one type of data was planned to match the other type of data collection, putting items in a similar order is preferable for efficiency, but not critical at the beginning. Look at both types of data. Can you find any gaps or missing information? Is there any additional information from other data sources you could bring into the analysis? If necessary, move the items around, but keep track of your changes. For example, you can retain original survey item numbers. To be mindful of the actual ordering from your instrument(s) and coding scheme, using a digital file, create a revised version each time you change ordering.

Variations in the Data Collection Inventory Workbox Structure

As noted in previous chapters, the workboxes should serve your needs. Rather than a static document, the data collection inventory may continue to evolve according to your needs. Variations (not illustrated) possible with this structure could include adding the study aim at the top. Alternatively, an additional column could be added on both sides for comments. This could allow notations about where the data are stored, dates of data collection, etc. Alternatively, a third comment column is appropriate for recording information such as the location of the files and dates data collection is projected to occur or has occurred already. Another option is to include a middle column that lists the elements of a theory that underlies and guides your project. In many projects, the order within each column may change across different versions. An initial version may reflect temporally the order of collection, while a later version may reflect areas of relatedness. Finally, for a sequential design you could consider the top half as the data collection during the first phase and the bottom half data collection from the second phase. The structure is there to help, not impede, so use and adapt as per the particular details of your project. The critical point is to begin the process of organizing the qualitative and quantitative data to understand how they relate to each other.

**Workbox 13.1.2: Conducting an Inventory of the
Mixed Methods Data**

Quantitative Sources	Qualitative Sources

STEP 2. FRAME THE ANALYSIS IN ACCORDANCE WITH THE STUDY PURPOSE

Your next step is to frame the analysis in accordance with the study purpose. Considering the analysis flows naturally from the content in Workbox 13.1.2. Begin by considering your mixed data relative to the specific hypotheses and questions.

Study Purpose/Objective

To get started, align the data analysis with the study purpose, objective, and aims. For reference, review the research aims or questions developed in Chapter 5. Determine if these have evolved. If you have not clearly defined your study purpose/objective, considering reviewing completing the Chapter 5 activities. The study purpose in mixed methods projects should reflect both the quantitative and qualitative intentions. Simply stated, what are you trying to accomplish with the quantitative strand? What are you trying to accomplish with the qualitative strand? Workbox Illustration 13.2.1 depicts the MPathic-VR trial, a medical education study examining effectiveness in a mixed methods intervention of a virtual human to teach communication skills, Kron et al., 2017). The illustration features the overarching quantitative purpose: Does the virtual reality module work better than a computer-based learning module for teaching communication skills? The illustration further provides the overarching qualitative purpose, namely, understanding why. The conjunction *and* helps to show that the quantitative and qualitative purposes are linked.

Study Questions/Hypotheses

For the quantitative strand of your MMR or evaluation project, you will be posing quantitative strand-based research hypotheses or questions. Similarly, you will pose research questions for the qualitative and the mixed methods strands. Workbox Illustration 13.2.1 illustrates how there were three hypotheses of the quantitative strand in the MPathic-VR medical education mixed methods trial (Kron et al., 2017). The qualitative strand question relates to understanding the participants' experiences with the virtual human simulation or the computer-based learning module based on their assignment to one or the other. The MMR question asked how the medical students' attitudes about their experience as measured on a Likert scale (Workbox Illustration 13.1.1) compared with their qualitative reflections about their experiences as reported through reflective essays.

Workbox Illustration 13.2.1: Merging Data for Integrated Mixed Methods Data Analysis From the MPathic-VR Mixed Methods Medical Education Study

General Objective/Study Purpose:

This research seeks to determine whether MPathic-VR is effective for teaching advanced communication skills and why.

Study Questions/Hypotheses:

Quantitative:

Hypothesis 1: Students randomized to learn with MPathic-VR will improve their communication performance after engaging in a communication scenario, receiving feedback on their performance, and then applying the feedback in a second run-through of two different virtual reality simulation scenarios.

Hypothesis 2: Knowledge acquired through MPathic-VR would be resilient, that is, students would incorporate learned materials into their manner of communication, and this would be evidenced by better performance of MPathic-VR-trained students than the control computer-based learning students, as assessed in a subsequent advanced-communication objective structured clinical exam.

Question: How do student attitudes about their experiences during the trial compare with those exposed to the virtual reality program and those exposed to the control?

Qualitative:

What are the experiences of medical students who use virtual human training to learn communication skills?

Mixed Methods Research Question:

How do qualitative findings from students' reflective comments and responses to a quantitative attitudinal survey compare with students in the interactive virtual human intervention and students who take a computer-based learning module?

Mixed Methods Data Analysis Process (choose one) and Rationale:

Independent Analysis Strategy:

The quantitative and qualitative data for merging will be collected at the same time, so there will be no opportunity or advantage for employing interactive analysis strategy.

Interactive Analysis Strategy:
Not applicable

Source: Kron et al. (2017).

Activity: Study Purpose/Objective and Study Questions/Hypotheses

For your next step, fill in the study questions/hypotheses and qualitative and MMR questions of your study. Using Workbox Illustration 13.2.1 as a reference, complete these sections in Workbox 13.2.2. If struggling with writing your research hypotheses and questions, review and complete the activities in Chapter 5. This will assist in writing and refinement of your quantitative, qualitative, and MMR questions and if applicable, hypotheses as you complete Workbox 13.2.2. If you have completed Chapter 5, copy your items into the box. It is possible (likely!) that your own thinking has evolved or become sharpened and you should update them.

Workbox 13.2.2: Merging Data for Integrated Mixed Methods Data Analysis

General Objective/Study Purpose:

Study Questions/Hypotheses:
Quantitative:

Qualitative:

Mixed Methods Research Question:

Mixed Methods Data Analysis Process (choose one) and Rationale:

Independent Analysis Strategy:

Interactive Analysis Strategy:

Mixed Methods Data Analysis Process and Rationale

For the mixed methods data analysis, decide whether to use an independent or interactive approach for the analysis. Moseholm and Fetters (2017) have referred to this as the **relational dimension** of the mixed methods analysis. This describes the extent to which researchers allow interfacing of the qualitative and quantitative strands during the analysis. **Independent data analysis** (they described this as the "separative approach") denotes the process of inferring the meaning of the mixed findings by first examining, exploring, and making interpretations separately within each of the qualitative and quantitative strands, and then comparing the two types of findings for an overall interpretation. In contrast, **interactive data analysis** (they referred to this as the "iterative approach") denotes the process of inferring the meaning of the mixed findings by examining, exploring, and making interpretations iteratively as data collection and analysis occurs based on an emerging understanding of findings of both the qualitative and quantitative data. As illustrated in Figure 13.1, these two approaches represent two poles on the spectrum of possibility. In actuality, the process often falls somewhere on the continuum. In my experience, the independent process is far more common.

FIGURE 13.1 ■ **The Spectrum Between Independent and Interactive Mixed Methods Data Analysis**

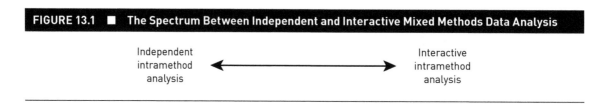

Independent Analysis

Independent data analysis refers to within strand, impartial, and rigorous examination of the qualitative data, and of the quantitative data, as a prequel to the merged analysis of qualitative and quantitative findings. Figure 13.2 depicts conceptually independent analysis. As shown, the qualitative data collection and analysis, and the quantitative data collection and analysis, occur separately from each other. Moreover, the figure illustrates through the double-headed arrow in the qualitative strand that the qualitative data collection and analysis occur iteratively. Once there are results from the data collection and analysis from both strands, the data are brought together in a descriptive analysis. This occurs most commonly, but not exclusively, in a convergent MMR design.

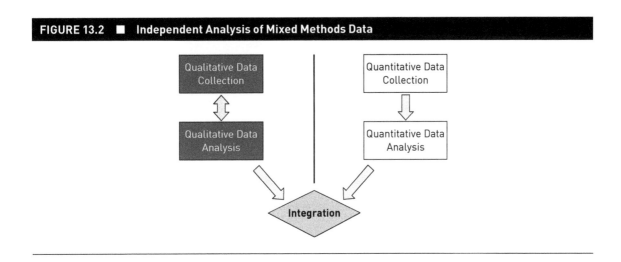

FIGURE 13.2 ■ Independent Analysis of Mixed Methods Data

Interactive Analysis

Interactive data analysis describes an iterative, interfacing, and rigorous examination of the qualitative and quantitative data while mixed methods data collection is ongoing. That is, researchers intentionally and iteratively allow the data to interact, or "talk" to each other, during data collection and analysis to make adjustments in data collection procedures and infer overall meaning. This approach can generate new mixed methods questions in consideration of emerging findings. Figure 13.3 illustrates conceptually interactive analysis (see Story From the Field 13.1). Rather than a hard line as in Figure 13.2, the dotted line emphasizes that with interactive analysis, examination and exploration occur simultaneously and iteratively within and between the qualitative and quantitative strands, as illustrated by the two laterally positioned two-headed arrows.

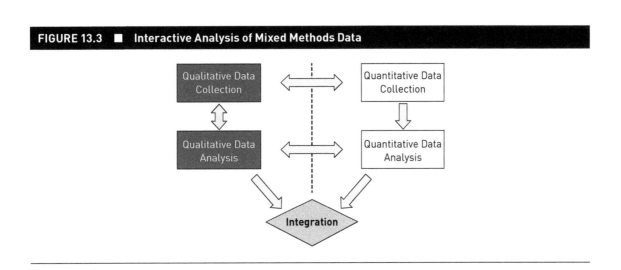

FIGURE 13.3 ■ Interactive Analysis of Mixed Methods Data

Considerations When Choosing Between Independent and Interactive Analysis Approaches

When conducting an interactive analysis, researchers must remain mindful of the research integrity considerations and not raise threats to validity or integrity of either type of data collection. Some methodologists use the language of qualitatively driven research where the precepts of research integrity will be driven by the qualitative strand (Johnson, 2015; Johnson, Grove, & Clarke, 2007; Moseholm & Fetters, 2017). In qualitative strands, iterative data collection and analysis are expected. Hence, it is natural for the interactive analysis to be more appealing. On the flip side, some scholars frame mixed methods studies as quantitatively driven (Johnson, 2015; Johnson et al., 2007; Moseholm & Fetters, 2017). As the research integrity issues relative to keeping data collection and analysis separated are heavily emphasized, the independent approach may be more apropos.

STORY FROM THE FIELD 13.1
ON INTERACTIVE MIXED METHODS DATA ANALYSIS

An example of the interactive process of MMR data analysis occurs in mixed methods case series studies. An early pioneer of MMR, Benjamin F. Crabtree, a medical anthropologist who moved into the health sciences, has conducted a number of mixed methods studies. These have included many mixed methods multiple case studies, trials, and evaluation studies. Crabtree and his colleagues have conducted studies looking at how primary care practices can provide the best quality care. His group also develops and tests practice interventions. He often speaks about how the quantitative data and quantitative data "talk to each other," and that this interaction generates iterative, critical revisions to survey instruments and qualitative assessments. That is, quantitative data collection instruments may expand in type or scope as his team conducts qualitative assessments. In evaluation studies, emerging patterns from qualitative data may influence quantitative inquiries. In addition, qualitative data collection in a practice might change depending on quantitative measures of performance. For example, a practice with very good or very poor immunization rates for certain vaccines might trigger a more in-depth qualitative assessment as to why this occurs.

Activity: Mixed Methods Data Analysis Process and Rationale

Using Workbox Illustration 13.2.1 as a reference, choose whether you will use an independent analysis process or an interactive analysis process in Workbox 13.2.2. To articulate your rationale, consider the following two points relative to an independent analysis or interactive analysis.

Rationale for Independent Analysis Process

For the most part, sequential designs, exploratory sequential, and explanatory sequential mixed methods designs will use an independent analysis process. Since the second phase will be building upon, connecting subjects, developing models or hypotheses for subsequent testing, by default, the second phase generally will not be conducted until there has been intramethod analysis of the first phase of the sequential design. In quantitatively driven studies in general, or convergent designs with quantitative studies where blinding of the investigators and/or subjects is particularly important for maintaining the validity of the study, intramethod analysis is critical. Pragmatically, this approach may be easier because analysis of the quantitative and qualitative data can proceed in the usual fashion without the qualitative or the quantitative analyst needing to consider the analysis of the other type of data.

Rationale for Interactive Analysis Process

This approach deserves consideration, especially in a convergent mixed method design. If one is conducting the qualitative strand of the research using an iterative process of data collection and analysis, then the research team will likely have information coming into the study in an ongoing way. In qualitatively driven studies in general, an interactive analysis process may be the most appropriate. While a less common approach, some of the more common examples include (1) conducting mixed methods multiple case studies, (2) developing an intervention, and (3) conducting a community or school-based intervention. In these cases, initial data collection is highly iterative and interactive with both forms of data informing the other type of data collection (see Story From the Field 13.1). There are pragmatic challenges, as this requires sufficient time and the expertise of the team to do both simultaneously.

Rationale for Using Both Independent and Interactive Analysis

Researchers conducting multiphase studies may have both sequential and convergent components, and similarly, quantitatively driven and qualitatively driven approaches. If your study is a multiphase study, and both are relevant, you can choose based on phase (usually the first phase), or you can write both. In this circumstance, be sure to identify clearly which phase the approach will be using.

STEP 3. DESCRIBE PATTERNS IN THE DATA

Mixed methods descriptive analysis follows from Table 13.1, as the next task is to identify commonalities between the two types of data and merge them together. This requires comparing and contrasting the data (Creswell & Plano Clark, 2018; Johnson & Christensen, 2017). Workbox Illustration 13.3.1 provides an illustration of the quantitative, qualitative, and mixed methods analysis procedures used in the MPathic-VR mixed methods trial to examine the impact of a virtual human simulation (Kron et al., 2017). **Descriptive mixed methods data analysis** refers to strategies useful for finding linkages between qualitative and quantitative data. Fundamentally, integrated analysis requires comparing and contrasting the two types of data. This is an area of MMR that is recognized as important but that lacks an agreed-upon terminology on how to portray this step. Various authors provide metaphors that can help conceptualize the process (Bazeley, 2012; Bazeley & Kemp, 2012; Fetters & Molina-Azorin, 2017c; O'Cathain, Murphy, & Nicholl, 2010). Here, I provide three approaches conceptualized using metaphors, though there are others, and it is important to understand this remains an area in MMR that continues to advance.

Workbox Illustration 13.3.1: Identifying Patterns From Mixed Data in the MPathic-VR Mixed Methods Medical Education Study

Descriptive Analysis Approach:

Quantitative Analysis:

We conducted descriptive statistics for the demographic variables and compared the intervention arm and control arm to examine for any differences between students in the intervention and control arm.

Hypothesis 1: We examined for changes in the mean scores obtained from the first to second run-through for two scenarios of the virtual human simulation intervention arm students, one on intercultural communication, and a second on interprofessional communication.

Hypothesis 2: We calculated mean student scores on the advanced communication objective structured clinical exam and compared the scores between the MPathic-VR computer simulation intervention arm and the computer-based learning module control arm.

Posttrial Attitudinal Survey: We calculated the mean scores on the 12 attitudinal survey items and compared the scores between the MPathic-VR computer simulation intervention arm and the computer-based learning module control arm.

Qualitative Analysis:

The qualitative data were combined into a single file and imported into the MAXQDA software, which was used for data management and support of the analysis. Two team members immersed themselves in the data and developed codes. Text segments were identified and assigned a code based on *de novo* coding scheme and creation of a preliminary codebook. By reviewing and discussing each code, we calibrated use of the codes and achieved intercoder agreement. The related codes were organized into primary themes. A third researcher reviewed the coded data.

Directional Dimension of the Mixed Data Analysis:

☑ Quantitatively driven

☐ Qualitatively driven

☐ Equivalently driven

(Continued)

(Continued)

> **Explain:** The lens framing this analysis is quantitatively driven. The trial was oriented primarily looking for statistical differences, as illustrated by the prominence of the hypotheses. In addition, the comparison of student experiences is organized by the attitudinal survey data.
>
> **Mixed Methods Data Analysis**
>
> ☑ Spiraled analysis: We cyclically considered the quantitative attitudinal scores and qualitative themes and quotes and descended continuously down to each common theme.
>
> ☑ Finding a common thread: Identified "experiences in system" as a linkage, a common area of interest in both datasets.
>
> ☑ Back-and-forth analysis: Iteratively considered the relevant QUAL textual data and relevant scales from QUAN attitudinal items.

Source: Kron et al. (2017).

As part of mixed methods analysis, *quantitative analysis* involves calculating descriptive statistics such as means, medians, and tabulations to depict descriptive information about the study population and research questions (Johnson & Christensen, 2017; Patton, 2015). As illustrated in Workbox Illustration 13.3.1, the MPathic-VR study initially involved calculation of descriptive statistics about demographics and survey items using means, medians, etc. In contrast, *qualitative analysis* involves a systematic approach for iteratively collecting and examining the collected text, observations, visuals or other media, and making sense of information to better understand a phenomenon of interest by segmenting text and coding iteratively as data are collected to construct and refine a coding scheme (Creswell, 2016; Miles et al., 2014; Patton, 2015). Typically, this process produces a coding scheme comprised of themes, codes, and exemplar text illustrations. Codes can be used to identify related material and even link different codes. Given the iterative nature of qualitative analysis, the coding scheme most likely will continue to evolve well into the project. A truncated version of the coding scheme for the MPathic-VR study can be seen in Table 13.2. With further searches and descriptions of the findings, this can lead to construction of a narrative that is primarily descriptive. Many qualitative papers finish with this level of descriptive analysis, though advanced qualitative researchers will move beyond this basic level of analysis to an advanced analysis.

TABLE 13.2 ■ Qualitative Coding Scheme Developed for the MPathic-VR Mixed Methods Medical Education Study (Kron et al., 2017)

Theme 1. Empathic Communication

1. Open mind
2. Working as a team
3. Cultural perspectives
4. Reflective language
5. Emotionally charged
6. Open-ended questions
7. Professionals in family politics

Theme 2. Interactive Learning

1. Objective evaluation
2. Be prepared
3. Be motivated to learn more
4. Method of instruction
5. Need more practice

Theme 3. Communication—General

1. Standard communication improves efficiency.
2. Communication depends on the situation.

3. "Speaker and listener" roles

4. Different manners of communicating

Theme 4. Useful Verbal and Nonverbal Communication Skills

1. Recognizing nonverbal cues

2. Method of communication

3. Choice of words

4. Connecting nonverbals to tense situations

5. Smiling and communication

6. Mirroring other's facial expressions

7. Remembering nonverbal communication

8. Connecting communication to errors

9. Standard way of team communication

10. Knowing a "mnemonic"

Source: Kron et al., (2017).

Three *mixed methods descriptive analysis* procedures presented here include spiraling, finding a common thread, and back-and-forth exchanges (Bazeley & Kemp, 2012; Fetters & Molina-Azorin, 2017c). Using any of these approaches can help identify mixed data linkages as constructs that can be weaved together to develop a coherent narrative about the findings.

Workbox 13.3.2: Identifying Patterns in the Data of Mixed Methods Research and Evaluation Studies

Descriptive Analysis Approach

Quantitative Analysis

Qualitative Analysis

Directional Dimension of the Mixed Data Analysis

☐ Quantitatively driven

☐ Qualitatively driven

☐ Equivalently driven

Explain:

Mixed Methods Data Analysis

☐ Spiraled analysis

☐ Finding a common thread

☐ Back-and-forth analysis

☐ Other

Activity: Mixed Methods Data Analysis Approach

Using Workbox Illustration 13.3.1 as a reference, complete your planning for analysis of your quantitative, qualitative, and mixed methods data in Workbox 13.3.2. While the workbook provides an order of quantitative, qualitative, and mixed methods, you can adjust the order as appropriate to your own project. Record with as much detail as you know, the process you anticipate (if in the planning stage), or in accordance with what you have done (if data collection is ongoing or is completed) for the analysis of your quantitative, qualitative, and mixed methods data.

Descriptions of the details of spiraled comparison, following a thread, and back-and-forth exchanges will help you choose one or more approaches.

As you approach your mixed methods analysis, consider the directional dimension of your analysis. Moseholm and Fetters (2017) described the **directional dimension** as whether the mixed data analysis occurs using a one-way directional approach, where either the quantitative data or qualitative data frame the analysis, or if there is a bidirectional approach, such that the data of both strands frame the analysis. If you have a quantitatively driven project as in the MPathic-VR virtual human exemplar study featured in this chapter, then your directional dimension will be quantitative, and this will be a good starting point for your mixed methods analysis. If you have a qualitatively driven project, then your directional dimension will be qualitative, and this will be a good starting point for your mixed methods analysis. If you have an equivalently driven project, either source of data can serve as a starting point, depending on your study.

Spiraled Comparing

Mixed methods descriptive analysis using spiraled comparison refers to cyclically considering the qualitative and quantitative findings derived from the intramethod analysis (Fetters & Molina-Azorin, 2017c). In this process, rather than just being cyclical, the diameter of the circle progressively narrows as the relationship between the qualitative and quantitative findings become increasingly clear. For MPathic-VR, the commonality of the linkages were found gradually by examining both types of data. The mixed methods analyst can hone in on common topics, ideas, or areas for comparison. This occurs at the broadest level. While there is spiraling at the broadest level, a key feature of a spiral is that the base comes to a tip. This tip symbolizes the discovery of related findings from the qualitative and the quantitative data. Once this process occurs for several themes, they can become a series of related findings (see Figure 13.4). In contrast to a cycle that repeats continuously, a spiral leads to a specific point. In the mixed data analysis, it produces a unifying construct.

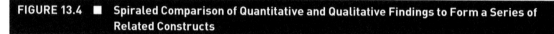

FIGURE 13.4 ■ Spiraled Comparison of Quantitative and Qualitative Findings to Form a Series of Related Constructs

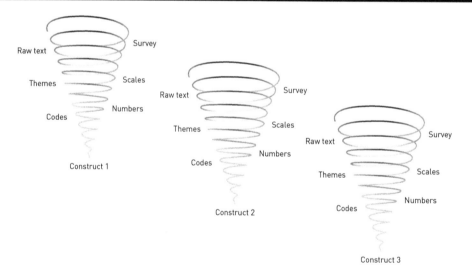

Following a Thread

Moran-Ellis et al. first depicted following a thread in 2004 in a presentation during the Economic and Social Research Council (ESRC) Research Methods Programme and published a paper using the approach two years later (Moran-Ellis et al., 2006). Their group collected quantitative, interview, narrative, visual (maps, photos), and multimedia (video) data to explore vulnerability in a town in the south of England. As explained in greater detail by Cronin, Alexander, Fielding, Moran-Ellis, and Thomas (2008), their approach used four steps. First, for each different type of data collected, the authors used "the analytic method appropriate to the data" (p. 576, cf. intramethod analysis described above) to conduct a within-paradigm analysis from which they identified emergent findings and questions for further analysis. Second, they explored a "promising finding" within a dataset that could be "picked up as a thread" (p. 576) and followed through into the other dataset(s). They characterize finding a common thread as being triggered or "sparked" by the study research question or by the thread's resonance with findings from one or more of the other data set(s). In their process, they subsequently placed their datasets alongside each other to identify key themes and analytic questions worthy of further exploration (in essence, a data inventory as above). Third, they involved their creation of a data repertoire (categories of findings) based on emergent findings, categories, and codes related to the thread (see Chapter 15). Fourth, they identified a thread and synthesized it with other threads that had similarly been identified and followed within the datasets (Cronin et al., 2008). In their vulnerability research, the common thread found and followed was "physical safety."

As characterized by Moran-Ellis et al. (2006), "The value of this integrative analytic approach lies in allowing an inductive approach to the analysis, preserving the value of the open, exploratory, qualitative inquiry but incorporating the focus and specificity of the quantitative data" (p. 54).

Exchanging Back-and-Forth

Back-and-forth exchanges (Bazeley & Kemp, 2012) basically conveys the idea of "the data talking with each other." While an overt anthropomorphism, conceptually this conveys the notion that ideas emerging from the analysis interact with the mind of the analyst. This process can help reach a greater understanding of what each type of data "has to say" about a phenomenon of interest. Practically speaking, this process involves looking "back-and-forth" at the qualitative and quantitative data. Citing Weiss, Kreider, Mayer, Hencke, and Vaughan (2005) as one example, Bazeley and Kemp (2012) describe an interactive search for related concepts that are found in both the qualitative and quantitative data. Bazeley explains that the back-and-forth exchange procedure can be conceptualized like a discussion between a team biostatistician and a team anthropologist who are trying to find something in common. Ultimately, the goal is to merge the data together according to related findings. Matching the qualitative questions, observations, or other sources of data collection to the quantitative scales, items, or other forms of measures collected in your study (see Workbox 13.1.2) will lead to related domains that can be analyzed in consideration of each other.

STEP 4. USE AN ORGANIZATIONAL STRUCTURE FOR SUMMARIZING THE FINDINGS

The next step of an MMR data analysis requires organizing the linked qualitative and quantitative findings. Organizing approaches can include a narrative approach (Fetters, Curry, & Creswell, 2013) or a visual means such as tables, figures, photos, or other representations. Increasingly, mixed methods researchers are turning to the use of joint displays (Guetterman, Fetters, & Creswell, 2015). Fetters et al. (2013) describe the intent of the joint display as "bringing the data together through a visual means to draw out new insights beyond the information gained from the separate quantitative and qualitative results" (p. 10) (see Chapter 14). The analogy to this step in qualitative research is the development of a table of themes or a figure to portray a model or theory. Often, especially in a table format, the mixed methods findings are portrayed and given more nuance by using illustrative quotes. With quantitative data, the analogy is arranging the findings in a series of tables according to major findings from items or scales and organizing the findings within the tables.

STEP 5. CHECK FOR INCONSISTENCIES, ANOMALIES, OR CONFLICTING FINDINGS

The next step in an integrated mixed methods analysis involves looking at the "fit" of the qualitative and quantitative data together for convergence, complementarity, expansion, and/or divergence (Fetters et al., 2013). Also sometimes called confirmation, in convergence, the qualitative and quantitative findings lead to the same interpretation. Some authors have begun reporting the fit as part of their mixed methods findings (Bustamante, 2017; Moseholm, Rydahl-Hansen, Lindhardt, & Fetters, 2017). Complementarity occurs when the compared qualitative and quantitative data illustrate different, yet nonconflicting interpretations. Expansion occurs when the qualitative and quantitative data provide both a central overlapping as well as a broader nonoverlapping, interpretation. Hence, expansion represents a hybrid of the confirmation and complementarity. Finally, divergence, also sometimes called discordance, occurs when the qualitative and quantitative data lead to conflicting interpretations (Fetters et al., 2013; Fetters & Molina-Azorin, 2017c).

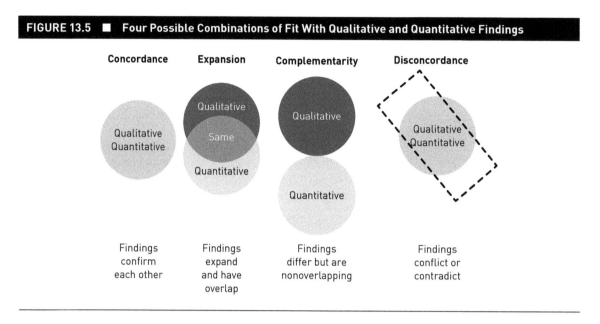

FIGURE 13.5   ■   Four Possible Combinations of Fit With Qualitative and Quantitative Findings

Approaches to Divergent or Discordant Qualitative and Quantitative Findings

MMR methodologists have considered various options for dealing with divergent or discordant findings (Figure 13.5). Under these circumstances, researchers can (1) collect additional data, (2) reanalyze existing databases to resolve the discrepancy, (3) turn to theory to find an explanation, (4) examine the validity of constructs, (5) identify potential sources of bias, or (6) pursue follow-up studies to explain (Moffatt, White, Mackintosh, & Howel, 2006; Pluye, Grad, Levine, & Nicolau, 2009).

STEP 6. ORGANIZE THE FINDINGS FOR DISSEMINATION

In this step, researchers refine or reconstruct the mixed findings using tables, figures, or graphs of their mixed methods findings. This step differs from Step 4, as the intent is now to organize the data in a format that best tells the story of the data. For example, at this stage, a mixed methods researcher may take the findings from the initial tables and create revised or new graphics or figures. A key to this step is asking, "How can I rearrange, reorder, visualize, or massage my mixed data for the understanding of the audience or reader?" In the course of reorganization, don't be surprised if you develop new insights or findings. This step has an analogous process for qualitative and quantitative studies. Qualitative researchers move beyond the initial coding scheme to develop multiple theme-based tables, figures, or graphics. The process may involve identifying more illustrative or different quotations or balancing the range of quotations from different groups of comparison. They may expand or combine codes to create new codes. Similarly, quantitative researchers may create reconfigured tables, figures, graphs, heat maps, and other visualizations of quantitative data. Many mixed methods researchers consider the joint display a critical tool for representing mixed data findings. Given its importance, Chapter 14 is devoted entirely to this topic.

STEP 7. INTERPRET AND ARTICULATE THE FINDINGS IN WRITING UP THE RESULTS

The last step of mixed methods analysis procedures involves writing an interpretation of the mixed findings using a logical organizational structure. This final step of interpretation is similar to the approaches for qualitative and quantitative studies where one writes a meaningful narrative or report based on key findings. There are two ways of writing up results within a publication using a separated, "contiguous" structure or a "weaving" structure (Fetters et al., 2013). A *contiguous structure* approach occurs when the qualitative and quantitative findings are reported in separate subsections of the results portion of a paper or dissertation. The interpretation may come in a third section of the results as the mixed methods findings or as a section in the discussion section. A second approach, a *weaving structure*, involves integrated presentation of the qualitative and quantitative findings on a theme by construct basis for each resulting finding. In this way, a series of constructs that have the qualitative and quantitative findings are presented sequentially in the results section of the paper. Chapter 18 provides more details on this process.

Application Activities

1. **Peer Feedback**. If working on your project as part of a class or in a workshop, pair up with a peer mentor, and one of you spend about 5 minutes talking about your mixed methods data analysis strategies. Take turns talking about your analysis strategies and giving feedback. Does an independent analysis or interactive analysis make more sense? Does an advanced analysis seem indicated? If you are working independently, share your completed workbox activities with a colleague or mentor.

2. **Peer Feedback Guidance**. As you listen to your partner, you hone the valuable skills of critiquing. Your goal is to help your partner refine the mixed methods data analysis strategy. Review the face value of each of the mixed methods data analysis steps chosen. Are there any strategies that don't make sense?

3. **Group Debrief**. If you are in a classroom or large-group setting, take volunteers to present the steps in their mixed methods data analysis plan. Reflect on how the strategies chosen help illuminate issues in the analysis strategy for your mixed methods project.

Concluding Thoughts

Use this checklist to assess your progress in achieving the Chapter 13 objectives:

☐ I applied seven primary mixed methods data analysis steps in my MMR or evaluation project.

☐ I assembled the mixed data, conducted a data collection inventory, considered gaps in the data sources, took steps to address deficiencies, and considered data reduction.

☐ I evaluated the mixed data relative to the specific hypotheses and questions, used an independent or interactive data analysis approach, and looked for new mixed methods questions given emerging findings.

☐ I identified commonalities between the two types of data using mixed methods analysis.

☐ I organized the linked qualitative and quantitative findings using a narrative approach or a visual means.

☐ I examined the "fit" of the qualitative and quantitative data together for convergence, complementarity, expansion, and/or divergence.

☐ I refined and/or reconstructed the mixed findings using tables, graphs, or figures.

☐ I interpreted and wrote out the findings using either a separate, "contiguous" structure or "weaving" structure with qualitative and quantitative findings presented together.

☐ I reviewed my mixed methods analysis procedures with a peer or colleague to refine my approach.

Now that you have completed these objectives, Chapter 14 will help you use joint displays for your MMR or evaluation project.

Key Resources

1. **FURTHER READING ON INTEGRATION THROUGHOUT THE MIXED METHODS PROJECT**

   • Creamer, E. G. (2018). *An introduction to fully integrated mixed methods research*. Thousand Oaks, CA: Sage.

   • Easterby-Smith, M., Thorpe, R., & Jackson, P. (2015). *Management and business research* (5th ed.). Thousand Oaks, CA: Sage.

   • Fetters, M. D., & Molina-Azorin, J. F. (2017). The *Journal of Mixed Methods Research* starts a new decade: The mixed methods research integration trilogy and its dimensions.

   Journal of Mixed Methods Research, 11(3), 291–307. doi:10.1177/1558689817714066

2. **FURTHER READING ON MIXED DATA ANALYSIS STRATEGIES**

   • Bazeley, P. (2012). Integrative analysis strategies for mixed data sources. *American Behavioral Scientist, 56*(6), 814–828. doi:10.1177/0002764211426330

   • Bazeley, P., & Kemp, L. (2012). Mosaics, triangles, and DNA: Metaphors for integrated analysis in mixed methods research. *Journal of Mixed Methods Research, 6*(1), 55–72. doi:10.1177/1558689811419514

- Bazeley, P. (2018). *Integrating analysis in mixed methods research*. Thousand Oaks, CA: Sage.
- Guetterman, T. C., Fetters, M. D., & Creswell, J. W. (2015). Integrating quantitative and qualitative results in health science mixed methods research through joint displays. *Annals of Family Medicine, 13*(6), 554–561. doi:10.1370/afm.1865
- Johnson, R. B., & Christensen, L. (2017). *Educational research: Quantitative, qualitative, and mixed approaches* (6th ed.). Thousand Oaks, CA: Sage.
- O'Cathain, A., Murphy, E., & Nicholl, J. (2010). Three techniques for integrating data in mixed methods studies. *BMJ, 341*, c4587. doi:10.1136/bmj.c4587

3. **FURTHER READING ON QUALITATIVE ANALYSIS**

- Creswell, J. W. (2016). *30 essential skills for the qualitative researcher*. Thousand Oaks, CA: Sage.
- Miles, M. B., Huberman, A. M., & Saldaña, J. (2014). *Qualitative data analysis* (3rd ed.). Thousand Oaks, CA: Sage.
- O'Reilly, M., & Kiyimba, N. (2015). *Advanced qualitative research: A guide to using theory*. Thousand Oaks, CA: Sage.
- Patton, M. Q. (2015). *Qualitative research and evaluation methods* (4th ed.). Thousand Oaks, CA: Sage.

4. **FURTHER READING ON QUANTITATIVE ANALYSIS**

- Carlson, K. A., & Winquist, J. R. (2017). *An introduction to statistics: An active learning approach* (2nd ed.). Thousand Oaks, CA: Sage.
- Salkind, N. J. (2017). *Statistics for people who (think they) hate statistics* (6th ed.). Thousand Oaks, CA: Sage.
- Tokunaga, H. T. (2016). *Fundamental statistics for the social and behavioral sciences*. Thousand Oaks, CA: Sage.

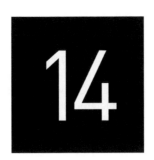

DEVELOPING A JOINT DISPLAY

Use of a joint display has increasingly become recognized as a state-of-the-art procedure for planning data collection, merging qualitative and quantitative data in mixed methods studies, and representing study findings. How to use a joint display for planning, analysis, and interpretation may seem like an enigma, but this chapter and its activities will help you understand features and applications of joint displays, distinguish how joint display structure varies with the mixed methods design, construct a joint display of mixed methods data collection, learn the overarching phases of joint display analysis, apply an approach for identifying linkages between qualitative and quantitative data, learn to create constructs from data linkages, consider both types of data together by drawing metainferences, and develop one or more joint displays for data representation. As a key outcome, you will develop one or more joint displays for illustrating mixed methods data collection procedures and/or mixed methods findings based on the specific design of your project.

LEARNING OBJECTIVES

To help you create a joint display as part of your mixed methods research (MMR) or evaluation project, this chapter illustrates key concepts and steps so you can

- Distinguish how a joint display structure varies with the type of mixed methods study design
- Construct a joint display of mixed methods data collection through joint display planning to match data collection and allow linkages between the qualitative and quantitative strands based on constructs held in common
- Learn overarching phases of joint display analysis to interpret mixed methods data
- Discover how linkages can be found between collected qualitative and quantitative data
- Acquire skills to create constructs from mixed data linkages to reflect an overarching idea, attribute, mental abstraction, working hypothesis, or theory for each construct
- Consider interpretations of both types of data together by drawing metainferences
- Develop one or more joint displays to represent your mixed data

WHAT IS A JOINT DISPLAY?

A joint display has become widely recognized as a highly effective tool for integrating qualitative and quantitative data (Creswell & Plano Clark, 2018). Joint displays and their development are a hot topic of discussion in the mixed methods literature. For example, Guetterman, Fetters, and Creswell (2015) examined key methodological and health science journals to illustrate the different types of joint displays and their application with various studies, as well as suggestions for developing joint displays. Johnson, Grove, and Clarke (2017) report on pillar integration as a joint display building technique to integrate data in mixed methods studies. Guetterman, Creswell, and Kuckartz (2015) provide details on how to create a joint display using software. Creswell and Plano Clark (2018) illustrate variations in joint displays according to core designs, convergent, exploratory sequential, explanatory sequential, as well as several complex (aka, advanced, scaffolded) designs, namely, mixed methods case study, evaluation, experimental (intervention), and participatory social justice designs.

Joint Display Definitions

As Creswell and Plano Clark (2018) describe:

A joint display (or integration display) is an approach to show the integration data analysis by arraying in a single table or graph the quantitative and qualitative data. This approach facilitates a more distinct and nuanced comparison of the results. In effect, the display merges the two forms of data. (p. 228)

Here, I use an expanded definition. A **joint display** is a table or a figure that can be used for organizing mixed data collection and analysis in a table, matrix, or figure that (1) can be used to represent juxtaposed data collection or findings of qualitative and quantitative strands of a project; (2) includes or implies specific linkages or areas of commonalities across the qualitative and quantitative strands that can be expressed as constructs or domains, and (3) contains an interpretation, often called metainferences, about the meaning of the two types of results when considered together.

Key Chapter Concepts

Joint display planning reflects the process of creating a table or matrix to juxtapose and match the constructs to be addressed through both the qualitative and quantitative data collection processes to ensure that two types of data will be linkable. A **joint display of mixed methods data collection** refers to a table or matrix depicting how both qualitative and quantitative data collection procedures have been matched to ensure collected data will address related study constructs, or for sequential designs, how the constructs of one type of data collection procedure were used to inform the constructs addressed in the subsequent, other type of data collection. **Joint display analysis** is the process of discovering linkages between the qualitative and quantitative constructs, organizing and reorganizing the findings into a matrix or figure to optimize the presentation as a finalized joint display. The process of building a joint display and developing different iterations yields new ways of thinking about the data, interpreting the meaning of the related data, and presenting the data (Fetters & Guetterman, forthcoming, 2020). The **joint display linkage activity** is a process of discovering commonalities between the qualitative and quantitative data and organizing the findings into a table, matrix, or figure. **Linking** is the active process of finding commonality between qualitative and quantitative data. **Linkages** represent content that is held in common between qualitative and quantitative data that forms a bond for associations, connections, or relations. A **construct** is an idea, attribute, mental abstraction, working hypothesis, or theory used to represent the linkages. Some authors may identify linkages as a **domain**, that is, an overarching area, sphere of activity, or thought. While constructs and domains are sometimes used interchangeably, domains suggest a broader range of ideas and typically comprise several constructs.

Variations in Joint Displays According to the Mixed Methods Design

Table 14.1 presents the options for creating a joint display for depicting mixed methods data collection according to the three core types of mixed methods designs (Chapter 7) and timing of the data collection.

TABLE 14.1 ■ Options for Creating a Joint Display of Mixed Methods Data Collection According to the Three Core Types of Mixed Methods Designs		
Design Type	**Timing Relative to Data Collection**	**Explanation**
Convergent mixed methods design	Before data collection begins	The researcher illustrates how mixed data collection will facilitate linking of the qualitative and quantitative strands *in advance*.
	After completing the sequential quantitative and qualitative data collection	In depicting the qualitative *and* quantitative data collection content or items, the researcher illustrates the specifics of how the mixed data collection was linked.

Design Type	Timing Relative to Data Collection	Explanation
Explanatory sequential mixed methods design	Before data collection begins	By depicting the constructs addressed in the first-phase quantitative data collection and the second-phase qualitative data collection *in advance*, the researcher illustrates the intended linkages *through* the two phases of data collection.
	After the first-phase quantitative findings are obtained, depicting the planned qualitative data collection of the second phase	By depicting the *completed* quantitative data collection source of the first phase and the *proposed* qualitative data collection during the second phase, the researcher illustrates how there *will be* linkages for specific constructs.
	After completing both first-phase quantitative and second-phase qualitative data collection	By depicting the constructs addressed during the completed first-phase quantitative data collection *and* second-phase qualitative data collection, the researcher illustrates how there were linkages for study constructs.
Exploratory sequential mixed methods design	Before data collection begins	By depicting the constructs addressed in the first-phase qualitative data collection and second-phase quantitative data collection *in advance*, the researcher illustrates the intended linkages *through* both phases of data collection.
	After the first-phase qualitative data findings are obtained, depicting the planned quantitative data collection of the second phase	By depicting the constructs addressed during the *completed* first-phase qualitative data collection and the proposed quantitative data collection during the second phase, the researcher illustrates how there *will be* linkages for specific constructs.
	After completing both the first-phase qualitative and second-phase quantitative data collection	By depicting the constructs addressed during the completed first-phase qualitative data collection *and* second-phase quantitative data collection, the researcher illustrates how there were linkages for specific constructs.

JOINT DISPLAY PLANNING

The variations in joint display planning can thus be best understood in consideration of the design, namely, convergent design, explanatory sequential design, and exploratory sequential design.

Creating a Joint Display of Mixed Methods Data Collection When Planning for a Convergent Mixed Methods Design

In the case of a convergent mixed methods design, the two possibilities for use of a data collection joint display are included before the initial mixed methods data collection begins or after both forms of data have been collected. The joint display can be used for representing the integration strategies depicted in Chapter 10 at a more detailed level. That is, the data collection joint display can show the integration relative to matching, expanding, diffracting strategies for data collection, or connecting procedures for an embedded sampling strategy (Chapter 10).

Before data collection begins in a mixed methods research or evaluation project. Prior to starting data collection in a convergent mixed methods design, a joint display can be used to plan the content of the qualitative and quantitative data collection for a convergent design. By considering the qualitative and quantitative constructs of convergent data collection in advance, the researcher illustrates explicitly how the mixed data collection will facilitate linking of the qualitative and quantitative strands after completing data collection.

After completing the sequential quantitative and qualitative data collection. A joint display of mixed data collection in a convergent mixed methods design can illustrate the linkages between the qualitative and quantitative constructs. By depicting mixed data collection using the constructs of both the qualitative *and* quantitative data collection in a joint display, the researcher illustrates the specifics of how the mixed data collection (e.g., qualitative interview questions or observation content and quantitative survey items or scales) were linked.

Creating a Joint Display of Mixed Methods Data Collection When Planning for an Explanatory Sequential Mixed Methods Design

In the case of an explanatory sequential mixed methods design, the three applications of a joint display of mixed data collection are (1) before the initial quantitative data collection begins, (2) after the initial quantitative data have been collected, or (3) after all data collection has been completed. Review Figure 10.1 as a conceptual model providing the basis for development of a joint display depicting the linkages of the quantitative constructs and development of qualitative questions to address related constructs. Considering the intents of integration depicted in Chapter 10, the focus may be on matching as one-to-one alignment of the content of data collection; diffracting, expanding, hypothesis generating quantitatively and validation qualitatively, or model development quantitatively and validation qualitatively. Adjunctive strategies of ascertaining (documenting) the need, optimizing, and monitoring can also be depicted in a joint display.

Before data collection begins. By depicting the data collection source (e.g., items or scales of the first-phase quantitative and the second-phase qualitative data collection research questions or observation content *before* data collection), the researcher illustrates how there will be data collection linkages *during* both phases of data collection that will lead to constructs addressed by both types of data.

After the first-phase quantitative findings are obtained, depicting the planned qualitative data collection of the second phase. By depicting mixed data collection the *completed* quantitative data collection source (e.g., items or scales of the first phase) and the *proposed* qualitative data collection during the second phase (e.g., interview questions or observation plans in a joint display), the researcher illustrates how there will be linkages for specific constructs.

After completing both first-phase quantitative and second-phase qualitative data collection. By depicting mixed data collection the constructs addressed in the completed first phase of quantitative data collection, e.g., survey items or scales, *and* in the completed qualitative data collection of the second phase, e.g., interview questions or observations in a joint display, the researcher illustrates how there were data collection linkages for study constructs. A joint display of mixed data collection in an explanatory sequential MMR or evaluation study can depict how the first-phase quantitative constructs were used to link to qualitative data collection addressing the same constructs.

Creating a Joint Display of Mixed Methods Data Collection When Planning for an Exploratory Sequential Mixed Methods Design

In the case of an exploratory sequential mixed methods design, the three applications of a joint display of mixed data collection are (1) before the initial qualitative data collection begins, (2) after the initial qualitative data have been collected, or (3) after both qualitative and subsequent qualitative data have been collected. Review Figure 10.2 as a conceptual model depicting how the constructs, in this case themes, are developed into scales, their related codes developed into variables, and associated quotations are developed into items. In consideration of the intents of integration depicted in Chapter 10, the focus may be on matching, diffracting, expanding, hypothesis generating qualitatively and validation quantitatively, or model development qualitatively and validation quantitatively. Adjunctive strategies of ascertaining (documenting) the need, optimizing, and monitoring can also be depicted in a joint display.

Before data collection begins. By depicting mixed data collection, the constructs addressed in the first phase of qualitative data collection (e.g., with interview questions or observation content) and the constructs of the second phase of quantitative data collection in a joint display, the researcher illustrates the intended linkages *through* both phases of data collection.

After the first phase of qualitative data findings are obtained, depicting the planned quantitative data collection of the second phase. By depicting the constructs addressed in a joint display of mixed data collection from the first phase of qualitative data collection (e.g., with interview questions or observation content) and the constructs of the second phase of quantitative data collection (e.g., items or scales), the researcher illustrates how there will be linkages *through* both phases of data collection. When initial qualitative findings have been analyzed, the use of a joint display of mixed data collection is appropriate for depicting systematically the specific data collection sources and questions to be used in the subsequent quantitative phase.

After completing both the first-phase qualitative and second phase-quantitative data collection. By depicting in a joint display of mixed data collection the constructs addressed during the qualitative data collection (e.g., interview questions or observation content) completed in the first phase *and* the quantitative data collection (e.g., survey items or scales) completed in the second phase, the researcher illustrates how there were linkages for specific constructs.

When Can a Joint Display of Mixed Methods Data Collection Be Used?

Before data collection for any three of the designs occurs, a joint display of mixed data collection is useful for a dissertation proposal, a contract proposal for an evaluation, or a grant proposal for funding. When data collection is completed, a joint display of mixed data collection can be used for inclusion in a dissertation, an evaluation report, a white paper, or an article for publication, as illustrated by the mixed methods study by Wu et al. (2018).

An Example of Joint Display of Mixed Methods Data Collection Used in a Multiphase Mixed Methods Investigation Focused on Improving Contraceptive Care for Women With Chronic Medical Issues

Concerned about the barriers for women with chronic medical problems (e.g., diabetes mellitus and hypertension) having access to contraceptive care, Wu et al. (2018) secured funding to design and implement a theory-driven, Web-based tool for women with chronic medical problems based on national recommendations for contraceptive care options (Workbox Illustration 14.1.1). In Phase I of the three-phase study, the authors proposed to conduct assessments in community medical offices with women affected by chronic medical diseases, their doctors, and staff members. They developed a theory-driven, joint display for data collection (Wu called it a mixed methods matrix) that featured the theoretical constructs and matching to the mixed methods data collection. Workbox Illustration 14.1.1, modified from the original more complex figure, illustrates one component of their data collection strategy. They used constructs (Column 1) from the transtheoretical model of behavior change (Prochaska, 2008) to identify questions for examination quantitatively on a 19-item survey for medical providers (Column 2), and qualitative data collection was based on variations in a clinical vignette (Column 3).

As illustrated by three constructs chosen from theory, Wu et al. (2018) developed specific quantitative and qualitative data collection strategies. This data collection joint display was used in the application for funding. As illustrated in the mixed methods data collection display, there is not an exact one-to-one match of quantitative and qualitative questions. This data collection joint display shows linkages of the quantitative survey questions and the qualitative interview questions about each of three constructs.

Workbox Illustration 14.1.1: Joint Display of Mixed Methods Data Collection (Wu et al., 2018)

Overarching Theoretical Construct	Quantitative Data Collection Source	Qualitative Data Collection Source
Knowledge: Familiarity with guidelines for contraceptive use for woman with chronic medical problems	Four hypothetical scenarios to assess if a clinician would recommend an intrauterine device under different medical circumstances (responses for the four scenarios: yes, no, I don't know).	Vignette: A woman with diabetes mellitus and obesity presents for a well exam. Question: "How you would typically approach this visit?"
	Four hypothetical scenarios to assess if a clinician would recommend oral contraceptive pills under different medical circumstances (responses for the four scenarios: yes, no, I don't know).	Scenario 2: The same woman from Scenario 1 comes for a visit to discuss her diabetes care and medications. Question: "How you would typically approach this visit?"
	Single question regarding whether the clinician has ever heard of national recommendations for birth control selection for women with different medical conditions	
Skills: Scope of contraceptive practice	Multiple-item question inquiring about the clinician's own scope of contraceptive practice, including provision of contraceptive devices, and referrals to other providers	Follow-up prompts about family planning.
Beliefs: About ability to deliver contraceptive care	Multiple-item question asking about how prepared a clinician feels to discuss specific contraceptive methods	What information would you need to discuss these methods?
		Are there clinical or medical conditions more challenging than others? Explain.

Source: Modified based on Wu et al. (2018) and Wu, J. (2017–22). *Improving Contraceptive Care for Women with Chronic Conditions: A Novel: Web-Based Decision Aid in Primary Care.* National Institute of Child Development and Human Health. 1 K23 HD084744-01A1 with permission.

Activity: Creating a Joint Display of Mixed Methods Data Collection

Workbox Illustration 14.1.1 provides an example of a joint display to depict and match mixed data collection to guide completion of your own joint display in Workbox 14.1.2. Follow the checklist in Workbox 14.2 to complete the activity.

Workbox 14.1.2: Creating a Joint Display of Mixed Methods Data Collection

Title. A Joint Display Depicting Data Collection in a(n) _____ Mixed Methods Design for the _____ Project on _____.		
Overarching Theoretical Construct	**Quantitative or Qualitative** (*choose one*) **Data Collection Source**	**Qualitative or Quantitative** (*choose one*) **Data Collection Source**

Workbox 14.2: Checklist for Creating a Joint Display of Mixed Methods Data Collection

Check off the steps while completing the joint display of mixed methods data collection planning:

☐ Complete the title

☐ Choose what phase from the three designs to represent from Table 14.1 based on your design and your current status of data collection

☐ Decide on the order of the quantitative and qualitative data collection sources in the top row

☐ Identify the constructs to use in Column 1, based on theory or a conceptual model

☐ Complete the quantitative data collection sources column to match the quantitative data collection for each construct in Column 1

☐ Complete the qualitative data collection sources column to match the qualitative data collection for each construct in Column 1

Steps for Completing the Workbox for Creating a Joint Display of Mixed Methods Data Collection

1. **Complete the title.** In the first blank, insert the type of your design. In the second blank, insert the title of your project. In the third blank, insert the topic of the study.

2. **Choose what stage you will be representing from Table 14.1 based on your design and your current status of data collection.** Based on whether you are currently in the design stage, the midst of data collection, or in a post-data-collection stage, determine the extent to which your entries in Workbox 14.1.2 will be projections or choices.

3. **Decide on the order of the quantitative and qualitative data collection sources in the top row.** If you are planning an explanatory sequential mixed methods design (QUAN to QUAL) or a quantitatively driven convergent design (QUAN + QUAL), use Workbox 14.1.2 as presented. If you are conducting an exploratory sequential mixed methods design (QUAL to QUAN) or a qualitatively driven convergent design (QUAL + QUAN), change the order of Columns 2 and 3 to "Qualitative Data Collection Source" and "Quantitative Data Collection Source," respectively.

4. **Identify the constructs to use in Column 1.** Theoretical models (social sciences) or conceptual models (health sciences) typically have multiple constructs. While somewhat arbitrary, it is good practice to follow the same order of the constructs as presented by developers of the theory or conceptual model.

5. **Complete the quantitative data collection sources column to match the quantitative data collection for each construct in Column 1.** Looking back at your quantitative data sources table from Chapter 6, and using other related documents (e.g., a diagram of the theory or conceptual model), fill in Column 2 with the qualitative data collection items that will address the construct in your mixed methods data collection. If you are using scales from an existing instrument, you can include the scale name. If you develop a more detailed version, you may add all the questions.

6. **Complete the qualitative data collection sources column to match the qualitative data collection for each construct in Column 1.** Looking back at your qualitative data sources table from Chapter 6, and using any other related documents (e.g., a diagram of the theory or conceptual model to guide you), fill in Column 3 with the qualitative data collection items that will be used to address the construct in your mixed methods data collection. If using multiple qualitative data collection sources (e.g., interviews, observations, existing documents), follow the same order (as it makes the most sense for your study) for each question/source and the related construct.

Optional Features for Data Collection Planning

The joint display activity Worksheet 14.1.2 illustrates the essential features of a joint display for data collection. Other features can be added. For example, Wu et al. (2018) added specific item and question numbers to their joint display. This format provided here is meant to be a basic framework. Based on project needs, you can alter it accordingly.

JOINT DISPLAY ANALYSIS

In addition to its utility for illustrating data collection sources in MMR and evaluation studies, the joint display can be used to organize, reorganize, and represent mixed methods findings. Now, you will learn to recognize the key elements of a joint display used for analyzing and portraying mixed methods findings. You will then learn how to identify linkages between the collected qualitative and quantitative data, and then label each resulting construct to reflect an overarching idea, attribute, mental abstraction, working hypothesis or theory, based on commonality in both types of data. Based on completion of this activity, you will be ready to develop a refined joint display to represent your mixed data findings.

Elements of Joint Display Analysis for a Mixed Methods Research or Evaluation Study

Figure 14.1 illustrates the elements of a joint display for analysis. Adapted from Legocki et al. (2015) and Fetters and Guetterman (forthcoming, 2020), this adaptation is one of six joint displays the authors used in the primary publication by Legocki et al. (2015). In this project, the team evaluated the process of multiple stakeholders developing randomized controlled trials using adaptive designs (Guetterman, Fetters, Legocki et al., 2015; Meurer et al., 2012). Adaptive designs remain controversial as some scholars support adaptive designs, while others are skeptical. The research team evaluated the development process and provided real-time suggestions for improving the process. One aspect of their evaluation involved assessing the attitudes of four groups engaged in the adaptive-trials-development process about ethical aspects of adaptive designs (Story From the Field 14.1). Ethical aspects are one area of contention among polarized camps of researchers, and for this evaluation, the investigators assessed the participants' attitudes and discussions/reflections about ethical aspects of adaptive designs (Legocki et al., 2015). The attitudinal scores of the four groups provided quantitative data, and discussions from mini-focus groups and comments from open-ended questions on the survey constituted the qualitative data.

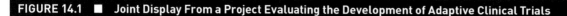

FIGURE 14.1   ■   Joint Display From a Project Evaluating the Development of Adaptive Clinical Trials

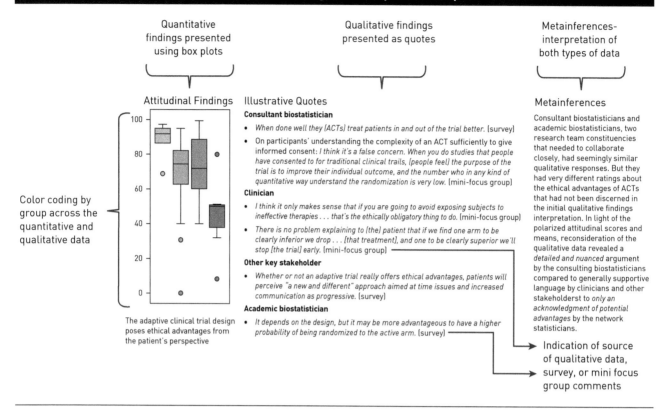

Source: Fetters, M. D., & Guetterman, T. C. (forthcoming, 2020) Development of a joint display as mixed analysis. In T. Onwuegbuzie & R. B. Johnson (Eds.), *Reviewer's guide for mixed methods research analysis.* Routledge.

Adapted from Legocki, L. J., Meurer, W. J., Frederiksen, S., Lewis, R. J., Durkalski, V. L., Berry, D. A., . . . Fetters, M. D. (2015). Clinical trialist perspectives on the ethics of adaptive clinical trials: A mixed-methods analysis. *BMC Medical Ethics, 16*(1), 27. doi:10.1186/ s12910-015-0022-z

Features of the Figure 14.1 Joint Display

As advised by Guetterman, Fetters, and Creswell (2015), this figure illustrates three key elements. The first two columns are labeled with the qualitative and quantitative findings and are consistent in ordering with the design and approach. The last column displays their interpretations/metainferences. From the left to right, the first component in this joint display is *quantitative results* that the authors represented with box plots representing combined responses to a single question on a 100-point visual analog scale. The middle component of the joint display depicts *qualitative illustrative quotes* from four key stakeholder groups: consultant biostatisticians, clinicians, other stakeholders, and academic biostatisticians. The source of the information, open comments from the survey, or comments from the mini-focus groups indicated in the parentheses provide transparency about the data source. The gray scale of the box plots correlates with the gray scale of the qualitative data of the four stakeholder groups. The right-most section *metainferences*, represents interpretations of the quantitative and qualitative data. Story From the Field 14.1 provides additional background about this innovative joint display. As illustrated by this example, the quantitative data were changed from their numerical form into a visual form that provides an example of how a joint display may involve structural change in the data, and hence meet the Bazeley and Kemp (2012) criteria for a type of advanced analysis (see also Chapters 13 and 15).

Example Illustrating Joint Display Analysis in a Mixed Methods Project

While not obvious by looking at a published joint display, the final table or figure often results from a process of multiple iterative back-and-forth reconfigurations of the quantitative and qualitative data, as depicted by Fetters and Guetterman (forthcoming, 2020). Commonalities between the two types of data have to be discovered (Kron et al., 2017). To build the joint display for the ADAPT-IT project, attitudinal scores were calculated and depicted with means and standard deviations. Then qualitative data from open comments and findings from mini-focus groups were organized. The quantitative data were reconfigured with box plots. These were then flipped from a lateral to a vertical axis. As there were four groups in the analysis, illustrative textual findings were linked by color with the box plots (see original for the color variations), and then the box plots were reorganized to illustrate a trend across the groups. A final step involved looking at both types of data to draw the metainferences (see Story From the Field 14.1).

STORY FROM THE FIELD 14.1

An Innovative Joint Display Depicting Quantitative and Qualitative
Data Linked With Color Shades and Metainferences Based on the Mixed Data Findings

While working on a National Institutes of Health grant with a mixed methods evaluation of Bayesian design development for randomized controlled trials, we collected qualitative data from mini-focus groups and open-ended questions on a baseline survey. We also collected quantitative data as scores from six visual analog scales with anchors ranging from 0 to 100 that allowed participants to rank their level of agreement about ethical advantages and disadvantages from the perspectives of three groups: patients, researchers, and society. The final joint display as illustrated in Figure 14.1 required six iterations. This figure quickly became an exemplar for presenting qualitative and quantitative

data together with features of box plots of the quantitative data and quotes from the qualitative data (Fetters, Curry, & Creswell, 2013). When writing about this joint display a process of data analysis for a book chapter, we decided to add a column for metainferences, as these were not in the orginal published joint display (Fetters & Guetterman, forthcoming, 2020), to emphasize fully state-of-the-art procedures of joint display analysis. When carefully considering both results together for the metainferences column, a new interpretation emerged. In short, creating the metainferences column also forced us to consider the meaning of both the qualitative and quantitative findings together from a new perspective.

DISCOVERING LINKAGES BETWEEN THE QUALITATIVE AND QUANTITATIVE DATA FOR JOINT DISPLAY ANALYSIS

Discovering linkages in mixed data can be achieved through a mixed methods data linking activity as depicted in Workbox Illustrations 14.3.1.1 and 14.3.1.2. The purpose of the mixed methods data linking activity in Workbox 14.3.2 is to organize the qualitative sources and the associated themes from these qualitative sources and to organize the quantitative sources and the associated quantitative findings, as measured by survey items. Upon doing so, the linkages between the qualitative themes and quantitative constructs can be identified.

Workbox Illustration 14.3.1.1: Linking Mixed Data in the MPathic-VR Mixed Methods Medical Education Study

Sources: Kron et al. (2017) and Fetters, M.D. and Kron, F.W. (2012–15). *Modeling Professional Attitudes and Teaching Humanistic Communication in Virtual Reality (MPathic-VRII).* National Center for Advancing Translational Science/NIH 9R44TR000360-04. Workbox Illustration created by the *Mixed Methods Research Workbook* author.

Workbox Illustration 14.3.1.2: Mixed Methods Data Linking in the MPathic-VR Mixed Methods Medical Education Project

Workbox Illustration 14.3.1.1 provides a completed example of an MMR linkage activity. This illustration is based upon the MPathic-VR virtual human mixed methods multisite randomized controlled trial comparing a virtual human computer simulation with training using a mixed media computer-based learning module (Kron et al., 2017).

Qualitative strand. The qualitative data collection sources for the project fill the first column. Relevant data were student reflections from an essay written after exposure to the intervention or control. Process observational notes from preceptors who were present during the training were also available. From these qualitative data collection sources came the qualitative data findings sources, a series of major themes found in the second column on empathetic communication, interactive learning, communications, useful verbal and nonverbal communication skills, and system features. Each of these themes had an additional 5–7 subthemes that were not included in the interest of space.

Quantitative strand. Inserted into the final fifth column are the quantitative data collection sources of information available from the study and attitudinal scales administered postexposure to the intervention and control. Additional sources not listed (due to the current focus on the mixed methods question on students' attitudes and experiences with the system) were objective-structured clinical examination (OSCE) scores (a simulated patient experience when students' skills are evaluated) and scores for the control students only from the MPathic-VR simulation achieved during the intervention (Kron et al., 2017). Illustrated in the fourth column, second from the right side, are the quantitative data findings sources, namely, the items from the survey. These include measures designed to understand the students' attitudes about their experiences relative to empathy, verbal, nonverbal, as well as items about the process and about interacting with the system.

Linking qualitative themes and quantitative survey items. The middle column features linkages between related qualitative themes and quantitative survey items. These linkages become study constructs. For example, the qualitative theme empathetic communication has commonality with the quantitative survey item "the training was effective for learning to handle emotionally charged situations." These two sources provided an appropriate match for juxtaposition in a joint display.

The second major theme from the qualitative findings about interactive learning has subthemes on "objective learning," "be prepared," "motivated to learn more," and "need more practice." Regarding interactive learning, there are related quantitative data findings with common meaning in several quantitative survey items, namely, Item 3: "Training was engaging," Item 7: "Improve clinical skills," and Item 10: "Interaction realistic." The lines from interactive learning to the survey items "Training was engaging," "Improve clinical skills," and "Interaction realistic" thus reflect linkages. The overarching construct to represent the linkage becomes interactivity. These two examples illustrate that there can be one-to-one linkages from a qualitative finding to a quantitative finding, or one-to-several items. The origins of this activity are depicted in Story From the Field 14.2.

Sources: Kron et al. (2017) and Fetters, M.D. and Kron, F.W. (2012–15). Modeling Professional Attitudes and Teaching Humanistic Communication in Virtual Reality (MPathic-VRII). National Center for Advancing Translational Science/NIH 9R44TR000360-04.

Activity: Mixed Methods Data Linking

The "Mixed Methods Data Linking" activity as seen in Workbox 14.3.2 has the qualitative data collection sources on the left and the quantitative data collection sources in the column furthest to the right. You can use this structure, or use a mirror image of the diagram by flipping the strand sides, if it better suits your project. Workbox 14.4 provides a checklist of steps to go through and complete this activity.

Workbox 14.3.2: Mixed Methods Data Linking

Qualitative Data Collection Sources	Qualitative Data Findings Sources	Connect With Lines	Quantitative Data Findings Sources	Quantitative Data Collection Sources

Workbox 14.4: Checklist for Completing the
Mixed Methods Data Linking Activity

Check off the steps as you complete the mixed methods data linking activity:

☐ Organize the information relative to the qualitative strand, including the data collection and findings sources, and the quantitative strand, including the data collection and findings sources

☐ Complete the qualitative data collection sources column

☐ Complete the qualitative data findings sources column

☐ Complete the quantitative data collection sources column

☐ Complete the quantitative data findings sources column

☐ Connect with lines the related qualitative data findings and quantitative data findings

MIXED METHODS DATA LINKING ACTIVITY

The following six steps will assist you in completing Workbox 14.4 Mixed Data Linking.

1. **Organize the information relative to the qualitative strand including the data collection and findings sources, and the quantitative strand including the data collection and findings sources.** For your qualitative and quantitative data collection sources, you may want to check your Chapter 6 data sources table and Chapter 13 data collection inventory. The project coding scheme may be the best organized source of information about the qualitative themes and subthemes for populating the qualitative data findings sources column. For the quantitative data findings sources, a good source of information is the survey items, or scales if you have multiple survey items.

2. **Complete the qualitative data collection sources column.** In the qualitative sources column, fill in the relevant qualitative data collection sources from your project with adequate space between each source entered. For example, this might include interviews, qualitative observations, or documents.

3. **Complete the qualitative data findings sources column.** For each qualitative data collection source, insert the relevant qualitative data findings. If you have used a comprehensive coding scheme for all data sources, the qualitative data findings may not match. However, in some cases, they can differ (e.g., observational findings or record review may have different, nonoverlapping findings from themes and subthemes coded from interviews). Starting with more overarching findings (e.g., themes rather than subthemes) generally is the easiest place to start. Start by adding the themes you have identified from your intra-method analysis of the qualitative data. After better understanding of the overall linkages, in a subsequent iteration, you may want to add subthemes.

4. **Complete the quantitative data collection sources column.** In the quantitative sources column, enter the different quantitative data sources from your project with adequate space between each source entered. For example, this might include instruments or scales.

5. **Complete the quantitative data findings sources column.** For each quantitative source, insert the relevant quantitative data findings source. Starting with more overarching findings (e.g., scales rather than items) generally is the easiest place to begin. As in the example, you might want to start with survey items. If you have collected multiple survey and scales, it may be easier to start at a more general level.

6. **Connect with lines-related qualitative data findings and quantitative data findings.** Examine the qualitative data finding sources and the quantitative data findings sources. Use a "linkage line" to connect related qualitative sources and the quantitative sources. Linkages reflect an overarching idea, attribute, mental abstraction, working hypothesis, or theory, based on commonality in both types of data. As illustrated in the discussion of Workbox Illustration 14.3.1.2, in some cases, a single theme may link with multiple constructs. Conversely, a single scale or item may link to qualitative themes. After you find general areas of linkages, you may wish to proceed with creation of additional linking activities featuring more detailed subthemes or items from the scales. The level of detail feasible and required is project dependent.

Having completed the linkage activity, you are now ready to create a joint display.

Organizing and Reorganizing the Linked Mixed Methods Data in a Joint Display Structure

Once linkages have been identified and labeled as a construct, the two types of data can be organized into the first iteration of a joint display. In the first iteration of the joint display, the analyst organizes the linked qualitative and quantitative data together in a logical way in a matrix, table, or figure as illustrated in Workbox Illustration 14.3.1.1. After you create the first joint display, you will most likely want to reorganize it with the intent of trying to make the content easier to understand. Try different ways of expressing the quantitative data, integers, graphs, pie charts, and bar graphs. I have found waiting several days between versions allows me to have new ideas for restructuring to be more effective. Use the criteria of "What organizational structure would be most easy for the reader to understand?"

Creating a Joint Display in the MPathic-VR Mixed Methods Medical Education Project

As illustrated in Workbox Illustration 14.5.1, a joint display table can be created from the linkage exercise (Kron et al., 2017). As a reminder, the MPathic-VR study sought to demonstrate the potential benefit of communication skills training through a virtual human. Medical students were randomized to the interventional arm featuring the virtual reality training module, or to the control arm featuring a standard computer-based learning module, to determine if exposure to the virtual reality training arm resulted in superior communication skills.

Choosing a logical ordering and structure. After reviewing the qualitative themes and quantitative constructs, consideration was given to ordering of the columns. In this study, the more logical choice was to place the qualitative findings in the first column and the quantitative findings in the second column. The third column is a place for recording a preliminary interpretation of the significance of the two types of findings relative to each other.

Qualitative findings. The qualitative findings are inserted into the first column. The ordering selected was verbal, nonverbal, engagement, effectiveness, and improve clinical skills. This made sense as a continuum from the kind of communication (verbal and nonverbal), which related to how the system did (or did not) engage the user, how effective the experience was, and finally, specific skills acquired, since these would apply in the future and would be the ultimate outcome of the training simulation.

Quantitative findings. The quantitative findings entry followed from the qualitative findings. The attitudinal items were the results of student rankings about their experiences with training on a 7-point Likert scale. Higher scores on the 7-point Likert scale were more positive. As there were two groups, the mean score and standard deviation for attitudinal items were entered into the appropriate row for both the intervention arm and control arm.

Interpreting Related Mixed Data

The third phase involves considering the findings of the two types of data together to draw metainferences, that is, an overall interpretation of both types of findings. Workbox Illustration 14.5.1 provides an example of the metainferences as added and serves as an example for your completion of Workbox 14.5.2. Metainferences require intensely comparing the two types of information together.

Interpreting the Two Types of Findings by Drawing Metainferences in the MPathic-VR Mixed Methods Medical Education Study

As illustrated, a preliminary assessment of the fit of the qualitative and quantitative data was made (see below, and also Chapter 13), as well as an interpretation of the meaning of the fit. In the MPathic-VR study, the authors found convergence for four of five constructs and discordance for one (Kron et al., 2017).

Workbox Illustration 14.5.1: Creating a Joint Display of Related Qualitative Themes and Quantitative Survey Items in the MPathic-VR Mixed Methods Medical Education Project

Qualitative Themes	Quantitative Survey Items mean (standard deviation)	Comment (metainferences)
1. Verbal communication	Item 4. Verbal communication Intervention: 5.02 (1.62) Control: 3.89 (1.67)	Convergence–intervention arm had a deeper understanding of the content compared to the control in qualitative data, confirmed by higher attitudinal scores.
2. Nonverbal communication	Item 5. Learn nonverbal communication. Intervention: 4.11 (1.85) Control: 2.77 (1.45)	Convergence–intervention arm qualitative data addressed the value of learning nonverbal communication, confirmed by higher attitudinal scores.

Qualitative Themes	Quantitative Survey Items mean (standard deviation)	Comment (metainferences)
3. Engagement of training/immediate reactions to learning experience	Item 3. Training was engaging. Intervention: 5.43 (1.55) Control: 3.69 (1.62)	Convergence–intervention data reflect engagement through the review, while the control comments suggested the need for interaction; difference confirmed by higher attitudinal scores.
4. Effectiveness in learning to handle emotionally charged situations	Item 6. Training effective for learning to handle emotionally charged situations. Intervention: 5.13 (1.48) Control: 2.34 (1.35)	Convergence–intervention arm comments indicate awareness of communication in emotionally charged situations, while control comments indicated need for additional training; confirmed by attitudinal scores.
5. Improve clinical skills	Item 7. Training will help me improve my clinical skills. Intervention: 4.93 (1.57) Control: 4.62 (1.40)	Discordance–intervention arm comments suggest the communication practice was more helpful in preparing for clinical work than the control arm; not supported by the attitudinal scores.

Source: Kron et al., (2017). Workbox Illustration adapted by the *Mixed Methods Research Workbook* author.

Activity: Conducting Joint Display Analysis

Having completed the linkage activity, and seen how joint display analysis occurred in a study, you are now ready to use joint display analysis to create your joint display. You will note the headers in Workbox 14.5.2 have you choose between qualitative and quantitative findings. Organize the linked data according to either the qualitative findings or quantitative findings in the order appropriate for your project. For simplicity, cross out the category you will not use in the top two rows of the second and third columns. Workbox 14.6 has a checklist of steps to follow to create your joint display.

Workbox 14.5.2: Using Joint Display Analysis to Create a Joint Display of Related Qualitative and Quantitative Findings

Overarching Constructs	Qualitative or Quantitative Findings (choose one)	Quantitative or Qualitative Findings (choose the other)	Comments (metainferences)
1.			
2.			
3.			
4.			
5.			
6.			
7.			

Workbox 14.6: Checklist for Using Joint Display Analysis to Create a Joint Display

Check off the steps as you complete the mixed data linkage activity:

☐ Confirm the underlying meaning of each type of data relative to the overarching construct

☐ Consider whether to organize the quantitative findings or the qualitative findings first in your display

☐ Label the constructs represented by the linkages

☐ Identify a logical ordering of the discovered constructs

(Continued)

(Continued)

☐ Place each construct into the table one row at a time for each construct created from pairing of qualitative and quantitative findings

☐ Reconsider the ordering of constructs created by the identified linkages

☐ Optimize the ordering of your columns

☐ Interpret collectively the qualitative and quantitative findings to draw metainferences

☐ Consider alternative presentations of your data

STEPS FOR CREATING A JOINT DISPLAY USING JOINT DISPLAY ANALYSIS

The following six steps will assist you in completing the Creating a Joint Display Workbox 14.5.2.

1. **Confirm the underlying meaning of each type of data relative to the overarching construct**. This requires ascertaining that the qualitative and quantitative findings are addressing the same construct. Take a moment to consider the degree to which both types of data have been collected with rigor from an intramethod perspective. If there are gaps where you would not have expected gaps, or findings that seem out of keeping, reconsider the rigor of your data collection and analysis procedures to determine if this could account for the discrepancy.

2. **Consider whether to organize the quantitative findings or the qualitative findings first in your display.** As described by Guetterman, Fetters, and Creswell (2015), organizing the joint display according to the design often makes sense. For example, in an explanatory sequential design or in a convergent design with a quantitatively driven component, listing the quantitative findings before the qualitative findings is effective. In an exploratory sequential design where qualitative findings lead to quantitative data collection, listing the qualitative findings first can be helpful. This holds as well for a convergent design that is qualitatively driven.

3. **Label the constructs represented by the linkages.** Having identified linkages between the qualitative and quantitative findings, the next step is to develop labels for the resulting constructs. Use a notepad or word processor to list the constructs represented by the linkages. In some cases, you may choose to use or adopt from an existing qualitative theme, as the overarching construct. Alternatively, if you have used a series of scales already reflecting certain constructs, you may choose these as the overarching constructs. Yet another option may be creating a new label to capture the construct. For examples, when one theme matches to multiple items, you should consider a construct label for each linkage. In studies that are qualitatively driven, the themes tend to become overarching constructs. In quantitatively driven research, the scales or survey topics tend to drive the overarching constructs. Ultimately, I recommend "listening to the data," that is, let the emerging findings drive your choices. Once you have identified the constructs with qualitative and quantitative data in common, you are ready to order the constructs for entry into a joint display.

4. **Identify a logical ordering of the linked constructs.** Having discovered a series of linked constructs on your notepad or in your word processor, you are ready to develop a logical ordering for insertion into a joint display. This requires judgment and creativity. If your project has an underlying theory, the theory may help provide an organizing structure to follow. As discussed, organization by the design may inform the order. For example, QUAN to QUAL explanatory sequential design logically lists the quantitative data first, and a QUAL to QUAN exploratory sequential design logically lists the qualitative data first.

5. **Place each construct into the table one row at a time for each construct created from pairing of qualitative and quantitative findings.** Having arranged the constructs in a logical order, the qualitative and quantitative findings can now be added into a joint display (see Workbox Illustration 14.5.1). Most researchers find they have options for multiple joint displays based on the volume of their data. For your first experience creating a joint display, I recommend you restrict your entries to no more than five to seven items. If several joint displays seem possible, begin with the one that is most intuitive. Over the course of many workshops, participants have found it easiest to follow the order of either the qualitative or the quantitative column if there are multiple joint displays.

6. **Reconsider the ordering of constructs created by the discovered linkages.** Does the order make sense for creating a narrative about the findings? Due to their iterative development, coding schemes of

qualitative data are often already organized in a logical fashion and can provide an overall organizational structure. There might be an underlying theory that could enhance the order. There may be a certain ordering of administration of quantitative instruments that suggest a logical order.

7. **Optimize the ordering of your columns.** Reconsider the ordering you have chosen relative to the qualitative and quantitative findings. Does it make more sense to have the qualitative or the quantitative findings listed first?

8. **Interpret collectively the qualitative and quantitative findings to draw metainferences.** Having satisfactorily found an order, that is, an overarching interpretation, a metainference is needed for each of the rows in the final column. The data comparison may lead to several interpretations (Fetters et al., 2013; Fetters & Molina-Azorin, 2017c; Greene, Caracelli, & Graham, 1989). Reconsider again the fit (Chapter 13). Convergence (also confirmation or concordance) denotes an interpretation when the two sources of data essentially confirm each other. Complementarity, as described by Greene et al. (1989), is an interpretation when the compared qualitative and quantitative data illustrate different, nonconflicting interpretations (see related concept of diffraction by Uprichard and Dawney, 2016). Expansion denotes an interpretation when the compared qualitative and quantitative data provide both a central overlapping, as well as a broader nonoverlapping interpretation (a hybrid of the situation of confirmation and complementarity). Discordance (or divergence) describes the situation when the qualitative and quantitative data lead to conflicting interpretations. When the metainferences conflict, the literature provides guidance on managing this outcome (Bazeley, 2018; Moffatt, White, Mackintosh, & Howel, 2006; Pluye et al., 2009) (see Chapter 13)

9. **Consider alternative presentations of your data.** Having created a draft joint display, now consider the overall appearance. Does the resulting joint display convey meaningfully what is found in the underlying data? Could you add representative quotes from the qualitative strand to help elaborate the qualitative findings? As illustrated in Story From the Field 14.1, you may go through multiple iterations of restructuring of your data presentation or restructuring of your figure. As part of this activity, participants often discover that a single joint display will not suffice, and they ultimately create several joint displays.

From Draft Joint Display to Polished Joint Display

The MPathic-VR findings are from a single blinded multisite randomized controlled trial (Kron et al., 2017). The joint display in Workbox Illustration 14.5.1 illustrates in the first column the overarching constructs. The second major column illustrates the findings from the intervention arm, but the quantitative findings as numerical scores, and the qualitative findings featuring representative quotes. In the third major column, the control findings are found, again featuring in parallel the quantitative scores and representative qualitative themes. The final column has the metainferences. For another joint display variation, review Figure 14.1 at the beginning of the chapter, as it illustrates how quantitative data can be presented using box plots. For additional examples of joint displays, see examples from Guetterman, Fetters, and Creswell (2015).

JOINT DISPLAY INNOVATIONS: A CIRCULAR JOINT DISPLAY

Mixed methods researchers are continuing to push the field forward with innovative methods, including the use of visualizations for data interpretation and presentation. One novel innovation in the realm of the joint display is the use of a circular joint display. Bustamante (2017) created a theory-driven joint display when she conducted a mixed methods case study (Figure 14.2). The unique presentation of this joint display involves progressive semicircular rings. At the core are overlapping circles and segments with the elements of theory as linked to the survey and its scales including the statistical significance. In addition, she created sections of related quantitative and qualitative data using "slices." By moving outward from the core, Bustamante added rings with the results of her qualitative analysis, first the qualitative themes and then, in another ring, illustrative quotes. In the outermost ring, she added her assessment of fit of the data, whether the qualitative and quantitative data confirm, expand, or are in discord. She illustrates the use of shading with quantitative data in black, qualitative data in white, and metainferences in gray. She has additionally used cross hatching to illustrate not significant or negative findings for the quantitative and qualitative findings, respectively. While not shown in this example, Bustamante could have added yet another ring containing written metainferences for each slice of the pie.

Workbox Illustration 14.7: Joint Display From the MPathic-VR Mixed Methods Medical Education Study

Domain	Intervention Arm		Control Arm		Metainferences
Domain	MPathic-VR		CBL		
	Attitudinal Item Mean (SD)	Qualitative Reflection Illustrative Quotes	Attitudinal Item Mean (SD)	Qualitative Reflection Illustrative Quotes	Interpretation of mixed methods findings
Verbal Communication	4.11 (1.85)	"How to introduce myself without making assumptions about the cultural background of the patient and the family"	2.77 (1.45)	"This educational module was useful for clarifying the use of SBAR and addressing ways that all members of a health care team can improve patient care through better communication skills"	Intervention arm comments suggest deeper understanding of the content than teaching using memorization and mnemonics as in the control, a difference confirmed by higher attitudinal scores.
Nonverbal Communication	5.13 (1.48)	"Effective communication involves non-verbal facial expression like smiling and head nodding"	2.34 (1.35)	None	Intervention arm comments address the value of learning non-verbal communication, the difference confirmed by attitudinal scores.
Training was engaging	5.43 (1.55)	"Reviewing the video review was a great way to see my facial expressions and it allowed me to improve on these skills the second time around"	3.69 (1.62)	"This experience can be improved by incorporating more active participation. For example, there could have been a scenario in which we would have to select the appropriate hand-off information per SBAR guideline"	Intervention arm comments reflect engagement through the after action review while the control comments suggested the need for interaction, the difference confirmed by higher attitudinal scores.

MPathic-VR: Modeling Professional Attitudes and Teaching Humanistic Communication in Virtual Reality; Computer-based learning; SBAR: Situation, Background, Assessment, Recommendation

Source: Adapted from Kron et al. (2017) with permission from Rightslink

FIGURE 14.2 ■ Illustration of a Circular Joint Display

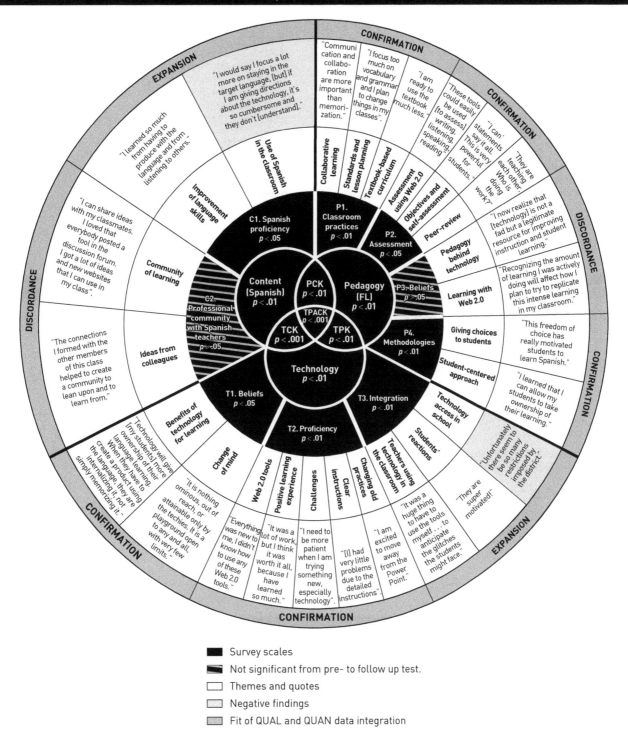

Survey scales

Not significant from pre- to follow up test.

Themes and quotes

Negative findings

Fit of QUAL and QUAN data integration

Source: Bustamante (2017). With permission.

Application Activities

1. **Peer Feedback.** If you are working on your project as part of a class or in a workshop, pair up with a peer mentor, and one of you spend about 5 minutes talking about your linkage activity and joint display. Take turns presenting and giving feedback. The helpful parts to discuss are those that you struggled with the most. In particular, focus on the ordering of your columns, the constructs and their order, and the metainferences you have drawn. Do they make sense to your partner? If working independently, share your worksheets with a colleague or mentor.

2. **Peer Feedback Guidance.** As you listen to your partner, you should focus on learning and honing the valuable skills of critiquing. Your goal is to help your partner refine the joint display. Focus on what section or area your partner needs feedback the most. Help him or her focus on effectiveness on the presentation. Does the order seem appropriate from left to right for the design? Does the organization of constructs from top to bottom make sense? Has your partner fully considered the meaning of both types of data in the metainferences cells? Can you think of alternative ways of presenting the joint display that may be more meaningful? Are there any sections that don't make sense, or seem infeasible?

3. **Group Debrief.** In a group setting, have each participant present in sequence the linkage figure, and then the resulting joint display. The participant can explain how the linkages were made, and how this transformed into the resulting joint display. Provide constructive feedback on alternative representations of the data. Reflect on how these same issues may play out in your own project.

Concluding Thoughts

Use this checklist to assess your progress in achieving the Chapter 14 objectives:

☐ I examined how a joint display structure varies with the type of mixed methods study design.

☐ I created a joint display of mixed methods data collection to ensure comparability of constructs found in common between the data collected in the qualitative and quantitative strands.

☐ I learned overarching phases of joint display analysis for mixed methods data.

☐ I discovered linkages between the data collected (or projected) in the qualitative and quantitative strands, and you labeled each to identify a construct to reflect an overarching idea, attribute, mental abstraction, working hypothesis, or theory, based on commonality in both types of my data.

☐ I labeled the linkages as constructs to reflect overarching ideas, attributes, mental abstractions, working hypotheses, or theory.

☐ I interpreted the two types of data together to draw out metainferences and examined for findings not otherwise obvious.

☐ I developed one or more joint display(s) or draft joint display to represent my mixed methods data collection or findings.

☐ I reviewed my Chapter 14 joint display activities and outputs with a peer or colleague to refine my joint displays.

Now that you have completed these objectives, Chapter 15 will help you consider additional advanced procedures of analysis for your MMR or evaluation project.

Key Resources

1. **USE OF JOINT DISPLAYS WITH DIFFERENT MIXED METHODS DESIGNS**

   - Creswell, J. W., & Plano Clark, V. L. (2018). *Designing and conducting mixed methods research* (3rd ed.). Thousand Oaks, CA: Sage.

2. **ILLUSTRATIONS OF VARIOUS JOINT DISPLAYS**

   - Guetterman, T. C., Fetters, M. D., & Creswell, J. W. (2015). Integrating quantitative and qualitative results in health science mixed methods research through joint displays. *Annals of Family Medicine, 13*(6), 554–561. doi:10.1370/afm.1865

3. **PROCEDURES FOR CREATION OF A JOINT DISPLAY**

   - Guetterman, T., Creswell, J. W., & Kuckartz, U. (2015). Using joint displays and MAXQDA software to represent the results of mixed methods research. In M. McCrudden, G. Schraw, & C. Buckendahl (Eds.), *Use of visual displays in research and testing: Coding, interpreting, and reporting data* (pp. 145–175). Charlotte, NC: Information Age Publishing.

   - Johnson, R. E., Grove, A. L., & Clarke, A. (2017). Pillar integration process: A joint display technique to integrate data in mixed methods research. *Journal of Mixed Methods Research.* doi:10.1177/1558689817743108

15

APPLYING ADVANCED PROCEDURES IN MIXED DATA ANALYSIS

To move beyond descriptive analyses, a growing number of mixed methods researchers are creating and applying advanced procedures in mixed data analysis. As many mixed data analysis procedures have only been emerging in the past several years, you may be unfamiliar with their potential utility for your mixed methods study. This chapter and its activities will help you learn three features of advanced procedures in mixed data analysis, examine multiple advanced procedures such as quantitizing, that is, data transformation of qualitative data into quantitative data; qualitizing, that is, data transformation of quantitative data into qualitative data; qualitative comparative analysis; geographic information system mapping; social network analysis; repertory grid analysis; and imitation game, and determine the relevance of the different procedures for application in your own mixed methods project. As a key outcome, you will choose one or more advanced mixed methods data analysis procedures for further exploration.

LEARNING OBJECTIVES

This chapter introduces seven additional advanced mixed methods data analysis procedures besides joint display analysis (Chapter 14), so you can

- Learn three features that characterize advanced mixed methods analysis procedures

- Explore the breadth of advanced mixed methods data analysis procedures

- Determine the relevance of the different procedures for your own mixed methods research (MMR) and evaluation projects

WHAT ARE ADVANCED MIXED METHODS DATA ANALYSIS PROCEDURES?

As discussed by Bazeley and Kemp (2012), categorizing different analysis procedures in MMR remains difficult due to lack of agreement about design typologies and the use of *a priori* and emergent designs. In addition, there is a lack of agreement for metaphors used for the mixed methods descriptive analysis. In reviewing the work of others and their own, Bazeley and Kemp (2012) characterized advanced mixed methods data analysis to have three key features. (1) Analysis goes beyond descriptive and focuses on drawing deeper inferences beyond descriptive work that includes higher-order theory building, or examination, exploration, evaluation for a deeper understanding through use of both types of data together. (2) The process involves or generates a change in the structure of the data form or entity such that the original identity is minimally or no longer recognizable. (3) The process involved is highly complex with extensive change and exchange between the two types of data. These dimensions illustrate the high level of integration possible and the potential complexity.

WHY USE ADVANCED MIXED METHODS DATA ANALYSIS PROCEDURES?

Many researchers are interested in going beyond the primary mixed methods analysis procedures that are essentially descriptive (Chapter 13). This chapter extends discussion beyond joint display analysis (Chapter 14) to address seven additional advanced mixed methods data analysis approaches. Increasing sophistication and advances in software now permit researchers to combine and explore data in ways that previously were not possible or very difficult. While use of fundamental integrated mixed analysis procedures are essential steps, advanced mixed methods data analysis procedures may be optional. In an MMR study, dissertation, or evaluation, the researcher will be unlikely to use more than one advanced mixed methods data analysis procedure in the same study, even though the fundamental procedures will generally apply.

DETERMINING THE NEED FOR ADVANCED ANALYSIS PROCEDURES

The first task of this chapter is to assess whether to pursue more advanced procedures to examine the mixed findings. Advanced levels of analysis may occur each for qualitative (Creswell, 2016; Miles, Huberman, & Saldaña, 2014; Patton, 2015), quantitative (Johnson & Christensen, 2017), and mixed methods data (Creswell & Plano Clark, 2018; Johnson & Christensen, 2017). Alternatively, there may be advanced procedures employed for two strands, one strand, or none at all.

Quantitatively driven mixed methods studies typically involve advanced inferential statistical analysis and modeling but have relatively less sophisticated qualitative analytics. Similarly, in **qualitatively driven mixed methods projects**, the qualitative analysis may be characterized by using a specific qualitative methodology (Creswell & Poth, 2018) or by using theory throughout the entire data collection and analysis process (O'Reilly & Kiyimba, 2015). In a qualitatively driven project, the quantitative analysis may not exceed simple statistics or two-group comparisons. With the third **equivalently driven mixed methods analysis**, both qualitative and quantitative data may be linked together based on an advanced mixed methods data analysis procedure (Moseholm & Fetters, 2017).

A Comparison of Advanced Analysis in Qualitative, Quantitative, and Mixed Methods Research

Advanced qualitative analysis uses specific methodological approaches (e.g., grounded theory, ethnography, and incorporates theory throughout, and/or creates new theories or models). **Advanced quantitative analysis** uses statistics to answer or model measurement, causality, and relationship-driven research questions. Advanced mixed methods analysis extends beyond descriptive interpretations and involves drawing metainferences by creating a higher-order understanding through examination, exploration, evaluation, or theory building that changes the structure of the data and is highly complex with extensive change and interaction between the mixed data. Workbox Illustration 15.1.1 illustrates the advanced analysis procedures in the MPathic-VR virtual human simulation trial. In the final steps, the authors used advanced quantitative data analysis for hypothesis testing. The qualitative data steps did not include use of theory or a particular qualitative methodology. The mixed methods advanced procedure employed joint display analysis.

Workbox Illustration 15.1.1: Advanced Analysis Approaches for the MPathic-VR Mixed Methods Medical Education Study

---

Advanced Analysis Approach*

Quantitative Data

The research team conducted the quantitative analyses using the SAS software, version 9.3. The outcomes were evaluated using an alpha level of 0.05.

Hypothesis 1*: To test for improvement during the MPathic-VR simulation, the researchers compared scores for each run-through of the intercultural and interprofessional scenarios with a repeated measures analysis of variance (ANOVA) to assess learning derived from additional interaction with the virtual human simulation system.

Hypothesis 2*: To compare the effect of MPathic-VR arm versus the control arm, the researchers conducted multivariate and univariate ANOVAs on the four objective structured clinical examination rating scale items with the intervention or control module as the independent variable.

Posttrial Attitudinal Survey: To compare student attitudes toward MPathic-VR learning and CBL learning, the researchers compared the mean scores for each module aggregated across rating scales with an independent *t*-test.

Qualitative Data:

The researchers used MAXQDA to identify text segments related to students' experiences while taking the MPathic-VR intervention module and the computer-based learning control module.

Mixed Data:

After completing the qualitative and quantitative analyses, the researchers linked the qualitative findings from learners' reflections on their experiences with the quantitative results of the attitudinal scale. Regarding the purpose of the MMR data analysis, they compared the two sources of data to gain a more complete understanding of learners' experiences and represented their mixed data analysis and interpretation in a visual joint display.

---

*Advanced analysis approaches according to criteria

Source: Kron et al. (2017).

Activity: Advanced Mixed Methods Data Analysis Approaches

Using Workbox Illustration 15.1.1 as a reference, add the planning for any advanced analyses of your quantitative and qualitative data. If you have already chosen any advanced procedures, add them to your mixed methods data section in Workbox 15.1.2. As illustrated in the example, advanced quantitative data analysis involved testing of three hypotheses using ANOVA/MANOVA. For the qualitative data analysis, the research question was answered by using qualitative data analysis software to organize the text and draw conclusions about medical students' experiences with the system. It did not use a more advanced approach such as using or creating theory. For the advanced MMR procedure, joint display analysis involved creating two columns that contained the quantitative and qualitative data from the intervention. Two more columns contained the quantitative and qualitative data from the computer-based learning module control. A final column was utilized to interpret the meaning of the two types of data for both the intervention and control (Chapter 14, Figure 14.1).

Workbox 15.1.2: Advanced Mixed Methods Research Data Analysis Approaches

Advanced Analysis Approach

Quantitative Data:

Qualitative Data:

Mixed Data:

WHAT ARE THE DIFFERENT TYPES OF ADVANCED MIXED DATA ANALYSIS PROCEDURES?

There are a number of advanced mixed methods data analysis procedures, and for *The Mixed Methods Research Workbook,* I have chosen eight. These are illustrated in Table 15.1 and include (1) joint display analysis (Chapter 14); (2) quantitizing (data transformation of qualitative data into quantitative data); (3) qualitizing (data transformation of quantitative data into qualitative data); (4) qualitative comparative analysis; (5) geographic information system (GIS) mapping; (6) social network analysis; (7) repertory grid analysis; and (8) imitation game. Workbox 15.2 provides an activity to assess the relevance of the eight advanced mixed data analysis procedures.

Table 15.1: Eight Advanced Mixed Methods Data Analysis Procedures for Use in Mixed Methods Research and Evaluation Studies

Technique	Process	Application	Example	How Used
1) Joint display analysis (see Chapter 14)	Bringing qualitative and quantitative findings together in a single table, matrix, or figure	Mixed methods projects with qualitative and quantitative data about related constructs	Moseholm and Fetters (2017) measured changes in health-related quality of life during the evaluation of patients presenting with nonspecific symptoms, possibly attributable to cancer.	Created three joint displays for the constructs of function, symptoms, and quality of life based on scales and qualitative quotes, assessed fit, and drew metainferences
2) Quantitizing—transformation of qualitative data into a quantitative form	Convert qualitative data into a quantitized format, and then integrate the converted quantitized findings with other quantitative findings	Merging transformed qualitative data into a quantitative database that can be used to conduct statistical modeling	Plano Clark et al. (2010) sought to understand how alumni of a STEM* graduate education program perceived the impact of their participation in the education program.	Quantitized qualitative themes to create a new variable incorporated into a statistical analysis
3) Qualitizing—data transformation of quantitative data into a qualitative format	Convert quantitative data into qualitative data and then integrate the qualitized findings with other qualitative data	Using quantitative data in a textual format that is compatible with the analysis or interpretation with other qualitative data from a project	Bradt et al. (2015) sought to compare the impact of music therapy versus music medicine interventions on psychological outcomes and pain in cancer patients and to enhance understanding of patients' experiences of the two types of music interventions.	Created a composite measure from four scales and then created a typology of four groups in research to compare music therapy (interactive choosing) and music medicine (prerecorded)
4) Qualitative comparative analysis	Solving research problems by identifying what causal contributions lead to a given outcome	Conducting statistical analysis to identify necessary and sufficient conditions for a particular outcome	Holtrop, Green, and Fetters (2016) endeavored to compare two novel care management programs using mixed methods.	Used fuzzy set QCA, and identified necessary and/or sufficient conditions for care management success
5) Geographic information system (GIS) mapping	Solve a geographic question by using digital technologies that store, manage, analyze, and represent spatial information (Elwood & Cope, 2009)	Using digital databases, technologies, and software to answer spatially driven questions	Jones (2017) used GIS procedures to map spatial relationships among distinct seed systems in Sahelian West Africa.	Identified five combinations of farmer decision making based on the type of system, seed, and access action
6) Social network analysis	Construct pictures and diagrams of social relations to reveal patterns not seen by observation, and examine structural properties and the implications for social action (Scott, 2017)	Investigating kinship patterns, community structure, and interlocking directories	Martinez, Dimitriadis, Rubia, Gómez, and de la Fuente (2003) introduced a project-based learning course on computer architecture and conducted a mixed evaluation by integrating quantitative statistics, qualitative data analysis, and social network analysis.	Used social network analysis in their mixed methods evaluation and demonstrated that the course encouraged collaboration through sharing of information
7) Repertory grid analysis	Elucidate personal constructs about a topic or phenomenon	Draw out different meanings, rationales, or choices based on participants' own views about a topic, question, or phenomenon	Marketing researchers Rogers and Ryals (2007) sought to understand how key account managers assess the effectiveness of long-term business-to-business relationships.	Used a 7-step repertory grid process to show that personal relationships were the best indicator of long-term account relationships with clients
8) Imitation game	Explores cultural understandings of a phenomenon by using "interactional expertise" to investigate the relationship between culturally or experientially different groups	A research method "game" that generates qualitative and quantitative data about a cultural phenomenon through an exercise of questioning and interpretation of responses	Collins and Evans (2014) conducted research with color-blind volunteers and sighted individuals to examine if minority affiliation could better describe living with color blindness.	Demonstrated blind volunteers can identify majority cultural parameters, while majority affiliation, sighted volunteers, could not distinguish features of color blindness

*Science, technology, engineering, and math

215

Activity: Choosing Among Advanced Mixed Methods Data Analysis Strategies for Potential Application in a Project

Using Workbox 15.2.2, consider each of the eight featured procedures for your project. Based on your MMR, dissertation, or evaluation project, choose the approach that will be most meaningful. You may ultimately decide you do not need to employ advanced mixed methods data analysis strategies. Ultimately, you should be prepared to justify your choice of an advanced procedure chosen or choice not to use an advanced approach. As you learn about each of the procedures, make a note to yourself in the potential relevance column such as likely, somewhat likely, or not at all likely, and use the comment box to record ideas you might want to explore or people you could contact for further information.

Workbox 15.2.2: Choosing Among Advanced Mixed Methods Data Analysis Strategies for Potential Application in a Project

Technique	Potential Relevance to My Project*	Comment
1) Joint display analysis (see Chapter 14)		
2) Quantitizing—transformation of qualitative data into a quantitative form		
3) Qualitizing—data transformation of quantitative data into a qualitative format		
4) Qualitative comparative analysis		
5) Geographic information system mapping		
6) Social network analysis		
7) Repertory grid analysis		
8) Imitation game		
Other		

*Suggested options likely, somewhat likely, not at all likely.

1. JOINT DISPLAY ANALYSIS

Chapter 14 is devoted completely to a comprehensive examination of joint display analysis. See Chapter 14 for details.

2. QUANTITIZING—DATA TRANSFORMATION OF QUALITATIVE DATA INTO A QUANTITATIVE FORM FOR AN INTEGRATED ANALYSIS

Quantitizing data in MMR involves converting qualitative data into a quantitative format (Tashakkori & Teddlie, 1998). It is a two-step process that involves conversion of analyzed qualitative data into categorical or continuous data (quantitizing), incorporating quantitized data with the quantitative database and conducting statistical analysis (Creswell & Plano Clark, 2018). Quantization can include transformation of qualitative data into nominal, ordinal, interval, and ratio data. Additionally emergent themes may be coded as present or absent for each participant (Driscoll, Appiah-Yeboah, Salib, & Rupert, 2007). Researchers may count codes associated with a particular theme. This process contributes an understanding of the salience, or importance of the theme, based on its emphasis by the participant (Collingridge, 2013). A variation of this process involves the frequency of themes within a sample (Driscoll et al., 2007). This strategy can also be used to identify patterns of relationships in the data, for example, "reveal the associative and dimensional structure of data," as noted by Bazeley (2018, p. 209). There are a number of multivariate techniques that can be used for this purpose, such as cluster analysis (Byrne & Uprichard, 2013), multidimensional scaling (Arabie, Carroll, & DeSarbo, 1987; Borg & Groenen, 2005), or correspondence analysis (Roux & Rouanet, 2009).

Core Concepts. Researchers typically use a quantitizing procedure when the intent is to conduct descriptive statistics or modeling using both the qualitative and quantitative data. Merging of qualitative and quantitative data provides an opportunity to supplement the qualitative analysis, rather than to replace it. A potential benefit is the ability to use volunteered information, rather than the researcher imposing choices upon subjects (Bazeley, 2018). Data transformation differs from content analysis by virtue of integrating the now-transformed-into-quantitative data with other quantitative data of the project in a statistical analysis. Untransformed qualitative data can be used to illustrate findings from transformed data, while merged data can be used in statistical analyses (Bazeley, 2018). Analyzing dichotomous data can proceed using tests of proportions, *t*-tests, correlating dichotomous themes with binary and continuous variables, and using a dichotomized theme as an outcome variable in binary logistic regression (Collingridge, 2013). For code counts, Collingridge (2013) suggests the use of permutation testing and is against traditional parametric and nonparametric testing. Still, Collingridge also advises caution with permutation testing, which may be unreliable for very small sample sizes and when qualitative data are collected in a nonsystematic way.

Example. Plano Clark, Garrett, and Leslie-Pelecky (2010) conducted a mixed methods investigation of individuals who had been graduate fellows in a National Science Foundation education program. The program was designed to raise awareness among future STEM (science, technology, education, math) leaders about the challenges of K–12 education. The researchers' primary research question was how graduates of the STEM graduate program perceived the impact of their participation in the program. The researchers distributed a Web-based survey with closed- and open-ended items. They had 36 (85.7% response rate) participants from the program. Their initial analysis identified the need for a new variable to address negative experiences that they found to be important in the qualitative analysis, but it was not present in the survey questions. They quantitized data by using two qualitative subthemes with a negative valence, "programmatic tensions" and "loss of disciplinary experience." These were combined as a new variable for the quantitative analysis. By adding this variable to their correlational analyses, they discovered a difference between individuals who rated their experiences as "very positive" from individuals rating it just as "positive." The latter group's enthusiasm was moderated by a perception of negative impacts that was detected only by quantitizing the negative themes that emerged and using them in the analysis.

Mixed Methods Considerations. In addition to the use of transformed data for descriptive statistics, Bazeley (2018) identifies four other approaches: (1) case by variable matrices that can stand alone or link with other data collected and attributed to each case; (2) profile matrices that use cross-tabulation with other categorical or scaled data; (3) pattern matrices that involve matching categories of one group with categories of another group; and (4) similarities matrices when dimensions or subcategories of a concept are cross-tabulated with dimensions or categories of another concept. A risk of quantitizing data comes from overreliance on content and losing sight of the meaning of the qualitative data.

3. QUALITIZING—DATA TRANSFORMATION OF QUANTITATIVE DATA INTO A QUALITATIVE FORMAT FOR AN INTEGRATED ANALYSIS

Qualitizing in MMR involves conversion of quantitative to qualitative data (Tashakkori & Teddlie, 1998). The data transformation and integration involves two steps: (1) converting analyzed quantitative data to qualitative text data as codes, themes, or descriptions, and then (2) using the transformed data (QUAN to QUAL) together with other qualitative data (Creswell & Plano Clark, 2018). This type of transformation is relatively less common and is most often used to create descriptive cases or typologies from complex quantitative data.

Core Concepts. Qualitizing entails converting quantitative data in a textual format that is compatible with the analysis or interpretation with other qualitative data from a project. The particular utility of this procedure comes from creating descriptive categories or cases from complex quantitative data.

Example. In a mixed methods randomized crossover trial comparing music therapy and music medicine on psychological outcomes and pain for cancer patients, Bradt et al. (2015) compared "music therapy," interactive choosing of music, versus "music medicine," that was prerecorded, to examine the effects on psychological outcomes and pain for 31 cancer patients. Quantitative data collection involved scales on mood, anxiety, relaxation, and pain, while qualitative data collection involved exit interviews after exposure. The authors wanted to explore if and why some patients derived greater benefit from music therapy versus music medicine sessions or vice versa. They calculated the Z score for both music therapy and music medicine for each participant. The QUAL-to-QUAN data transformation resulted from conversion of the resulting combinations into a typology of four groups. Imagine using a 2 × 2 table with music therapy high and low, and music medicine high and low to create four groups. Integration of the transformed QUAN-to-QUAN data with qualitative interview data then occurred. The authors used joint display analysis matching to each of the four groups' representative qualitative responses from the interviews. They represented these results in a final joint display showing the quantitatively created four typologies and the patient experiences.

Mixed Methods Considerations. Researchers most commonly use qualitizing to convert complex datasets into descriptive or narrative formats that are more easily understood. Saint Arnault identifies five procedures for qualitizing analyses: (1) Creation of new variables using data transformation; (2) factor analysis; (3) cluster analysis; (4) multidimensional scaling; (5) and latent class analysis (Saint Arnault, personal communication, April 25, 2019). The approach can be used to profile different cases or groups (Bazeley, 2018). The primary limitations of the procedure are that it is much less intuitive for many researchers, especially qualitative researchers, and that qualitized information looks more like themes or variables that lack characteristic features of qualitative findings of stories or thick rich description.

4. QUALITATIVE COMPARATIVE ANALYSIS

Qualitative comparative analysis (QCA) is a theory-driven approach designed to look for solutions to problems by examining the contributions of various conditions and understand how they lead to a given outcome. QCA relies on both quantitative and qualitative methods, while ultimately conducting statistical analysis to identify necessary and sufficient conditions for a particular outcome. After documenting different conditions associated with an observed outcome, minimization procedures are used to identify the simplest set of conditions that can account for the presence or absence of observed outcomes (Kahwati & Kane, 2020).

Core Concepts. In QCA, the researcher must specify both an outcome and one or more conditions (variables) that could be associated with the outcome that are used for the analysis (Ragin, Shulman, Weinberg, & Gran, 2003). QCA is useful for moderately sized datasets, that is, "a number considered by most social scientists to be too few for the application of commonly used multivariate statistical procedures (e.g., multiple regression) but too many for in-depth, case-oriented analysis" (Ragin et al., 2003). Both the outcome and the conditions must be quantified (data transformation). In crisp set QCA (csQCA), the conditions are dichotomized as either not present (0) or present (1). In fuzzy set QCA (fsQCA), conditions exist in degrees of set memberships, and values can range from 0 to 1. QUAL and QUAN data are used to create component "conditions" with a 0/1 value. In fsQCA, researchers transform variables into sets. In multivalue QCA (mvQCA), conditions account for multiple values of data. QCA accepts the possibility of equifinality, meaning that multiple pathways can lead to the same outcome. Set membership is assigned based on whether/what degree a case satisfies criteria for each outcome or condition. QCA contrasts with regression analysis that discovers the effect of the variable on an outcome, magnitude, and direction of effect of variables, and the net effect of other variables in the model. Researchers commonly present results using Boolean notation.

Example. Holtrop et al. (2016) conducted a mixed methods investigation examining novel care management programs. They compared care managers based in a practice with care managers situated centrally who were employees of health insurance programs. The investigators conducted medical record extraction and obtained claims data from 2,592 practice-delivered care management patients, 1,128 health plan–delivered care management practices and patients, and surveys of clinicians and patients from 51 pilot practices. Moreover, they conducted qualitative interviews with 10 practice organization leaders and 25 practice members; 70 observations; and 3 health plan–delivered care management interviews. Using fsQCA, they conducted a necessary and sufficiency analysis, and identified complex, parsimonious, and intermediate solutions. The main outcome of the research was identification of practice features (i.e., environment, care management program, and implementation) that were necessary and/or sufficient for care management success.

Mixed Methods Considerations: QCA involves data transformation of both qualitative data to quantitative data as well as quantitative data to another quantitative format (Kahwati & Kane, 2020). Bazeley (2018) considers QCA an inherently mixed data analysis approach. While QCA uses qualitative and quantitative data, the output is primarily statistical. Analysis requires software from the developer of the procedure.

5. GEOGRAPHIC INFORMATION SYSTEM MAPPING

Geographic information system mapping describes the process of solving a spatial question by using digital technologies that store, manage, analyze, and represent spatial information (Elwood & Cope, 2009). GIS can be used to create integrated searches, analyze spatial information, and edit data. Mixed methods GIS incorporates qualitative data with maps to provide context about a locality.

Core Concepts. It is an information system that integrates, stores, edits, analyzes, shares, and displays geographic information (Elwood & Cope, 2009). The typical outcome will be a map of variables of interest. The addition of qualitative data to geographic information can be used to create a mixed methods interpretation.

Example. Jones (2017) sought to better understand how and why farmers in Sahelian West Africa incorporated new seed varieties, how decisions varied with different social/spatial characteristics, and how a market-oriented approach impacts different environmental and social contexts. She used multilevel data sampling and simultaneously gathered qualitative, quantitative, and spatial data. Jones conducted semistructured interviews, participatory mapping procedures, GPS coordinates in villages, secondary data sources, and publicly available geographic coordinates. The study had a theoretically informed approach to code qualitative data to identify patterns and structural equation modeling to test the hypothesis that distinct seed systems could be characterized over time based on engagement and decision making within the systems. Jones used digital GIS procedures to map spatial relationships of the seed systems and corroborated these with maps drawn by farmer participants. She identified five combinations of farmer decision making based on the type of system, seed, and access actions useful for seed system development in rural areas. Her mixed methods approach examining changing seed systems in Sahelian West Africa illustrates the potential for mixed methods GIS to investigate complex social, spatial, and temporal phenomena.

Mixed Methods Considerations. GIS procedures use multiple ways of knowing to enhance quantitative calculations and distributions produced by traditional mapping, and they add value by bringing in stories, interpretations, multiple meanings, identities, and characteristics of geographic locations. Mixed methods GIS is indicated when there are geospatial considerations, as well as local conditions and context that require consideration.

6. SOCIAL NETWORK ANALYSIS

Social network analysis (SNA) refers to the process of researchers constructing pictures and diagrams of social relations to reveal patterns not seen by observation and examining structural properties and the implications for social action (Scott, 2017). In mixed SNA, researchers create sociograms, or maps illustrating various social patterns or networks, and then explore the relationships qualitatively.

FIGURE 15.1 ■ Sociogram Created Using Social Network Analysis That Demonstrates Collaboration Through Sharing of Information Martinez et al.'s (2003)*

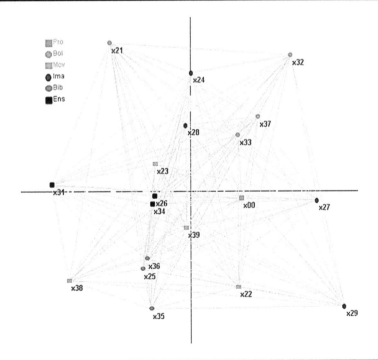

Source: Martinez et al. (2003) with permission by Elsevier and Copyright Clearance Center.

*Their SNA demonstrates collaboration through sharing of information beyond the teacher (x00) to four other student pairs (x26, x34, x23, x39) in a computer architecture course.

Core Concepts. SNA uses two main types of data: attribute data and relational data. Attribute data represent attitudes, opinions, and behaviors as properties, qualities, or characteristics. Relational data represent the contacts, ties, connections, group attachments, and meetings that relate one agent to another agent. SNA may also include ideational data, namely, meanings, motives, definitions, and typifications associated with actions (Scott, 2017).

Example. Over three years, Martinez et al. (2003) introduced project-based learning in a course on computer architecture designed to provide contextualized, integrated, and meaningful knowledge, and to promote active, intentional, and collaborative learning. They conducted a mixed methods evaluation to understand *collaboration as sharing information* during an upper-level undergraduate course, and they used questionnaires with open- and closed-items, student post-hoc comments, focus groups, and nonparticipant observations. Their sociograms revealed connectivity not evident from their other sources of data. As illustrated in Figure 15.1, in addition to the teacher as the most central actor (node x00), there were other actors, in this case pairs of students (x26, x34, x23, x39), who took central positions in the diagram, as they were publishing notes and became information sharers with others. Their SNA demonstrated that writing of a joint report as a class activity increased collaboration through sharing information that they corroborated with qualitative interview findings.

Mixed Methods Considerations. Bazeley (2018) provides six potential mixed methods applications of social network analysis. These include (1) using qualitative approaches to understand cultural and linguistic context to gather data on social ties, (2) using different methods to create maps of a single phenomenon, (3) gathering qualitative data to understand idiosyncratic aspects of ties within a network such as who initiated the tie, (4) using a mapped network in an elicitation interview to prompt a participant to discuss a created network or a participant's place in the network, (5) using a network map to prompt discussion about related topics, and (6) using these methods to explain change that occurs over time in networks. SNA can be used for a variety of MMR and evaluation studies when there is a need to understand varied patterns of social relationships that need to be connected or mapped and then explained with contextual qualitative information.

7. REPERTORY GRID ANALYSIS

Repertory grid analysis refers to a type of cognitive mapping tool. The method utilizes an interview to elicit people's ideas or opinions using their own words to understand how they construe reality. George Kelly, a psychologist and counselor, originally developed personal construct theory as a technique for use in counseling to interpret emotional triggers of clients (Kelly, 1955). A constructivist approach, individuals interpret and understand experiences and anticipate future events through their own "personal construct system" (Bernard & Flitman, 2002). Since the 1960s business researchers have adapted the tool for research in human resources, marketing, and organizational behavior and management development, for example, evaluating the impact of training and career counseling (Rogers & Ryals, 2007).

Core Concepts

A **repertory grid** (or **RepGrid**) is a written structure used to elucidate what people think about a certain topic as a cognitive mapping tool. An interviewer uses the RepGrid template as an infrastructure during interviews to elicit people's ideas or opinions using their own words to understand how they construe reality.

Constructs are the dimensions examined and are formulated as bipolar dimensions that allow clients to formulate understandings, organize, and understand elements (Caputi & Reddy, 1999; Rogers & Ryals, 2007). **Elements** are examples or instances of the topic (i.e., people, objects, or events). **Linkages** represent the way an element is described relative to each construct. Constructs must have bipolar dimensions, or two anchoring ideas with descriptions on both ends of the spectrum. Personal constructs can be elicited using a triadic or dyadic approach. In the **triadic approach**, the interviewee compares three elements and explains how two are similar and the third, is different. In the **dyadic approach**, the interview contrasts only two elements.

Once a range of elements and constructs with bipolar dimensions is elucidated, a RepGrid is constructed (Figure 15.2). The RepGrid features a series of elements across the top, where each element forms a column. Consider marketing interviews with consumers about where to shop for groceries. The interviewee would list out elements—the stores for comparison. The interviewer then asks the person to define constructs (e.g., cleanliness, quality, cost, warmth of staff, size, parking, restroom cleanliness) for comparison. Each construct is situated in rows at opposite sides of the grid, and each row is populated by the interviewee who develops bipolar dimensions (e.g., cleanliness bipolar dimensions would be store is clean, or store is dirty). Finally, the interviewee uses a Likert scale rating in each cell for each construct (clean–dirty, etc.) for each element (the stores). The interviewer elicits the rationale for the choices. Across multiple participants, the choices by element and by construct can be compared.

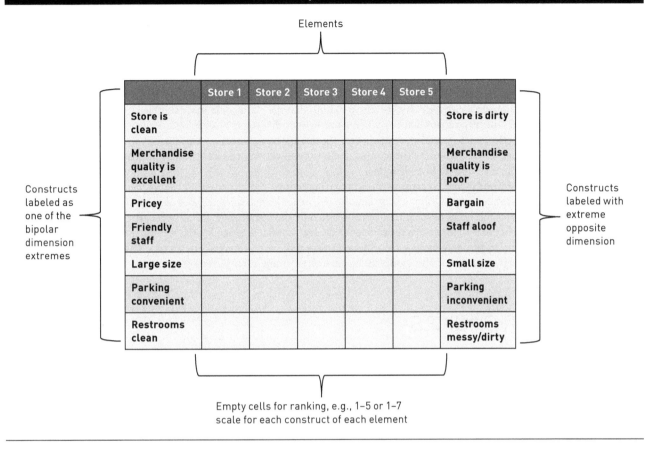

FIGURE 15.2 ■ Repertory Grid Partially Completed by an Interviewee Using Hypothetical Study to Understand Preferred Features of Various Grocery Stores

Elements

Constructs labeled as one of the bipolar dimension extremes

Constructs labeled with extreme opposite dimension

	Store 1	Store 2	Store 3	Store 4	Store 5	
Store is clean						Store is dirty
Merchandise quality is excellent						Merchandise quality is poor
Pricey						Bargain
Friendly staff						Staff aloof
Large size						Small size
Parking convenient						Parking inconvenient
Restrooms clean						Restrooms messy/dirty

Empty cells for ranking, e.g., 1–5 or 1–7 scale for each construct of each element

Example. Rogers and Ryals (2007), marketing researchers, wanted to understand why long-term, key account relationships are effective. They conducted 10 repertory grid interviews and identified 39 constructs. Their analysis revealed that key account managers identified a close personal relationship to be the best indication of effectiveness. Second, they found simple product requirements to be more effective than complex interorganizational products or process design. The most important ranked items did not include the most frequently mentioned, thereby demonstrating the value of both measured ranking and interviewing.

Mixed Methods Considerations. From the repertory grids, a series of mixed analysis procedures are possible. For example, a researcher can aggregate repertory grids across individuals to create simple frequency accounts of mentions of a particular construct. For larger samples, lumping the constructs into categories may become necessary. Next, the analysis examines variability in the constructs, for example, the spread between constructs. Third, the researcher can aggregate ratings. With any of these processes, interviews can be incorporated to give context to the personal constructs. The constructs may have different meanings for different people (Rogers & Ryals, 2007). The process involves conducting multiple interviews, and challenges involve how to analyze mixed findings across multiple individuals.

8. IMITATION GAME

Imitation game refers to an inherently mixed methods approach developed in sociology that allows researchers to explore cultural aspects of a phenomenon. The approach uses a technique that generates qualitative and quantitative data (Collins et al., 2017). The imitation game is inspired by the "Turing test" designed to examine intelligence of computers (Collins & Evans, 2014). Part of the appeal of this method is that before collecting data, the investigator does not have to be an expert in the culture of exploration.

Core concepts. Each imitation game has three participants who are linked by a computer and who don't know the others' identities. A participant from the target group of investigation acts as "interrogator/judge" who composes questions and sends them to the other two—one a member of the target group of study, a "nonpretender," who answers naturally, and the other a "pretender," who is not a member of the target group but is tasked with answering questions as if he or she is a member of the target group. The judges ask a series of 6–8 questions and has the task of identifying who is the pretender, and who is the bona fide member of the target cultural group. In a variation, the interrogator/judge position can be filled by two people, one the interrogator and one the judge.

Example. Collins and Evans (2014) recruited five blind volunteers. Sighted judges were advised to develop questions pertaining to adult life experiences that a blind person could not have practiced or watched. Judges were advised that one of the other two participants was pretending and that the task was to identify the person who was pretending based on the answers. Judges were told to develop questions on their own that they thought could distinguish between seeing and nonsighted adults. Responses to the questions were shown simultaneously on the judge's screen. The judge then assessed with a level of confidence who was/wasn't blind and could ask another question or end the game. In a second phase, judges only saw the transcripts. Based on a specific quantitative scoring system, the investigators demonstrated conclusively ($p < 0.000$) that the blind could pass as sighted, but the sighted could not pass as blind. The investigators have conducted testing for other topics of sociological interest as well, based on color blindness, perfect pitch, sexuality, religion, etc. The qualitative component of testing involves analyzing transcripts, questions asked, and responses. The authors demonstrated varying results based on affiliation or lack of affiliation with the group targeted for investigation.

Mixed Methods Considerations. Participants' questions and responses and subsequent interviews will supply many answers about the cultural group, and the researcher learns characteristics of the study group iteratively. The game generates five kinds of data: (1) questions asked by the interrogator, (2) answers provided by the two players, (3) the decision of the judge, (4) a measure of the judge's confidence, and (5) the reasons for the judge's decision. In addition, participants may provide other data, demographic data, responses to surveys/scales, etc. The participants become "proxy researchers." The game can be conducted online or in person using various group sizes.

OTHER CHOICES

A full treatise of the advanced procedures of mixed data analysis are beyond the scope of this book. Two other known "mixed strategies" that are similar to repertory grid analysis (RepGrid) are concept mapping (Windsor, 2013) and Q-methodology (Franz, Worrell, & Vögele, 2013), which can both be used for the identification and measurement of constructs. The book by Pat Bazeley (2018) called *Integrating Analyses in Mixed Methods Research* contains both depth and breadth about other possibilities. Many advances in analysis continue to occur with new software and digitally based computing strategies. The field continues to grow and develop. Be bold and consider what your own work has to offer for advancing the field and procedures in mixed data integration.

Application Activities

1. **Peer Feedback**. If you are working on your project as part of a class or in a workshop, please pair up with a peer mentor, and one of you spend about 5 minutes talking about your advanced mixed methods data analysis. Take turns talking about your advanced mixed methods data analysis strategy and giving feedback. If you are working independently, share your table with a colleague or mentor to get feedback.

2. **Peer Feedback Guidance**. As you listen to your partner, you should focus on learning and honing the valuable skills of critiquing. Your goal is to help your partner refine the mixed data analysis planning.

3. **Group Debrief**. If you are in a classroom or large-group setting, take volunteers to present their advanced mixed methods data analysis plans. Reflect on how these same issues may play out in your own project.

Concluding Thoughts

Use this checklist to assess your progress in achieving the Chapter 15 objectives:

☐   I learned three features that characterize advanced mixed methods analysis procedures.

☐   I explored a broad range of advanced mixed methods data analysis procedures.

☐   I assessed the potential relevance of the different procedures for my own project.

☐   I reviewed my advanced mixed methods data analysis considerations with a peer or colleague to refine my project planning.

Now that you have completed these objectives, Chapter 16 will help you consider research integrity issues for your MMR or evaluation project.

Key Resources

1. **FURTHER READING ON DATA INTEGRATION DURING ANALYSIS**

   - Bazeley, P. (2009). Integrating data analyses in mixed methods research. *Journal of Mixed Methods Research, 3*(3), 203–207. doi:10.1177/1558689809334443

   - Bazeley, P. (2018). *Integrating analyses in mixed methods research.* Thousand Oaks, CA: Sage.

   - Fielding, N. G. (2012). Triangulation and mixed methods designs: Data integration with new research technologies. *Journal of Mixed Methods Research, 6*(2), 124–136. doi:10.1177/1558689812437101

   - Plano Clark, V. L., Garrett, A. L., & Leslie-Pelecky, D. L. (2010). Applying three strategies for integrating quantitative and qualitative databases in a mixed methods study of a nontraditional graduate education program. *Field Methods, 22*(2), 154–174. doi:10.1177/152 5822X09357174

2. **FURTHER READING ON DATA TRANSFORMATION USING QUANTITIZING OF QUALITATIVE DATA**

   - Collingridge, D. S. (2013). A primer on quantitized data analysis and permutation testing. *Journal of Mixed Methods Research, 7*(1), 81–97. doi:10.1177/1558689812454457

   - Driscoll, D. L., Appiah-Yeboah, A., Salib, P., & Rupert, D. J. (2007). Merging qualitative and quantitative data in mixed methods research: How to and why not. *Ecological and Environmental Anthropology, 3*(1), 19–28.

3. **FURTHER READING ON DATA TRANSFORMATION USING QUALITIZING OF QUANTITATIVE DATA**

   - Bazeley, P. (2018). Integration through transformation 2: Exploratory, blended and narrative approaches. In *Integrating analyses in mixed methods research* (pp. 208–234). Thousand Oaks, CA: Sage.

4. **FURTHER READING ON GEOGRAPHIC INFORMATION SYSTEMS**

   - Albrecht, J. (2007). *Key concepts and techniques in GIS.* Thousand Oaks, CA: Sage.

   - Elwood, S., & Cope, M. (2009). Introduction: Qualitative GIS: Forging mixed methods through representations, analytical innovations, and conceptual engagements. In *Qualitative GIS: A mixed methods approach* (pp. 1–12). Thousand Oaks, CA: Sage.

5. **FURTHER READING ON SOCIAL NETWORK ANALYSIS**

   - Scott. J. (2017). *Social network analysis* (4th ed.). Thousand Oaks, CA: Sage.

   - Yang, S., Keller, F. B., & Zheng, L. (2017). *Social network analysis: Methods and examples.* Thousand Oaks, CA: Sage.

6. **FURTHER READING ON QUALITATIVE COMPARATIVE ANALYSIS**

   - de Block, D., & Vis, B. (2018). Addressing the challenges related to transforming qualitative into quantitative data in qualitative comparative analysis. *Journal of Mixed Methods Research,* 1–33. doi:10.1177/1558689818770061

   - Holtrop, J. S., Potworowski, G., Green, L. A., & Fetters, M. D. (2016). Analysis of novel care management programs in primary care. *Journal of Mixed Methods Research,* 1–28. doi:10.1177/1558689816668689

   - Kahwati, L., & Kane, H. (2020). *Qualitative comparative analysis in mixed methods research and evaluation.* Thousand Oaks, CA: Sage.

7. **FURTHER READING ON REPERTORY GRID ANALYSIS**

   - Bernard, T., & Flitman, A. (2002). Using repertory grid analysis to gather qualitative data for information systems research. *ACIS 2002 Proceedings,* 98.

   - Kington, A., Sammons, P., Day, C., & Regan, E. (2011). Stories and statistics: Describing a mixed methods study of effective classroom practice. *Journal of Mixed Methods Research, 5*(2), 103–125. doi:10.1177/1558689810396092

8. **FURTHER READING ON THE IMITATION GAME**

   - Collins, H., & Evans, R. (2014). Quantifying the tacit: The imitation game and social fluency. *Sociology, 48*(1), 3–19. doi:10.1177/0038038512455735

   - Collins, H., Evans, R., Weinel, M., Lyttleton-Smith, J., Bartlett, A., & Hall, M. (2017). The imitation game and the nature of mixed methods. *Journal of Mixed Methods Research, 11*(4), 510–527. doi:10.1177/1558689815619824

16

ENSURING MIXED METHODS RESEARCH INTEGRITY: QUALITY CONSIDERATIONS FOR MIXED METHODS RESEARCH AND EVALUATION STUDIES

Mixed methods integrity encompasses the research quality issues relevant to qualitative and quantitative methods as well as to mixed methods and mixed methods methodology. You may be uncertain about how to conceptualize and assess the threats to the quality of your mixed methods project. This chapter and its activities will help you assess for threats to the quality of the qualitative strand from the perspective of trustworthiness; assess for threats to the quality of the quantitative strand from perspectives of validity, reliability, generalizability and replicability; identify possible threats to the quality of the mixed methods based on the particular design; determine the elements of legitimation that could be relevant to the project; and choose among different approaches for considering quality in the project. As a key outcome, you will systematically consider quality issues for the qualitative, quantitative, mixed methods, and methodology issues relative to your mixed methods research or evaluation project.

LEARNING OBJECTIVES

To help you apply the salient issues relevant to ensuring quality and rigor in mixed methods studies, the ideas presented here will help you

- Assess for threats to the quality of your project's qualitative strand from a trustworthiness perspective
- Assess for threats to the quality of your project's quantitative strand from perspectives of validity, reliability, generalizability, and replicability
- Identify possible threats to the quality of your mixed methods based on your mixed methods design
- Determine the elements of legitimation, a set of quality criteria for mixed methodology, that could be relevant threats to quality in your project
- Choose among different approaches for considering quality in your mixed methods project

QUALITY AND MIXED METHODS RESEARCH

Mixed methods scholars unequivocally agree on the importance of taking measures to ensure quality in mixed methods research (MMR). Beyond this key point of agreement, there are multiple views on how to conceptualize and assess for quality in mixed methods studies. Bryman developed one of the early typologies empirically through mixed methods survey research with social scientists (Bryman, Becker, & Sempik, 2008). Some interpretations emerged from early explorations of the field in classic textbooks or editions in the field (Teddlie & Tashakkori, 2009). One proposed framework, legitimation, has evolved from the original account (Onwuegbuzie & Johnson, 2006), to a more holistic account with five frameworks (Collins, 2015), to a comprehensive account (Johnson & Christensen, 2017). Differences stem in part from the frame of reference. For example, the legitimation typology focuses on methodology, while Creswell and Plano Clark (2018) take a methods orientation. O'Cathain (2010) considers the entire investigation under a single framework. Another category relates to development and application of quality criteria for synthesizing studies as a systematic mixed studies review (Fàbregues, Paré, & Meneses, 2018; Hong & Pluye, 2018; Pluye & Hong, 2014). The latter is a special category and beyond the scope of this chapter.

THREE CONCEPTUALIZATIONS OF MIXED METHODS QUALITY

A straightforward conceptualization of quality in mixed methods comes from the work of Alicia O'Cathain, who lays out three perspectives (O'Cathain, 2010). (1) The generic questions approach to quality means that there are certain features of any design that can be considered with particular quality criteria. (2) The individual components approach to quality means attending to rigor and quality of the individual qualitative and quantitative strands will ensure quality in the mixed methods. (3) **The mixed methods approach to quality** signifies there are unique features to MMR and evaluation that require attention for ensuring quality. Increasingly, a consensus is emerging for attending to the quality of both the qualitative and quantitative strands, as well as the specifics of the mixed methods procedures (Collins, 2015; Johnson & Christensen, 2017).

MIXED METHODS RESEARCH INTEGRITY

For the purposes of this chapter, **mixed methods research integrity** represents the attributes of rigor and quality with regard to conceptualization, implementation, and interpretation with respect to the qualitative strand, quantitative strand, the mixed methods, as well as the integration in mixed methodology dimensions. Figure 16.1 illustrates the concept of research integrity in MMR and evaluation using three ellipses. The three ellipses inside the larger circle encompass the quantitative strand quality, the qualitative strand quality, and the mixed methods quality. The larger external ellipse of mixed methodology quality encompasses the quantitative, qualitative, and mixed methods procedures, while also extending to the level of mixed methodology to incorporate philosophical and theoretical dimensions. The MMR integrity means that mixed methods researchers must consider the intramethod quality issues of the quantitative, the qualitative, and mixed methods. Second, mixed methods researchers must also consider the mixed methodology quality.

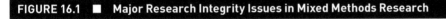

FIGURE 16.1 ■ Major Research Integrity Issues in Mixed Methods Research

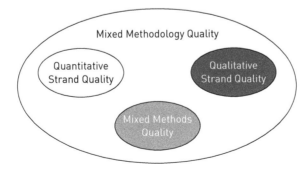

CONSIDERATION OF THE RESEARCH QUALITY ISSUES RELATIVE TO THE QUALITATIVE AND QUANTITATIVE RESEARCH

Despite the lack of agreement about details, mixed methods researchers agree about many of the overarching threats or criteria for quantitative, qualitative, and MMR. For quantitative data collection, the concepts of validity and reliability are particularly salient. In qualitative research, many scholars use the overarching concept of trustworthiness (Lincoln & Guba, 1985).

In MMR, Creswell and Plano Clark (2018) address quality using the language of mixed methods validity. The following two sections aim to address quality in qualitative and quantitative research sufficiently for you to consider the relevance to your own project, but not in substantial depth, as many references contain information about these topics. Moreover, the details and differences become discipline specific, so these short overviews and the tables serve primarily as a starting point for considering the quality criteria. Subsequent to identifying areas of relevance from the qualitative strand and quantitative strand, the remainder of the chapter will go into more depth relative to mixed methods.

ASSESSING FOR THREATS TO QUALITY IN QUALITATIVE RESEARCH: TRUSTWORTHINESS

The research quality issues of qualitative research have been addressed extensively. Many researchers cite the work of Lincoln and Guba (1985) who laid substantive groundwork for the consideration of quality. Table 16.1 provides a published list from Creswell (2016), supplemented with additional concepts that commonly arise in the qualitative literature. The variations in interpretation of quality derive in part from having many rich traditions of qualitative research (Creswell & Poth, 2018). In this section, I seek to provide sufficient information for you to identify potential threats to the quality of the quantitative strand of your project. Note that threats to integrity in qualitative research are contextually based and identified within the context of the research. You may require supplemental readings to understand and fully assess relevant issues.

Creswell's (2016) Framework for Considering Quality in Qualitative Research: The Researcher's, the Participant's, and the Reader/Reviewer's Lens

Many qualitative researchers use the language of trustworthiness. While not the only author to do so, Creswell prominently speaks of validity as the overarching concept of qualitative as well as MMR. In his book *30 Essential Skills for Qualitative Researchers*, Creswell (2016) conceptualizes quality in qualitative research from three lenses: that of the researcher, the participant, and the reader/reviewer. Table 16.1 summarizes the eight aspects, plus two additional criteria from O'Cathain (2010) and Bryman, Becker, and Sempik (2008).

TABLE 16.1 ■ Strategies for Assessing Quality Criteria in Qualitative Research From the Perspective of the Researcher, Participant, and the Reviewer/Reader		
Category	**Aspect**	**Process**
Researcher's Lens	Reflexivity	Reflecting or conducting a personal inventory of one's own values and beliefs for potential impact on the study
	Triangulation	Triangulating or bringing together data from multiple sources to assess for consistency of interpretation
	Disconfirming evidence	Looking for evidence that contradicts or disconfirms preliminary findings
Participant's Lens	Collaborate with participants	Engage participants of your research so that they contribute to the study
	Prolonged engagement	Spending extended or prolonged periods of time in the field investigating through interviewing, observing, and other forms of data collection

Category	Aspect	Process
	Member checking	Presenting findings back to participants in the study to assess if the research findings adequately include their perspectives on the phenomenon of interest
Readers' or Reviewers' Lens	Rich description	Providing a compelling account of the phenomenon of investigation in great depth and detail
	Peer debriefing	Engaging colleagues or experts in content or the field of study to read the accounts you have developed and to challenge you on your findings
	Transparency (O'Cathain, 2010)	Portraying the steps and procedures of the research clearly enough that the reader can understand in depth how the research/evaluation was conducted
	Relevance to users (Bryman et al., 2008)	Conducting research that delves into subject matter or problems that are understandable and meaningful to a wide constituency of the research

Source: Adapted from Creswell's (2016) *30 Essential Skills for the Qualitative Researcher* with permission with expansion by *Mixed Methods Research Workbook* author.

Activity: Identifying Threats to and Strategies to Promote Trustworthiness of the Qualitative Strand

After reviewing the elements of trustworthiness in Table 16.1, use Workbox Illustration 16.1.1 as a reference to complete Workbox 16.1.2. Use the three lenses suggested by Creswell—the researcher's, the participant's, and the reader/reviewer's—to systematically consider the potential threats to trustworthiness. Fill in the elements as they apply to your project and the strategies your plan to use (or actually used) to minimize the threat. In more qualitatively focused projects, you should have more comprehensive consideration, while more quantitatively focused projects may have less.

Workbox Illustration 16.1.1: Assessment of Trustworthiness in the Qualitative Strand From the MPathic-VR Mixed Methods Medical Education Project

Type	Process Used to Minimize Threat in the MPathic-VR Project
Reflexivity	Reviewing of coding by an independent third person beyond the two primary coders
Triangulation	Collecting student experiences, proctor notes, and field notes
Disconfirming evidence	Looking for alternative interpretations during the analysis
Collaboration with participants	Honing fidelity of the virtual human characters through interviews with real-life individuals
Prolonged engagement	Not applicable
Member checking	Offering to participants, though the medical schools declined
Rich description	Using student narratives in a joint display
Peer debriefing	Submitting to external peer review
Transparency	Focusing on clarity in the narrative in resulting papers
Relevance to users	Collecting posttrial reflections
Other	Developing open-ended questions and multiple researchers reviewing the questions Analyzing specific grant questions, while also remaining open to new questions emerging from the data

Source: Kron et al. (2017).

**Workbox 16.1.2: Assessment of Threats to Quality
in the Qualitative Strand in Your Project**

Type	Process to Minimize Threat in Your Project

ASSESSING FOR THREATS TO QUALITY IN QUANTITATIVE RESEARCH: VALIDITY, RELIABILITY, GENERALIZABILITY, REPRODUCIBILITY, AND REPLICABILITY

As with qualitative research, various researchers have considered threats to quality in quantitative research (Johnson & Christensen, 2017; Salkind, 2017; Teddlie & Tashakkori, 2009). As with qualitative research, among the many disciplines using quantitative research, researchers have agreement about overarching considerations relative to ensuring quality and rigor, but different fields have different foci and some variations in terminology. In this section, I seek to provide sufficient information for you to identify potential threats to the quality of the quantitative strand of your project. You may require supplemental readings to understand and fully assess the relevant issues. There are many resources, and if you are a graduate student, you will likely be required to take at least one biostatistics class.

Two of the most commonly discussed criteria in qualitative research are validity and reliability. Validity refers to whether the research or a test measures what it is intended to measure. Reliability refers to whether a tool or instrument measures a phenomenon of interest consistently and provides the same result.

Measurement validity addresses the extent that "your data collection instrument actually measures what you intend it to assess" (Teddlie & Tashakkori, 2009). As illustrated in Table 16.2, Teddlie and Tashakkori (2009) present six aspects of measurement validity appropriately considered when executing the quantitative strand of your study.

Measurement reliability reflects the extent that "the results of a measurement consistently and accurately represent the true magnitude or 'quality' of a construct" (Teddlie & Tashakkori, 2009). As illustrated in Table 16.3, Teddlie and Tashakkori (2009) describe five aspects of measurement reliability for consideration in your mixed methods project.

There are additional potential internal and external invalidities such as confounding variables or threats for consideration when conducting quantitative research, as illustrated in Table 16.4.

Generalizability, also sometimes called external validity, reflects the extent that quantitative findings from the study population can be extrapolated to a broader population. As illustrated in Table 16.5, Johnson and Christensen (2017) identify six generalizability or external validity considerations for your mixed methods project.

TABLE 16.2 ■ Aspects of Measurement Validity in Quantitative Research Methods (Teddlie & Tashakkori, 2009)

Aspect	What to Consider?
Internal validity	Can a causal relationship be determined?
Historical validity	Did any events precede the study that could influence the findings?
Content validity	To what degree does an instrument measure a specific attribute?
Convergent validity	To what degree are measures of a construct that should be related, similar to another/different measure of that construct?
Concurrent validity	To what degree does a measure correlate with other measures of the same construct (type of convergent validity)?
Predictive validity	To what degree does an instrument correlate highly with an outcome that it is supposed to measure (a type of convergent validity)?
Instrumentation validity	Does a research instrument measure what it is supposed to measure during the course of the study?
Construct validity	Do(es) the variable(s) fully measure the construct that it is (they are) supposed to measure?
Criterion validity	To what extent does a chosen measure predict the same outcome of another measure?
Face validity	Is there a logical association between a variable and that which is being measured?
Maturation validity	Did any changes occur to participants during the research that could influence the outcomes?
Discriminant (divergent) validity	To what extent a can measure distinguish between groups that are supposed to be different?
Known group validity	To what extent are groups that are expected to be measured differently actually measure differently (type of discriminant validity)?
Conclusion validity	To what extent are conclusions based on the data about relationships between variables reasonable?

Source: Teddlie and Tashakkori (2009).

TABLE 16.3 ■ Threats to Measurement Reliability in Quantitative Research Methods (Teddlie & Tashakkori, 2009)

Type	What to Consider?
Test-retest reliability	To what extent repeated assessment does a measure consistently distinguish between groups?
Split-half reliability	When a group is split into two halves, to what extent do the measures of the two halves correlate?
Parallel forms reliability	Do two forms of the same test correlate?
Internal consistency	When examining the correlation of all items on a test, to what extent does the scoring of all correlate?
Interrater (interobserver) reliability	To what degree do two or more raters have the same ratings?

Source: Teddlie and Tashakkori (2009).

Activity: Identifying Threats to the Quality in the Quantitative Strand of Your Mixed Methods Research and Evaluation Projects

After reviewing the potential threats to quality in your quantitative strand using Table 16.2 on measurement validity, Table 16.3 on measurement reliability, Table 16.4 on internal and external validity threats, and Table 16.5 on generalizability, use Workbox Illustration 16.2.1 as a reference to complete Workbox 16.2.2. You should consider each of these features, and then express in Workbox 16.2.2, how you plan (or already have) to address it.

TABLE 16.4 ■ Internal and External Threats to Validity of Quantitative Research (Johnson & Christensen, 2017)

Type	What to Consider?
Confounding variable	Could a variable be related to both the independent and dependent variable?
Selection bias	Could individuals selected for the study differ systematically from individuals not selected for the research?
Selection–maturation interaction	Could the selection of comparison groups interact with changes that occur during the research, to influence the outcomes?
Testing bias	Could baseline testing or pretesting affect how participants perform in a subsequent test?
Statistical regression	To what extent do the findings occur from regression to the mean of outlying values?
Reproducibility	Would another researcher who analyzes your data have the same findings and reach the same conclusions as reported in your analysis?
Replicability	Would similar findings be found when testing is conducted under similar circumstances by others?

Source: Johnson and Christensen (2017).

TABLE 16.5 ■ Threats to Research Generalizability in Quantitative Research Methods (Johnson & Christensen, 2017)

Type	What to Consider?
External validity	Do findings from the study population extrapolate to a target population, settings, times, outcomes, or variations in treatment (cf. generalizing in Chapter 10)?
Population validity	Can study findings be inferred to individuals who did not participate in the study?
Ecological validity	To what extent can study findings be generalized across multiple settings?
Temporal validity	To what extent do study findings extrapolate across time?
Treatment variation validity	To what extent can treatment findings be inferred to individuals who were not treated and are not in a controlled setting?
Outcome validity	To what extent can study findings be generalized across different but related dependent variables?

Source: Johnson and Christensen (2017).

Workbox Illustration 16.2.1: Assessment of Threats to Quality in the Quantitative Strand Using the Example of the MPathic-VR Mixed Methods Medical Education Project

Type	Strategy Used to Minimize Threat in the MPathic-VR Project
Validity	Using face validity Considering content validity
Reliability	Conducting internal consistency reliability testing
Generalizability	Conducting study in three sites chosen for regional differences (e.g., one Midwest medical school and two Southern medical schools)
Replicability	Assessing for replicability by comparing results of three different sites, that is, three different medical schools separately, as well as in aggregate
Reproducibility	Did not apply

Source: Kron et al. (2017).

Workbox 16.2.2: Assessment of Threats to Quality in the Quantitative Strand in Your Project

Type	Strategy to Minimize Threat in Your Project
Validity	
Reliability	
Generalizability	
Replicability	
Reproducibility	

ASSESSING FOR THREATS TO QUALITY IN MIXED METHODS RESEARCH AND EVALUATION PROJECTS

Consideration of the research integrity in MMR extends beyond the methods. Having identified issues specific to your mixed methods design with guidance from Creswell and Plano Clark (2018), the next step requires focusing on the quality of the methodology. Johnson and Christensen's (2017) framework expands into the methodology of mixed methods at a more comprehensive level. O'Cathain's (2010) approach expands comprehensively into the entire investigation process, from conceptualization and arguably funding, through the final publication stage. Depending on your project, you can selectively choose how comprehensively to consider these levels. You have a chance to consider each perspective systematically through the following activities.

RESEARCH INTEGRITY: QUALITY ASSESSMENT IN THE METHODS

Creswell and Plano Clark (2018) take a methods design orientation throughout their work. They call for using the construct of "validity in mixed methods research" (p. 249).

They propose the use of validity as an overarching and unifying language for discussing quality across quantitative, qualitative, and MMR. They argue for validity as a unifying term because people in general are familiar with the concept and accept it (Creswell & Plano Clark, 2018). Further arguments for using the concept include that various methodologists have used parallels with specific aspects of validity from quantitative research, which can be beneficial by allowing others to build their understanding based on concepts already familiar to them.

TABLE 16.6 ■ Three Tactics for Considering Quality Assessment in Mixed Methods Research and Evaluation Projects by Focus, Discipline, Research Quality Concept and Expert Source			
Focus	Discipline	Research Quality Concept	Mixed Methods Expert Source
Methods	Educational psychology, physics, and educational psychology	Validity	Creswell and Plano Clark (2018)
Methodology	Research, evaluation, measurement, and statistics; psychology; sociology; public administration; and psychology	Validity/Legitimation	Johnson and Christensen (2017)
Program of investigation	Health services research	Quality domains in mixed methods research	O'Cathain (2010)

Activity: Identifying Research Quality Threats in Your Methods for Your Research and Evaluation Project

To identify research quality threats occurring in the methods of your MMR and evaluation study, choose from among the workbox illustrations, Workbox Illustration 16.3.1.1 for a convergent mixed methods design, Workbox Illustration 16.3.1.2 for an explanatory sequential design, Workbox Illustration 16.3.1.3 for an exploratory sequential mixed methods design, and Workbox Illustration 16.3.1.4 for a mixed methods evaluation design. If you are using a more advanced/scaffolded/complex mixed methods design, use the core design that best fits you project. You can also review Creswell and Plano Clark's (2018) material for criteria about mixed methods experimental designs, mixed methods case study designs, and mixed methods participatory justice designs. After reviewing the illustration appropriate for your project, complete Workbox 16.3.2.

Convergent Mixed Methods Design

In Workbox Illustration 16.3.1.1, examine the threats and the strategies to minimize threats. The example features a mixed methods multisite randomized controlled trial by Kron et al. (2017) comparing a virtual human simulation and a computer-based learning module conducted with medical students (Appendix 1). The intervention and control learning modules were evaluated posttrial when students answered attitudinal survey questions and wrote reflective essays about their experiences. After reviewing Workbox Illustration 16.3.1.1, complete Workbox 16.3.2 based on your convergent mixed methods design.

Workbox Illustration 16.3.1.1: Research Integrity Threats in a Convergent Mixed Methods Design: An Example Using the MPathic-VR Mixed Methods Medical Education Study

Design Type: Convergent Mixed Methods Study		
Type of Threat	**Strategy to Minimize Threat**	**Example From the MPathic-VR Study**
Not using parallel concepts in data collection for both the quantitative and qualitative databases	Create parallel questions addressing the same concept	Matched the qualitative and quantitative data collection to address the same constructs
Having unequal sample sizes	Use the same sample size for qualitative and quantitative strands if you're comparing data for each participant or acknowledge different intents of sample size (e.g., to compare group means with individual experiences).	The sample for the qualitative and the quantitative data collection were identical. The two arms of the randomized controlled trial had a similar number of participants: n = 210 for the intervention and n = 211 for the control.
Keeping results from the different databases separate	Use convergent data analysis integration strategy (e.g., a joint display or comparing quantitative and qualitative results side by side).	Constructed a joint display to represent key findings about students' experiences during the trial and compared the qualitative and quantitative findings for both arms of the trial in a joint display, which further included study metainferences (p. 7).
Failure to resolve disconfirming results	Engage in strategies to understand disconfirming results (e.g., new analyses).	While the investigators found no disconfirming results, for the domain of "improve clinical skills," they noted that attitudinal scores did not reflect as a significant difference, though this was supported by the qualitative results.

Sources: Table structure: Creswell and Plano Clark (2018) with permission by SAGE Publications; content from Kron et al., 2017 adapted with permission.

Explanatory Sequential Mixed Methods Design

In Workbox Illustration 16.3.1.2, examine the threats and the strategies to minimize threats. The example features Harper's (2016) study to examine how the culture of academic optimism in schools relates to academic achievement when he assessed this relationship in 26 of Alabama's 218 middle schools stratified by socioeconomic status using correlation, regression, and recursive partitioning analyses (Appendix 2). To explain the findings, he explored qualitatively how three dimensions of academic optimism were related to student achievement using interviews with 11 principals of high-achieving middle schools. After reviewing Workbox Illustration 16.3.1.2, complete Workbox 16.4.2 based on your explanatory sequential mixed methods design.

Workbox Illustration 16.3.1.2: Threats to Quality of the Methods in an Explanatory Sequential Mixed Methods Design: An Example Using the Culture of Academic Optimism in Schools Study

Design Type: Explanatory Sequential Mixed Methods Study		
Type of Threat	**Strategy to Minimize Threat**	**Example From Harper's (2016) Academic Optimism and Academic Achievement Study**
Failing to identify important quantitative results to explain	Consider all possibilities for explanation of results (e.g., significant and nonsignificant predictors).	The survey questions in the quantitative strand of this study were asked of teachers, and their results helped develop the protocol for principals with the intent to explore how principals fostered high achievement through their impact on the dimensions of academic optimism. In this manner, the quantitative questions and results guided the development of the principal interview protocol (p. 88).
Not explaining surprising, contradictory quantitative results with qualitative data	Design qualitative data collection questions to probe into surprising or contradictory qualitative results.	The quantitative results, which revealed only a small to moderate link between academic optimism and student achievement, but a strong association between academic emphasis and student achievement, helped refine the qualitative research questions, inform the sample of principals to be interviewed, and guide the principal interview protocol development (p. 86).
Not connecting the initial quantitative results with the qualitative follow-up	Purposefully select the qualitative sample using quantitative results to identify participants from the sample of quantitative participants who can provide the best explanations.	Principals were purposefully selected from high-achieving schools with different levels of socioeconomic status, geographic location, and a broad range of academic optimism scores to achieve maximal variation and help the researcher understand the quantitative results from as many perspectives as possible (p. 86).

Sources: Table structure: Creswell and Plano Clark (2018) with permission by SAGE Publications; content from Harper (2016) adapted with permission.

Exploratory Sequential Mixed Methods Design

Review Workbox Illustration 16.3.1.3 to examine the threats and the strategies to minimize threats. The example comes from the Sharma and Vredenburg (1998) study to examine corporate environmental responsiveness to organizational capacity and performance where they conducted 19 in-depth interviews with senior and middle management executives to create case studies, and then they longitudinally interviewed additional executives before distributing a mail-based survey (Appendix 3). Based on Sharma and Vredenburg's (1998) mixed methods approach, they demonstrated that strategies of proactive responsiveness to uncertainties of the interface between business and ecological issues were associated with unique organizational capabilities that had implications for firm competitiveness. After reviewing Workbox Illustration 16.3.1.3, complete Workbox 16.3.2 based on your exploratory sequential mixed methods design.

Workbox Illustration 16.3.1.3: Research Integrity/Validity Threats in an Exploratory Sequential Mixed Methods Design: An Example Using the Corporate Environmental Responsiveness to Organizational Capacity and Performance Study

Design Type: Exploratory Sequential Mixed Methods Study		
Type of Threat	**Strategy to Minimize Threat**	**Application to Your Mixed Methods Project**
Not building the quantitative feature based on the qualitative results	Make explicit how each major qualitative finding is used to inform the development of specific elements of the quantitative features.	The items constituting the scale were based on the 11 dimensions identified and used in the exploratory research (p. 743).
Not developing rigorous quantitative features	Use systematic procedures to design the quantitative feature (e.g., use good psychometric design steps or pilot test intervention materials).	The instrument was vetted and pretested. Reliability checks (using Cronbach's alpha) with high reliability. Factor analysis using oblimin rotation demonstrated three constructs were a single variable (pp. 743-744).
Selecting participants from the quantitative test that are the same individuals as the qualitative sample	Use a large sample of individuals for the quantitative sample who are different from those in the qualitative sample.	Qualitative interviews were conducted with senior and middle management executives. While not clear in the article, it appears that the respondents were managers, supervisors, and CEOs of sufficient numbers such that it would not likely be a threat to the validity of the conclusions (p. 746).

Sources: Table structure: Creswell and Plano Clark (2018) with permission by SAGE Publications; content from Sharma and Vredenburg 1998 adapted with permission.

Evaluation Mixed Methods Design

Review Workbox Illustration 16.3.1.4 to examine the threats and the strategies to minimize threats. The example features Martinez, Dimitriadis, Rubia, Gomez, and de la Fuente's (2003) mixed methods evaluation of a computer-supported collaborative learning system to examine their program's effectiveness for promoting collaboration as information sharing in an upper-level undergraduate computer architecture course. The researchers collected and analyzed data from questionnaires with open- and closed-items, student post-hoc comments and criticisms, focus groups, and nonparticipant observations, as well as a social network analysis. After reviewing Workbox Illustration 16.3.1.4, complete Workbox 16.3.2 based on your evaluation mixed methods design.

Workbox Illustration 16.3.1.4: Threats to Quality of the Methods in an Evaluation Mixed Methods Design: An Example Using the Computer-Supported Collaborative Learning System Study (Martinez et al., 2003)

Design Type: Evaluation Mixed Methods Study		
Type of Threat	**Strategy to Minimize Threat**	**Application to Your Mixed Methods Project**
Lacking an evaluation model to frame the project	Clearly articulate an overall objective and the evaluation steps in the project.	Used the DELFOS (a Description of a Tele-educational Layered Framework Oriented to Learning Situations) curriculum development model for structuring the computer-supported collaborative learning system, and used a mixed methods case study approach, including social network analysis for the evaluation

Design Type: Evaluation Mixed Methods Study		
Type of Threat	**Strategy to Minimize Threat**	**Application to Your Mixed Methods Project**
Failing to link the steps in the evaluation process so that one step builds on the previous step	Be clear as to how the steps in the evaluation process connect and build toward a common objective.	Used an elaborate approach to data collection involving open questionnaires, observations, focus groups, close-ended questionnaires, and social network analysis, where data collection iteratively informed subsequent investigation in longitudinal fashion
Failing to identify the core design(s) embedded within the stages of the evaluation process	Draw the core design(s) into the evaluation process to make their use explicit and to highlight the points of integration where connection and building occurs.	Demonstrated elaborate integration of data collection and analysis procedures, though integration strategies not explicitly identified

Sources: Table structure: Creswell and Plano Clark (2018) with permission by SAGE Publications; permission from Elsevier and Copyright Clearance Center for the content from Martinez et al. (2003).

Workbox 16.3.2: Assessment of Threats to Quality in the Methods of Your Mixed Methods Project

Design Type:		
Type of Threat	**Strategy to Minimize Threat**	**Application to Your Mixed Methods Project**

CONSIDERATION OF RESEARCH INTEGRITY ISSUES FROM THE METHODOLOGICAL PERSPECTIVE: THE LEGITIMATION FRAMEWORK

Another approach to MMR expands consideration beyond the methods to the full methodology of MMR. Scholarship about legitimation has evolved among several authors over time. For example, compare Onwuegbuzie and Johnson (2006), Collins, Onwuegbuzie, and Johnson (2012), and Johnson and Christensen (2017). While full examination of these criteria extends beyond the scope of this chapter, the information here provides sufficient information to understand the concept and consider its relevance for your research and evaluation projects.

THE LEGITIMATION PERSPECTIVE ON QUALITY IN THE METHODOLOGY OF MIXED METHODS RESEARCH AND EVALUATION PROJECTS

To the original nine legitimation criteria of Onwuegbuzie and Johnson (2006), two more criteria have been added. Despite their innovative work, a consistent definition has been elusive, and the authors use the language interchangeably with validity (Johnson & Christensen, 2017). Table 16.7 presents features of the 11 aspects of legitimation for mixed methods methodology.

TABLE 16.7 ■ Illustration of Eleven Research Quality Features of Legitimation for Mixed Methods Methodology Based on Johnson and Christensen Typology (2017)		
Aspect	**Description**	**Comment**
1. Inside-outside legitimation	Refers to the extent to which a researcher accurately understands, uses, and presents the participants' subjective insider or "native" views (emic) and the researcher's objective outsider view (etic)	Another metaphor is stepping in and out of the two viewpoints. The mixed methods researcher needs to represent both viewpoints and create a third mixed methods research (MMR) viewpoint. This emphasizes the need to draw metainferences, that is, interpretations based on both types of data.
2. Paradigmatic/ philosophical legitimation	Addresses the degree that a mixed methods researcher explains his or her mixed methods paradigm	Seven articulated worldviews or philosophical perspectives include pragmatism, participatory/ transformative, critical realism, postmodernism, yinyang, dialectical pluralism, and performative paradigm. Chapter 4 activities will help clarify your own stance.
3. Commensurability approximation legitimation	Addresses the degree to which a mixed methods researcher can make Gestalt switches between the lenses of a qualitative researcher and a quantitative researcher and integrate the two views into an "integrated" or third viewpoint	Highlights the imperative to become a mixed methods researcher by moving back and forth between the qualitative and quantitative strands. Commensurability approximation validity may require working in teams with qualitative, quantitative, and MMR expertise.
4. Weakness minimization legitimation	Describes the extent to which limitations from one research strand, method, or approach are compensated by the strengths from another research strand, method, or approach	Mixed methods researchers can minimize weaknesses by utilizing the QUAN and QUAL strands to avoid nonoverlapping weaknesses. This may include using both QUAL or QUAN strands to address gaps not addressed by the other.
5. Sequential legitimation	Represents the extent that a mixed methods researcher appropriately addresses and/ or builds on effects, understandings, knowledge, or findings from earlier qualitative and quantitative phases	It applies in both types of sequential mixed methods designs (Chapter 7). Consider the extent the results would have been different, in a negative way, if the sequencing of data collection and analysis had been done in reverse. Ask how a subsequent phase builds upon the previous phase.
6. Conversion legitimation	Applies under the circumstance in mixed methods studies when the mixed methods researcher converts one form of data into the other to evaluate the accuracy/quality of data transformations	Conversion validity applies when quantitizing qualitative data, and in unusual cases when there is qualitizing of quantitative data. Under these circumstances, there should be appropriate interpretations made on the transformed data (see Chapter 15).
7. Sample integration legitimation	Reflects the degree to which a mixed methods researcher makes appropriate conclusions, generalizations, and metainferences from mixed samples, that is, combinations of QUAN and QUAL samples	Statistical generalizations are achieved from randomly collected samples. In contrast, examining meaning and experiential aspects of research can best be achieved with intentional or purposive samples, while also considering transferability when there are smaller sample sizes.
8. Pragmatic legitimation	Implies the degree to which the researchers achieve their research purpose, answer the research or evaluation of questions posed, and elucidate results that can be acted upon	This criterion applies particularly in applied research and seeks to know from a practical perspective the extent the purpose, questions, results, and resulting actions added value.

Aspect	Description	Comment
9. Integration legitimation	Means the degree to which a researcher achieves integration throughout the project and can occur at multiple dimensions from the philosophical, the rational, the specific MMR questions, the design, sampling, data analysis, interpretation, and conclusions	Mixed methods researchers can achieve integration validity by drawing interpretations or so-called metainferences based on both types of data.
10. Sociopolitical legitimation	Conjures the degree to which a mixed methods researcher addresses the interests, values, and viewpoints of multiple standpoints and stakeholders in the research process	Mixed methods researchers attentive to sociopolitical validity will consider and value the positions and viewpoints of the oppressed or victims of injustice. The researcher will be sensitive to the needs of stakeholders without a voice, or for those with a compromised voice (see relevance to social justice/participatory designs, e.g., Chapter 15).
11. Multiple validities legitimation	Describes the degree to which the mixed methods researcher has addressed the quality issues of the qualitative research (e.g., trustworthiness), quantitative research (e.g., validity, reliability, generalizability), and MMR quality	This concept closely approximates the notion of MMR integrity.

For any particular research or evaluation study, usually only a subset of the features for legitimization will apply. Johnson and Christensen (2017) emphasize multiple validities legitimation as the most important, an emphasis substantiating the notion of MMR integrity. As you may recall, Harper (2016) sought to understand the relationship between academic optimism and school performance in middle schools. Workbox Illustration 16.4.1 illustrates how six of the 11 criteria apply to Harper's (2016) mixed methods study on the role of the principal in creating a culture of academic optimism.

Workbox Illustration 16.4.1: Example of Study Legitimation in a Mixed Methods Study on the Role of the Principal in Creating a Culture of Academic Optimism (Harper, 2016)

Type and Description	Strategies to Minimize Threat	Explanation
Sample integration: "The extent to which the relationship between the quantitative and qualitative sampling design yields quality metainferences" (Onwuegbuzie & Johnson, 2006).	Qualitative strand sample taken from the quantitative sample; purposive qualitative sampling for maximal variation utilized; fidelity to sample qualifications	The smaller sample of principals was selected from the larger quantitative sample of schools to provide opportunities for in-depth discussion of questions and topics. Only teachers and principals working in the school at the time of the SA tests were eligible to participate.
Inside-outside: "The extent to which the researcher accurately presents and appropriately utilizes the insider's and the observer's views for purposes such as description and explanation" (Onwuegbuzie & Johnson, 2006).	Etic viewpoint: dissertation committee audit review, review, by outside principal Emic viewpoint: member checking	A review by dissertation committee members ensured an accurate emic perspective and viewpoint. The principal interview protocol was piloted and revised based on feedback from a nonparticipating principal, strengthening its legitimacy. Principals member-checked their verbatim transcripts of their interview. Teacher respondents completed the survey privately online with enough time to avoid inaccuracies. These strategies raised the credibility of the survey data and strengthened the legitimacy of metainferences.

(Continued)

(Continued)

Type and Description	Strategies to Minimize Threat	Explanation
Weakness minimization: "The extent to which the weakness from one approach is compensated by the strengths from the other approach" (Onwuegbuzie & Johnson, 2006).	The sequential QUAN QUAL design uses complementary strengths to balance the weaknesses of each strand.	The qualitative open-ended principal interview was created to overcome the inability of the teacher survey to generate insight and knowledge about how AO is created through the actions of the principal to influence the three dimensions of AO (FT, CE, AE). Conversely, the quantitative teacher survey identified and summarized the degree to which AO was present in schools and its influence on student achievement in ways the qualitative survey could not.
Paradigmatic mixing: "The extent to which the researcher's epistemological, ontological, axiological, methodological, and rhetorical beliefs that underlie the quantitative and qualitative approaches are successfully a) combined or b) blended into a usable package" (Onwuegbuzie & Johnson, 2006).	Assumption and maintenance of a pragmatic stance on paradigmatic mixing to reveal inferences that will be considered legitimate	As stated in a previous section, the researcher has carefully considered and stated the philosophical assumptions that underlie this study. Moderate, rather than extreme, views characterize these assumptions.
Commensurability: "The extent to which the metainferences were made reflect a mixed world-view based on the cognitive process of Gestalt switching and integration" (Onwuegbuzie & Johnson, 2006).	Accepting a nonexclusive approach to the MMR process, which recognizes the ability of both the qualitative and quantitative worldviews to yield knowledge, and thus bring forth a third, mixed worldview	Once the study accepted pragmatism as its philosophical foundation (which it did at the start), only a mixed worldview could be admitted and the compatibility thesis accepted.
Multiple validities: "The extent to which addressing legitimation of the quantitative and qualitative components of the study result from the use of quantitative, qualitative and mixed validity types, yielding high quality metainferences" (Onwuegbuzie & Johnson, 2006).	Relevant strategies are used to maximize the validity and legitimation of both quantitative and qualitative methods and techniques to make metainferences that can suggest answers to the research questions.	Relevant procedures were used to promote quantitative reliability and validity, as well as qualitative trustworthiness, credibility, and validity.

Source: Harper (2016). Adapted with permission.

Activity: Identifying Legitimation Threats and Strategies to Minimize the Threat

Consider the relevance of legitimation (Table 16.7) to your own MMR or evaluation project using Workbox Illustration 16.4.1 as you complete Workbox 16.4.2. As shown in Workbox Illustration 16.4.1, enter the type and description of the legitimation criteria. Second, enter your planned or already utilized strategies for minimizing the effect. In the last column, provide an explanation. Importantly, Harper (2016) only identified six of the nine as relevant to his own project. To assess relevance to your own study requires systematically considering each carefully and addressing only those that apply.

Workbox 16.4.2: Legitimation Threats to Your Mixed Methods Research or Evaluation Project

Type and Description	Strategies to Minimize Threat	Explanation

A PROGRAM APPROACH TO MIXED METHODS QUALITY: O'CATHAIN'S RESEARCH AND EVALUATION QUALITY

O'Cathain (2010) expands the discussion about quality to consideration of the entire investigation. Informed by a comprehensive search of various mixed methodology experts and examples, her work considers six dimensions of an investigation: planning, undertaking, interpreting, integrating, reporting, and applying in the real world (Workbox Illustration 16.5.1). From the six dimensions, she synthesized eight domains meriting consideration of quality issues. Inherent with the strengths of this comprehensive approach, comes a downside of being too comprehensive. This more comprehensive framework may be particularly relevant to individuals developing large-scale projects for funding. Depending on your study scope, only a limited number of domains may have relevance and you may choose to consider only those with relevance to your research or evaluation project.

Workbox Illustration 16.5.1: Illustration of Eight Domains of Mixed Methods Research Quality (O'Cathain, 2010)

Stage	Domain	Description
Planning	1. Planning quality	Foundational element, rationale transparency, planning transparency, and feasibility
Undertaking	2. Design quality	Design transparency, design suitability, design strength, design rigor
	3. Data quality	Transparency, rigor/design fidelity, sampling adequacy, analytic adequacy, integration rigor
Interpreting	4. Interpretive rigor	Interpretative transparency, interpretative consistency, theoretical consistency, interpretive agreement, interpretive distinctness, interpretive efficacy, interpretive bias reduction, interpretive correspondence
Integrating	5. Interference transferability	Ecological transferability, population transferability, temporal transferability, theoretical transferability
Reporting	6. Reporting quality	Report availability, reporting transparency, yield
Application in real world	7. Synthesizability	Fifteen quality criteria: six applied to the qualitative component, six applied to the quantitative component, and three applied to the mixed methods study component
	8. Utility	Utility quality, that is, the degree results inform change in policy or practices

Activity: Identifying Domains of Mixed Methods Research Quality for Your Mixed Methods Research or Evaluation Project

Consider the relevance of the eight domains of quality to your own MMR or evaluation project using Workbox Illustration 16.5.1 as a reference, and complete Workbox 16.5.2. This activity should serve as a "screener" for you to think about the potential relevance. To complete the activity, choose the stages that have immediate relevance. Then consider the domains and record as applicable to your own study. Once you have identified relevant domains, you can dive deeper if necessary, based on the immediacy of the relevance.

Workbox 16.5.2: Relevance of Eight Domains of Mixed Methods Research Quality to Your Project (O'Cathain, 2010)

Stage	Domain	Your Study
Planning	1. Planning quality	
Undertaking	2. Design quality	
	3. Data quality	
Interpreting	4. Interpretive rigor	
Integrating	5. Interference transferability	
Reporting	6. Reporting quality	
Applying in the real world	7. Synthesizability	
	8. Utility	

Application Activities

1. **Peer Feedback**. If you are working on your project as part of a class or in a workshop, pair up with a peer mentor, and one of you spend about 5 minutes talking about the threats to quality in your mixed methods study or evaluation project. Take turns talking about your project's threats to quality and your strategy to minimize the threat and giving feedback. If you are working independently, share your protocol with a colleague or mentor.

2. **Peer Feedback Guidance**. As you listen to your partner, you should focus on learning and honing the valuable

skills of critiquing. Your goal is to help your partner refine consideration of quality issues. Help them reflect on their assessments to the threats to quality. Focus on the section or area where your partner needs feedback the most. Are there any sections that don't make sense or seem infeasible?

3. **Group Debrief**. If you are in a classroom or large-group setting, take volunteers to present their assessments of the threats to quality in their MMR or evaluation projects. Reflect on how these same issues may play out in your own project.

Concluding Thoughts

Use this checklist to assess your progress in achieving the Chapter 16 objectives:

☐ I assessed for threats against the quality of my project's qualitative strand from a trustworthiness perspective.

☐ I assessed for threats against the quality of my project's quantitative strand from perspectives of validity, reliability, generalizability, and replicability.

☐ I identified possible threats to quality of my mixed methods based on my specific mixed methods design.

☐ I determined the elements of legitimation that could be relevant as threats to quality in my project.

☐ I ascertained the relevance of an overall investigation approach to considering quality in my mixed methods project.

☐ I reviewed my Chapter 16 research integrity threats and strategies to mitigate threats with a peer or colleague to strengthen my mixed methods procedures.

Now that you have completed these objectives, Chapter 17 will help you prepare for the submission of your MMR or evaluation project articles.

Key Resources

1. **FURTHER READING ON QUALITY IN MIXED METHODS STUDIES**

   - Collins, K. M. T. (2015). Validity in multimethod and mixed research. In S. N. Hesse-Biber & B. Johnson (Eds.), *The Oxford handbook of multimethod and mixed methods research inquiry* (pp. 240–256). New York, NY: Oxford University Press.

   - Creswell, J. W. (2016). Implementing validity checks. In *30 essential skills for the qualitative researcher* (pp. 190–195). Thousand Oaks, CA: Sage.

   - O'Cathain, A. (2010). Assessing the quality of mixed methods research toward a comprehensive framework. In A. Tashakkori & C. Teddlie (Eds.), *SAGE handbook of mixed methods in social & behavioral research* (2nd ed., pp. 531–558). Thousand Oaks, CA: Sage.

   - Teddlie, C., & Tashakkori, A. (2009). Considerations before collecting your data. In *Foundations of mixed methods research: Integrating quantitative and qualitative approaches in the social and behavioral sciences* (pp. 197–216). Thousand Oaks, CA: Sage.

2. **FURTHER READING ON LEGITIMATION**

   - Collins, K. M. T., Onwuegbuzie, A. J., & Johnson, R. B. (2012). Securing a place at the table: A review and extension of legitimation criteria for the conduct of

   mixed research. *American Behavioral Scientist, 56*(6), 849–865. doi:10.1177/0002764211433799

   - Johnson, R. B., & Christensen, L. (2017).Validity of research results in quantitative, qualitative and mixed methods research. In *Educational Research Quantitative, Qualitative, and Mixed Approaches* (6th ed., pp. 281–313). Thousand Oaks, CA: Sage.

   - Onwuegbuzie, A. J., & Johnson, R. B. (2006). The validity issue in mixed research. *Research in the Schools, 13*(1), 48–63.

3. **FURTHER READING ON SYSTEMATIC MIXED STUDIES REVIEWS**

   - Hong, Q. N., & Pluye, P. (2018). A conceptual framework for critical appraisal in systematic mixed studies reviews. *Journal of Mixed Methods Research*, 1–15. doi:10.1177/1558689818770058

   - Pluye, P., & Hong, Q. N. (2014). Combining the power of stories and the power of numbers: Mixed methods research and mixed studies reviews. *Annual Review of Public Health, 35*(1), 29–45. doi:10.1146/annurev-publhealth-032013-182440

   - Sandelowski M., Voils, C. I., & Barroso, J. (2006). Defining and designing mixed research synthesis studies. *Research in the Schools, 13*(1), 29–44.

PREPARING FOR SUBMISSION OF MIXED METHODS RESEARCH AND EVALUATION ARTICLES FOR PUBLICATION

Conducting a mixed methods research or evaluation project opens multiple venues for publication. In the throes of conducting your mixed methods project, you may be preoccupied with just conducting the project, and you may have given limited thought to a publication plan. This chapter and its activities will help you recognize the variety of publication options, conduct a project inventory to organize a publication strategy, develop a list of candidate journals, rate identified candidate journals as potential submission destinations, and develop a comprehensive mixed methods publication plan. As a key outcome, you will complete a mixed methods paper organizer, identify journals for submission of mixed methods articles, and complete a comprehensive mixed methods paper publication plan.

LEARNING OBJECTIVES

The ideas presented here will help you

- Recognize publication options open to mixed methods research (MMR) and evaluation studies

- Conduct a project inventory to organize a publishing strategy based on the project strengths, limitations, and relevant publication types, and to develop a rationale for order of submission

- Develop a list of candidate journals organized as "stretch," "good fit," and "safety," which can be pursued for publication of mixed methods articles

- Identify candidate journals and rate them as submission destinations for manuscripts of your MMR and evaluation studies

- Develop a comprehensive mixed methods publication plan

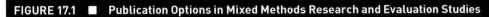

FIGURE 17.1 ■ Publication Options in Mixed Methods Research and Evaluation Studies

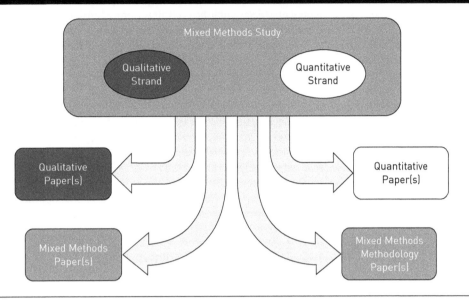

PUBLISHING OPPORTUNITIES WHEN CONDUCTING MIXED METHODS RESEARCH AND EVALUATION PROJECTS

Most individuals engaged in academic or applied research and evaluation outside of, or within, the halls of academia relish the opportunity for, and success in, publishing their research. There are many reasons to publish. Upon completing a dissertation or postdoctoral training program, publications are the ticket to a job. Publishing establishes one as a scholar and authority within a field. Publishing is the opportunity to disseminate information that can inform change in current practices or bring to light issues needed to inform or change policy. A variety of academic institutions utilize publication records promoting individuals for higher ranking in the organization and even for their compensation. If you are conducting an MMR or evaluation study, then the publication of an empirical mixed methods paper will (or at least should!) be a high priority.

Conducting an MMR or evaluation project creates excellent opportunities for publication (Stange, Crabtree, & Miller, 2006). Publication venues include journals, chapters, or monographs. Mixed methods researchers and evaluators have the opportunity to create four categories of publications (Figure 17.1). Mixed methods empirical papers incorporate the mixed findings developed through the use of fundamental analysis procedures (Chapter 13), a joint display (Chapter 14), or from an advanced mixed data analysis (Chapter 15). Moreover, MMR and evaluation studies create opportunities for two types of monomethod papers: papers from the qualitative strand and papers from the quantitative strand. If you have completed the Mixed Methods Data Linking Activity Workbox in Chapter 14, you may have found qualitative themes or quantitative constructs that did not have analogous data from the other method. In such cases, these are opportunities for empirical qualitative-only papers and empirical quantitative-only papers. When possible, I encourage you to write mixed methods papers, but when the two types of content are not linkable in a meaningful way, writing monomethod papers will help advance your writing portfolio. A fourth category of publication involves a mixed methods methodological paper.

SHOULD I WRITE EMPIRICAL OR METHODOLOGICAL PAPERS?

To the question of "Should I write empirical articles/chapters or methodological articles/chapters?" the answer is a resounding yes. That is, write both if you can! If you have collected and analyzed both qualitative and quantitative data, then you should be writing one or more empirical mixed methods articles/chapters. Empirical mixed methods papers and mixed methods methodological papers have many similar features but also have some important differences. Empirical mixed methods papers include articles publishing integrated qualitative and quantitative data. Methodological mixed methods papers represent articles published to inform procedures, theory, or methodological aspects in the field of MMR. Many researchers and evaluators don't recognize the opportunity to publish a methodological paper. In the process of conducting your project, if you encounter a methodological challenge for which you cannot find clear guidance from existing literature, consider writing a methodological/theoretical article. Methodological/theoretical articles/chapters can be written when you have developed an innovative way of approaching any of the numerous dimensions of integration in mixed methods inquiry.

Discerning whether you have done something novel or not depends on whether you have developed a unique approach at the philosophical level relative to conceptualization of the field, a new theoretical conceptualization, an innovative approach to methodology, or a novel approach to the methods (e.g., data collection, analysis, or representation of MMR and evaluation). Methodological articles require more detail about the study methodology than empirical articles. Moreover, methodological articles, when published first, can allow authors to truncate the methods section of an empirical paper, and they also benefit from having citable, previous successful peer review of the methodology. With so many options available for publication of mixed methods articles and papers also comes the challenge for identifying journals for publication of these various types of papers. A project inventory can help with organization.

CONDUCTING A PROJECT INVENTORY FOR PUBLISHING MIXED METHODS RESEARCH AND EVALUATION STUDIES

In planning for your publications from MMR and evaluation studies, taking an inventory of the project strengths, limitations, order of publications pursuit, and the rationale for the ordering can be very helpful to organize. A **project inventory for publication** is a written activity to organize study strengths, limitations, order of publications pursuit, and the rationale for the ordering of submission. Workbox Illustration 17.1.1 provides an example based on the MPathic-VR project using a virtual human intervention in a mixed methods intervention trial with medical students. This particular project received funding through two grants, and unfunded projects were used to obtain the first small business grant to demonstrate feasibility of the product. This led to publications useful as "pilot data" for an even larger grant. The illustration documents the strengths, limitations, and publication strategies pursued, as well as the rationale.

Workbox Illustration 17.1.1: Project Inventory for Mixed Methods Publication Planning: Example From the MPathic-VR Line of Research

What are the strengths of your project for publication?
The study conducted a series of pilot studies prior to funding, during funding of a Phase I study, and through acquired additional funding. This provided many opportunities for publishing papers that have included those on medical student attitudes about gaming (Kron, Gjerde, Sen, & Fetters, 2010), nursing student attitudes about gaming (Lynch-Sauer et al., 2011), a construct validity paper (Guetterman et al., 2017), a mixed methods research trial (Kron et al., 2017), and a methodological paper (Fetters, Guetterman, Scerbo, & Kron, 2017). The strength of this study was the team's success in implementing a multisite, single-blinded mixed methods randomized controlled trial.
What are the limitations?
Publication of the early findings, especially qualitative findings relative to development of the intervention, were not pursued due to limited resources and concern early on about compromise of a potential technological advantage in a competitive field.
What order of publication would best tell the story of your work (e.g., qualitative, quantitative, mixed methods, methodological)?
The most important paper from this study is about the findings of the trial itself. However, the order of publication involved first preliminary studies that could be cited in a grant application for funding. The pilot studies conducted in preparation for the study involved three pilot studies, all quantitative, examining medical student and nursing student attitudes about the use of serious games in medical education, as well as a third study examining construct validity conducted with medical residents. The first two studies demonstrated need in a population segment. The third study demonstrated rigor of the system and expanded the population of demonstrated use and utility into a population of medical residents.

Why this order?

The survey findings about medical student attitudes (Kron et al., 2010) and nursing student attitudes about serious gaming (Lynch-Sauer et al., 2011) were published first because the data were available in that order, and we needed to publish data appropriate as pilot data for our grant proposal. While the project was about medical student education, the team partnership included a private start-up entity that was eager to develop a track record of publication. In addition, from a business perspective, the publication track record was valued for establishing the credibility of the business. These objectives were all enhanced with publication of an additional study regarding the construct validity conducted with higher-level learners, medical residents, to further expand the study portfolio (Guetterman et al., 2017). Publication of the findings of the trial (Kron et al., 2017) was the first publication to disseminate information about the research from an academic perspective, while it was further clearly a benefit from a business perspective given the goals of the start-up company. Since that time, a mixed methods methodological paper was developed (Fetters et al., 2017). While we would have preferred to publish the methodological paper sooner, we were waiting for the publication of the trial data first.

Activity: Project Inventory for Mixed Methods Publications

While using Workbox Illustration 17.1.1 as a reference, fill in the four sections of Workbox 17.1.2, so you can consider the publication strengths of your MMR or evaluation project. For the first *strengths section*, consider your ability to publish each of the different types of publications: empirical qualitative only, empirical quantitative only, empirical mixed methods papers, and methodological papers. Can you first publish a methods paper or a protocol paper that can be referred to in subsequent papers? Do you have a collaborator on a paper who may have limited availability or have a planned away such that you want to prioritize a specific paper? Is one of your papers competitive about a cutting edge topic? Do you have skill sets that set you up for more quick publication of one type of paper rather than another? Are you trying to reach a specific audience or conference where a certain type of paper would be a better fit?

For the second *limitations section*, consider what might be limitations relative to publication. Is your work cutting edge such that publication could compromise other work that is ongoing? Do you have an advisor or colleague on the team who is on sabbatical or does not carry through with correspondence? Does your institution prevent doctoral students from publishing before they complete their defense? Is there confusion about authorship?

For the third *publication order section*, consider the publication order. Is there a logical order for publication (e.g., a sequential design where one form of data is available before the other)? Are there considerations about the optimal order of publication? Will publication of the mixed methods paper take place last since the data collection and analysis of the qualitative and quantitative strand occur first?

In the fourth *rationale for order section*, describe if there is a particular rationale for the order. Perhaps you are following the order that you have followed for the conduct of your research. Alternatively, you have a scientific meeting that will be instrumental for dissemination early of a paper that involved data collection later in the process. Or, maybe a certain paper would be pivotal for a change in job, for acquiring a postdoctoral position, or for landing your first teaching job.

Workbox 17.1.2: Project Inventory for Mixed Methods Publication Planning

What are the strengths of your project for publication?

(Continued)

(Continued)

What are the limitations relative to publication?

What order of publication would best tell the story of your work (e.g., qualitative, quantitative, mixed methods, methodological)?

Why this order?

SELECTING TARGET JOURNALS FOR SUBMITTING MIXED METHODS RESEARCH AND EVALUATION STUDIES

During the course of conducting MMR consultations individually, and during workshops, I am often asked how to choose a target journal and for a recommendation about where to submit. **Target journals** represent publishing venues chosen as destinations for dissemination of MMR and evaluation papers or articles. If you are still starting your research career, this is an opportunity to explore for journals of interest and look for matches to their work and methodology. When you're ready to write, you will need a framework for choosing where to submit. Table 17.1 provides three levels of journals to consider when getting ready to choose journals. I often spend 2 or 3 hours studying the journals where an article could be submitted. For researchers only publishing in a single content area, the usual journals and their rankings may be well known. But if you are more junior and/or less familiar with the publications in your field, you will likely have some work to do. An advisor or committee member is an excellent resource for recommendations on choosing a journal. People seeking advice from me often are surprised that I create a list of target journals, as per Table 17.1, with a minimum of three levels (see also Story From the Field 17.1). This approach was developed, in part, based on my observation that researchers new to publication often do not fully understand the challenges and strategies of choosing target journals for submission.

TABLE 17.1 ■ Conceptualizing Three Categories of Target Journals for Mixed Methods Papers				
Relative Fit	Tier	Difficulty	Assessment of Success	Probability of Acceptance
Stretch journal	Upper	High	Not highly likely	10%–30%
Good fit journal	Mid to top	Moderate	Good chance	40%–60%
Safety journal	Lower	Low	Very good chance	70+%

When you embark on your search for journals, the most important task is to create a list of three to four choices when you finish your session. Rather than choose only one journal, prioritize your list. The only thing worse than spending 2 to 3 hours up front identifying a journal for your submission is spending 2 to 3 hours a second time if you get a rejection from the first journal.

The publication goal of most researchers is for the article's acceptance at the most prestigious journal possible. I like the maxim, "if you do not submit to the best journals, you will never be published in the best journals." The corollary is that when submitting to the best journals, the odds are high that your paper will be rejected. The advantage of choosing several journals up front—for each paper category—eliminates time spent reconsidering for an additional 1 to 2 hours where a paper should be sent if rejected by a top-tier journal (see Chapter 18). If you have a rejection from a journal, your goal will be to turn the paper around as quickly as possible for submitting elsewhere. By creating a ranked list of journals at the outset, most papers can be reformatted and resubmitted within a week or less.

IDENTIFYING CANDIDATE JOURNALS AND RATING THEM AS SUBMISSION DESTINATIONS

Having developed a sense about the papers that you could produce and a relative prioritization, the challenge of where to submit the paper emerges. **Candidate journals** refer to the publishing venues for dissemination of MMR and evaluation papers or articles.

As above, the time that goes into evaluating the destination for a submission destination is time well spent, especially if you are willing to identify three or four journals. As to why it can take a long time to consider, glance at Workbox Illustration 17.2.1, which includes multiple criteria that experienced authors often consider when developing a publication strategy. This illustration was filled out with reference to the MPathic-VR randomized controlled trial (Kron et al., 2017). The rating for submission refers to the order of where the journal will be submitted. The second row indicates the actual journal name, and this is followed by the *categorization of fit*: stretch, good, or safety. The *impact factor* describes the influence of the journal. The impact factor is a simple calculation as a ratio where the numerator is the current-year citations of articles from the journal, and the denominator is the number of articles published in that journal in the previous 2 years. Knowing if the article is *online, paper*, or *both* is a factor to consider, especially given the increasing number of online publication options. Some online journals have a fee after acceptance or may offer open access for payment. If there is a charge, but the amount is not explicit, this is a red flag for a possible predatory journal (see Story From the Field 17.2, and below). *Word limit* is a very important consideration, because if you need to resubmit to another journal (odds are high if you go to a stretch journal), then you will not want to spend an inordinate amount of time editing the text down. Ideally, the ranked choices will have the same number of words, but that is unusual. If possible, keep the differences to no more than 500–1,000 words. For the MPathic-VR submission list, as the rank goes down, the word count limits actually goes up. The description of each journal (e.g., *aims* and *audience* come from the journal website and, as illustrated, each has a somewhat different focus). The question as to whether there are *similar papers* is important, and it should be answered from the perspective of the content and from a mixed methods perspective. The *website link* will help you go back, and *comments* provide flexibility for your thoughts/ideas or concerns.

Finding Candidate Journals

When you are a new researcher, or working as a methodologist, identifying journals can be challenging. JANE is an acronym for Journal/Author Name Estimator, and it is a website (http://jane.biosemantics.org) where the user can type in a title, abstract, or other information, and find journals, authors, or similar articles with just a click of a button (The Biosemantics Group, 2007). The outputs for "find journals" lists up to 40 journals that are a potential match and rates them with a confidence level, rating of article influence, and a link to related articles. The journal listing even includes notices if the article is high-quality open access or Medline-indexed and if the journal is in PubMed Central. It is a website supported by the Netherlands Bioinformatics Center, which is "the Dutch network of bioinformatics experts active in research, education and support" (The Biosemantics Group, 2007).

Another general resource for exploring journal options is the Scimago Institutions Rankings website (https:// www.scimagojr.com/journalsearch.php). This portal is an evaluation resource designed to search and assess the world's universities and research institutions (Scimago, 2007). Scimago Lab developed the website and utilizes information from Scopus. Based on scientific indicators and scientific domains, users can compare or analyze journals from the database. This portal allows researchers to search 27 major thematic areas and 313 subject categories, even by country. On its website, the Scimago organization is self-described as a research group from the Consejo Superior de Investigaciones Científicas, University of Granada, Extremadura, Carlos III (Madrid) and Alcalá de Henares, dedicated to information analysis, representation, and retrieval by means of visualization techniques.

A commercial resource is now available to EndNote users through Clarivate Analytics (n.d.). Its tool is called Manuscript Matcher. It claims that the matching function will identify top candidate journals for a manuscript based on the topic and references.

Activity: Identifying Journals and Ranking Them as Submission Destinations

Complete Workbox 17.2 to identify and rank journals to identify submission destinations. You may want to duplicate this sheet and use each of the article types: empirical qualitative, empirical quantitative, empirical mixed methods, and mixed methods methodology. Select one journal and complete the entire column. In most cases, the full information is available from the Internet. The final rating for submission will likely be the last row to complete after considering other factors. Enter the journal name. If there is no impact factor listed, then the journal probably does not have one. Be cautious about journals claiming to have a high impact factor, especially if it is a new journal, or one you have never heard about. There are many predatory journals and a high impact factor with a new journal is generally inconceivable. Some journals do not have a word count limit, especially in the case of online journals. The way words are counted varies by the journal—some use a total word count, while others allow a set number of figures and tables, often five, while others yet have a word count and assign a word count equivalent for each figure or table. Yet others use page counts. If necessary, make a note in the comment section at the bottom, or if word processing your worksheet, add a comment note under the row.

The journal aims can be somewhat long and redundant, so you may only need the essential information. The audience may need to be inferred if not stated explicitly. Clues can be if it is an official journal of a professional organization. Examination of similar content and methods usually takes the longest. If the journal website has a search function, a search using keywords from your own paper can be very productive. Don't be surprised if you find a couple of articles of interest! Reading through the past 2–3 years is usually sufficient—looking further back in time may be unproductive, as the content area may no longer be of interest to the editors. Similarly, searching for mixed methods may return methodologically similar articles, but be aware that not all articles self-described as mixed methods are truly mixed methods articles, and some articles that use mixed methods may not have this term in the article. For both content and methods, the journal focus can change if there is a change in editors. After copying the link to the online instructions to authors, add any final comments or ideas. Noting articles with similar content or methods can be helpful if you ultimately choose to submit to the particular journal. After completing each column, consider the rating for submission.

Workbox 17.2: Identifying Journals and Ranking Them as Submission Destinations

Rating for submission				
Journal name				
Relative fit				
Impact factor				
Online/Paper				
Payment?				
Word limit				

Journal aims				
Audience				
Similar content and methods?				
Link to instructions for authors				
Comments				

Predatory Journal Behaviors: Beware!

With the developments of online publication and the opportunity for revenue have come an explosion in the number of predatory publishers and journals (Berger, 2017). Publication predators represent publishing organizations or journals that charge exorbitant fees for dissemination with only thinly veiled peer review, if at all. In some cases, the entity never even posts the article for access by the public. One early resource exposing predatory journals and publishing practices was an online list created by librarian Jeffrey Beall, who started tracking these ("Beall's List of Predatory Journals and Publishers," 2018). Unfortunately, the number of publishers and stand-alone journals was so great that the original list became difficult to keep updated, though there are still interval updates to the list. Additionally, the list became controversial as some journals may have been unfairly classified as predatory. Fortunately, major professional organizations have started taking steps to prepare researchers to recognize the predatory journals, but steps for actually mitigating the practice seem very difficult to achieve (Federal Trade Commission, 2016).

STORY FROM THE FIELD 17.1
Watch Out for Publication Predators

The online predatory journal racket is a true threat. Just as predatory journals were emerging, we almost got caught in 2014. After receiving an email that sounded like a good fit for a paper that we were working on, we sent the paper to the journal. It was pay to publish, but that was common for online journals, and the team was eager to have an initial publication for the project quickly. I was the senior author on this paper so the correspondence was through an emerging but savvy junior scholar. We got reviews back very quickly, *surprisingly quickly*, and the reviews were quite short, very glowing, and included the pay-to-publish charge. My junior colleague was skeptical that our paper was that good and frankly disappointed by the lack of sophistication of the reviews. He had heard of predatory journals. Upon investigation, he found the journal on Beall's list and immediately wrote back to the journal and advised we were withdrawing the manuscript from further review.

Two years later, another colleague wrote me desperately seeking advice. She discovered she had unwittingly submitted to a predatory journal. I advised her to immediately write and withdraw the article. The journal then wrote back to her that the journal was billing for the cost of their peer-review process and demanded a fee after her team had withdrawn the article. We discussed the situation again, and she wrote a terse letter refusing and fortunately did not hear back again.

In addition to predatory journals, there are additional needs for precaution (see Story From the Field 17.1). Hijacking involves predators using material from a real print journal and creating a false website to charge outrageous fees without the paper ever getting published. Predatory journals create false metrics. Berger lists 15 points to consider when evaluating a journal as predatory (Berger, 2017). In my experience, some of the most important red flags for caution are (1) the journal is not produced by an established publisher; (2) an invitation to publish from the journal arrives as spam; (3) the invitation has glowing honorifics or misspellings; (4) the publication fees are unspecified or unclear; (5) the peer-review process is unclear; (6) the journal offers editorial positions while requesting contributions or theme issues at the same time; (7) the journal is new or debuting an issue. If intuitively you have any doubts, consult with colleagues, peers, advisors, and mentors. An information science colleague can assist if you have access to a library/media center.

Journal "Safe" Lists

The best resource are "Safe Lists" that indicate the journal has been vetted and demonstrated not to engage in predatory publication practice (Oren, 2017). Unfortunately, the language commonly used to depict lists of safe journals has become "White List" and predatory journals "Black List." I try to avoid this language as it can be offensive to individuals of diverse backgrounds. The Directory of Open Access Journals (DOAJ) is an excellent resource for checking on the predatory status (DOAJ, n.d.). An independent organization, the DOAJ website features various search strategies for identifying legitimate journals and articles. The National Institutes of Health has released a document on precaution measures (NIH, 2017), and there is a resource called "Think. Check. Submit." that also provides guidance ("Think. Check. Submit.," 2018).

DEVELOPING A COMPREHENSIVE PUBLICATION PLAN

Having conducted an inventory of your project strengths for publication, potential limitations, an order, and a rationale, your next step is to develop a comprehensive publication plan for the actual writing. In many projects, especially large projects, experienced researchers develop a publication strategy plan early. An example of a publication for the MPathic-VR virtual human grant is found in Workbox Illustration 17.3.1. Constructing such a plan will help guide your publication progress. While the MMR or evaluation project may have the potential for multiple publications, the publications do not write themselves. As illustrated, there were multiple papers under consideration for publication.

Workbox Illustration 17.3.1: Developing a Comprehensive Mixed Methods Publication Plan: An Example from the MPathic-VR Mixed Methods Medical Education Line of Research

Article Types	Content	Lead Author[1]	Journal Genre	Stretch, Good Fit, Safety Journals[2]
Qualitative	Medical student and educator views on how to incorporate virtual human teaching into the medical school curriculum	NG	Medical education	ST *Acad Med* GF *Teach Learn Med* SA *BMC Med Educ*
Quantitative	Medical student attitudes toward video games and new media medical education	GL	Medical education	ST *JAMA* ST *Acad Med* ST *Teach Learn Med* ST *Med Teach* GF *BMC Fam Pract* GF *BMC Med Educ* (Kron et al., 2010) SA *Adv Med Educ Pract*
Quantitative	Nursing student attitudes toward video games and new media technology	HM	Nursing education	ST *J Nurs Educ* (Lynch-Sauer et al., 2011) ST *Nurse Educ Today* GF *J Contin Educ Nurs* SA *Nurs Educ Perspect*
Quantitative	Construct validity of virtual human application for competency assessment in breaking bad news to a cancer patient	UH	Medical education	GF *Med Teach* SA *Adv Med Educ Pract* (Guetterman et al., 2017)
Mixed methods	Findings of the trial, difference between intervention and control students on the objective structured clinical examination	GL	Medical education	ST *JAMA* ST *Acad Med* GF *Patient Educ Couns* (Kron et al., 2017) SA *Med Teach*

Article Types	Content	Lead Author[1]	Journal Genre	Stretch, Good Fit, Safety Journals[2]
Methodology	Use of joint displays for analysis: The MPathic-VR mixed methods randomized controlled trial	UH	Family medicine	ST *Ann Fam Med* GF *Fam Med* SA *BMC Fam Pract* SA *BMC Med Educ*
Methodology	Scoring of interactive video games with branching choice patterns	NT	Gaming	ST *J Med Internet Res* GF *Simul Healthc* SA *Games Health J*
Methodology	A two-phase mixed methods project illustrating development of a virtual human intervention to teach advanced communication skills and a subsequent blinded mixed methods trial to test the intervention for effectiveness	NG	Mixed methods	GF *Int J Mult Res Approaches* (invited submission)

[1]Initials are for pseudonyms
[2]ST, stretch journal; GF, good fit journal; SA, safety fit journal

Source: Fetters, M.D. and Kron, F.W. (2012–15). *Modeling Professional Attitudes and Teaching Humanistic Communication in Virtual Reality (MPathic-VRII).*National Center for Advancing Translational Science/NIH 9R44TR000360-04.

Activity: Developing a Comprehensive Mixed Methods Publication Plan

Using Workbox Illustration 17.3.1 as a reference, complete Workbox 17.3.2. The Workbox Illustration includes the article types, the content, who will serve as the lead author, the journal genre, and the fit. The Workbox features an addition: the target date to submit. This could be an actual date or a chronological ordering. It is valuable to begin thinking as soon as possible about not only the types of publications but what will be the particular content.

The Workbox arbitrarily contains two rows each for potential qualitative, quantitative, mixed methods, and mixed method methodological papers. This can be adapted for individual projects from more or less of any category. Considering at least two papers in each category may trigger candid discussions or ideas. Dividing up the content can be challenging, as specific topics often overlap with each other, and if not carefully planned, two different lead authors may envision papers that have too much overlap.

Moreover, authors are needed to write the papers. For a dissertation, the graduate student will (and generally should) take the lead on the papers coming from the dissertation. On mixed methods teams, that often include graduate students or postdoctoral faculty, delineating early who will lead which papers can greatly help headaches later if two different team members both believe they should take the lead on the paper about a particular topic. Assigning the author then clarifies who will take the lead. After that, this work will include identifying the journal genre, and finally, the stretch, good fit, and safety journals.

Workbox 17.3.2: Developing a Comprehensive Mixed Methods Publication Plan

Article Types	Content	Lead Author	Journal Genre	Stretch, Good Fit, Safety Journals	Target Date to Submit
Qualitative					
Qualitative					
Quantitative					
Quantitative					
Mixed Methods					
Mixed Methods					
Methodology					
Methodology					

Application Activities

1. **Peer Feedback**. If you are working on your project as part of a class or in a workshop, pair up with a peer mentor, and one of you spend about 5 minutes talking about your comprehensive publication plan. Take turns talking about your publication plan and giving feedback. The helpful parts to discuss are those that you struggled with the most. If you are working independently, share your publication plan with a colleague, mentor, project team members, or dissertation committee members.

2. **Peer Feedback Guidance**. As you listen to your partner, you should focus on learning and honing the valuable skills of critiquing. Your goal is to help your partner refine the comprehensive publication plan. Focus on the component that your partner needs feedback on the most. Are the target journals realistic for the level of the project?

3. **Group Debrief**. If you are in a classroom or large-group setting, take volunteers to present the types of papers and target journals under consideration. Reflect on the relevance of the discussion for your own project.

Concluding Thoughts

Use this checklist to assess your progress in achieving the Chapter 17 objectives:

☐ I recognize my MMR and evaluation study publication options to include empirical qualitative, empirical quantitative, empirical mixed methods, and mixed methods methodological articles.

☐ I conducted a project inventory to organize my publishing strategy based on my project strengths, limitations, relevant publication types, and to develop a rationale for order of submission.

☐ I developed a list of candidate journals organized as "stretch," "good fit," and "safety" that can be pursued for publication of my mixed methods articles.

☐ I identified candidate journals and rated them as submission destinations for manuscripts of my MMR and evaluation studies.

☐ I developed a comprehensive mixed methods publication plan.

☐ I reviewed my mixed methods publication plan with a peer mentor, colleague, or advisor.

Now that you have completed these objectives, Chapter 18 will help you publish one or more articles from your MMR or evaluation project.

Key Resources

1. **FURTHER READING ON PUBLISHING MULTIPLE STUDIES FROM A SINGLE PROJECT**

   - Stange, K. C., Crabtree, B. F., & Miller, W. L. (2006). Publishing multimethod research. *Annals of Family Medicine, 4*(4), 292–294. doi:10.1370/afm.615

2. **FURTHER READING ON DIFFERENCES BETWEEN EMPIRICAL, THEORETICAL, AND PHILOSOPHICAL MIXED METHODS PAPERS**

   - Fetters, M. D., & Freshwater, D. (2015). Publishing a methodological mixed methods research article. *Journal of Mixed Methods Research, 9*(3), 203–213. doi: 10.2147/AMEP.S138380

3. **FURTHER READING ON AVOIDING PREDATORY PUBLISHERS AND JOURNALS**

   - Bowman, D. E., & Wallace, M. B. (2017). Predatory journals: A serious complication in the scholarly publishing landscape. *Gastrointestinal Endoscopy, 87*(1), 273–274. doi:10.1016/j.gie.2017.09.019

   - Hunziker, R. (2017). Avoiding predatory publishers in the post-Beall world: Tips for writers and editors. *American Medical Writers Association Journal, 32*(3), 113–115. doi:10.3389/fmars.2018.00106

   - Pisanski, K., Sorokowski, P., & Kulczycki, E. (2017). Predatory journals recruit fake editor. *Nature, 543*, 481–483.

   - Vence T. (2017). On blacklists and whitelists. Retrieved from https://www.the-scientist.com/?articles.view/articleNo/49903/title/On-Blacklists-and-Whitelists/.

WRITING A MIXED METHODS ARTICLE USING THE HOURGLASS DESIGN MODEL

Writing a mixed methods publication poses unique challenges that can be overcome by attention to structure and application of the hourglass model of mixed methods publication. You may feel uncertainty about whether to write qualitative, quantitative, or mixed methods papers, and you may even be wondering if your work has the makings of a methodological paper. This chapter and its activities will help you consider your writing strengths, utilize four elements for writing a mixed methods title, apply the hourglass model for writing of publications, utilize one of two writing templates for writing, evaluate for the inclusion of essential elements of mixed methods in the article's abstract and body, and apply a mixed methods writing template for a dissertation or thesis as applicable. As a key outcome, you will develop an article composed to best represent your mixed methods empirical article or chapter, and, if working on a dissertation or thesis, an overall writing strategy.

LEARNING OBJECTIVES

The ideas and writing activities will help you

- Identify your writing strengths and develop a strategy for writing your article

- Recognize and utilize four elements for writing a mixed methods research (MMR) article title

- Apply the hourglass model of writing to compose MMR and evaluation study articles

- Choose and utilize an appropriate template for writing mixed methods articles/chapters

- Evaluate and confirm inclusion of essential elements of mixed methods inquiry into your abstract in preparation for submission for peer review

- Evaluate for the incorporation of essential elements of mixed methods inquiry into your article or chapter in preparation for submission

- Utilize a template for writing a mixed methods dissertation or thesis

WHAT ARE THE PUBLICATION FORMATS FOR MIXED METHODS ARTICLES?

Mixed methods research and evaluation studies can produce empirical qualitative, empirical quantitative, empirical mixed methods, and mixed methods methodological articles (Chapters 17). Regardless of the empirical or methodological genre, articles, chapters, white papers, theses, and dissertations have similar features. In this chapter, as a convention, I use the term *article* to reflect parsimoniously all these formats. While each has unique characteristics, as related to writing, the strategies and approaches still generally apply.

RECOGNIZING YOUR WRITING STRENGTHS AND IDENTIFYING STRATEGIES TO WRITE: WRITE EARLY AND WRITE OFTEN

Getting started can seem daunting (See Story From the Field 18.1). I often ask very prolific writers, "How do you write?" The answers vary a lot (which is one reason I enjoy asking!). Some respond that they write best in the morning when distractions are minimal. Others report writing at night after the emails stop coming, the dog is walked, and the kids are asleep. Yet others describe their long sessions sitting in a favorite coffee shop during the day with a double latte keeping quiet company. Writing styles vary dramatically, and you will become more efficient when you find what works best for you. My favorite advice comes from a pioneer in MMR, David Morgan, who advised, "Write when you are ready." Ultimately, you have to find your own approach, as there is no one recipe for writing.

STORY FROM THE FIELD 18.1
Write Early and Write Often

I can recall many instances when working on a project when I was very junior. After getting results back, I would hear, "OK, time to write it up!" It seemed like such a monumental task. Now, rather than waiting for results to come back, I advise all my mentees to write as early as possible. One of the best predictors of long-term academic success is early publication, especially predoctoral degree publication (von Bartheld, Houmanfar, & Candido, 2015), and the more top-tier journals where you publish, the better your pay (Gomez-Mejia & Balkin, 2017)! (If you haven't written anything yet, don't worry, early is all relative!)

UNIQUE FEATURES AND STRATEGIES FOR WRITING A MIXED METHODS TITLE

The title of your project is the most important component of your paper as it will be the most frequently read written representation of your MMR or evaluation project. Many authors revise their study title multiple times, as they desire a very catchy and finessed title that can catch the eye of potential readers. The best titles are concise, a point that can be difficult considering the complex topics and methods of an MMR or evaluation project. Creswell and Plano Clark (2018, p. 144) recommend keeping the title to no more than 12 words and include four elements: the topic, participants, site, and the mixed methods design.

Activity: Elements for Inclusion in Your Mixed Methods Title

Using the other titles in Workbox 18.1 as a reference, fill in the four sections of the workbox, so you can identify the key elements for inclusion in your mixed methods title.

**Workbox 18.1: Identifying Study Elements for a
Mixed Methods Title With Examples From Mixed Methods
Publications in Multiple Disciplines**

Authors	1. Topic	2. Participants	3. Site	4. Mixed Methods Methodology
Sharma and Vredenburg (1998) (Business)	Proactive environmental strategies and competitively valuable corporate strategies	Middle- and senior-level managers	Major oil corporations	Exploratory sequential mixed methods design
Harper (2016) (Education)	Role of the principal in creating a culture of academic optimism	Principals, teachers	Middle schools	A sequential QUAN to QUAL mixed methods study
Kron et al. (2017) (Health sciences)	Using a virtual human computer simulation for teaching communication skills	2nd-year medical students	Multisite	A mixed methods randomized controlled trial
Your study				

Activity: Developing a Mixed Methods Title

Referencing the information in Workbox 18.1, create an alternative title in column three of Workbox 18.2 as the featured studies do not include all four title elements. After writing the three examples, draft a title for your own project in the last row of Workbox 18.2.

**Workbox 18.2: Creating a Mixed Methods Title With
Examples From Mixed Methods Publications in
Multiple Disciplines**

Author(s)	Actual Title	Potential Revised Title* (Based on Workbox 18.1)
Sharma and Vredenburg (1998) (Business)	*Proactive corporate environmental strategy and the development of competitively valuable organizational capabilities*	
Harper (2016) (Education)	*Exploring the role of the principal in creating a culture of academic optimism: A sequential QUAN to QUAL mixed methods study*	
Kron et al. (2017) (Health sciences)	*Using a computer simulation for teaching communication skills: A blinded multisite mixed methods randomized controlled trial*	
Your study		

*See answers in Workbox Answers at the end of the chapter

WHAT IS THE HOURGLASS MODEL OF WRITING?

As introduced in Chapter 5 the hourglass model of writing provides a metaphor for a writing structure based on the timepiece containing sand with broad shaped bulbs on the top and bottom, and a narrow funnel connecting them. The overarching structure of the hourglass model can guide your writing regardless of whether you are authoring an empirical or methodological/theoretical article. There are minor differences, as illustrated in Figure 18.1. The

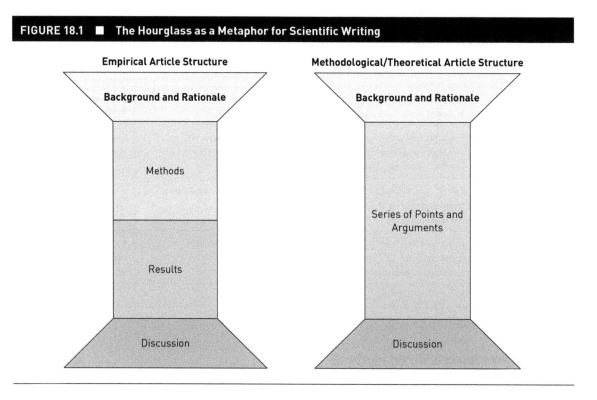

FIGURE 18.1   ■   The Hourglass as a Metaphor for Scientific Writing

top of the hourglass symbolizes writing about the broader context and rationale of your topic. Just as the bulb narrows, the text then focuses on a specific context and aim for the paper. The hourglass then has a narrow section. For the empirical article, this neck symbolized the methods and results. For a methodological paper, the narrow neck represents a series of points and arguments. Just as the neck of the inverted bottom bulb starts expanding, the text begins expanding to a discussion of the study findings. There are of course other possible writing structures, but the hourglass structure can be found in many articles across the educational, social, and health sciences. As Fetters and Freshwater (2015b), editors of the *Journal of Mixed Methods Research*, have previously provided detailed advice for writing a methodological mixed methods article, the remainder of this chapter will focus on empirical articles.

Using the Hourglass Model to Write Empirical Mixed Methods Articles

Figure 18.2 provides a more detailed illustration of the hourglass model of writing. This expanded figure features two headers straddling the hourglass: abstract on the left, and article on the right. The model contains the top bulb of the hourglass, the introduction (or background) with the relevant overarching context, specific context, rationale prompting MMR or evaluation study, and study objectives. The methods section equates to the top half of a long neck that comprises the mixed methods design, data collection, and integrated analysis. The results section follows as the bottom half of a long neck and includes Paragraphs 1–5 of the results. These roughly correspond to explanations of study tables and figures. Many journals restrict authors of empirical articles to five figures or tables in total. Generally, one paragraph each is dedicated to these findings. The bottom bulb of the hourglass represents the discussion, where the author reflects on key mixed methods findings from the study and, in consideration of the published literature, expounds the broader implications for the field, hence the broad base. Authors typically include a paragraph on limitations of the study and a final paragraph on broader implications and future research.

The Mixed Methods Abstract

Your abstract is really important as it typically becomes the first written representation of the overall study. The quality of the abstract can determine acceptance to the conference and placement in particular sections of the conference. The abstract represents a critical part of any article submitted for publication. As illustrated in Figure 18.2, abstracts for scientific meetings commonly include four sections: the introduction (or background), methods, results, and discussion (or conclusions). The introduction, methods, and discussion all have a ratio of approximately

FIGURE 18.2 ■ The Hourglass Model for an Empirical Mixed Methods Abstract and Article

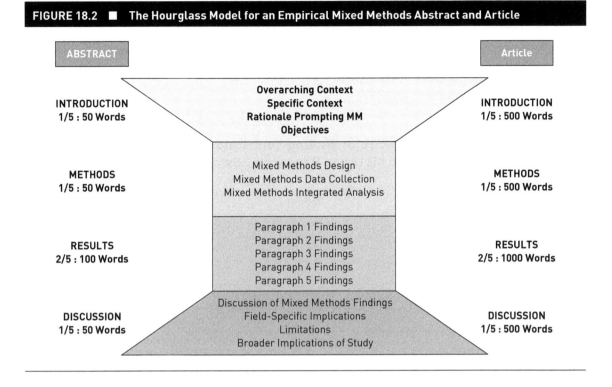

1:5 of the total word count, or about 50 words for a 250-word abstract. In contrast, the results have about a 2:5 ratio with about 100 words for a 250-word abstract. Depending on the scientific venue, I have seen the abstract total word counts range from 100 to 500. Using the ratios can help with the general structuring. Your goal is to avoid overwriting. *Overwriting* describes drafting substantively more text than can be used in the projected submission venue. This requires extensive editing to bring the text volume to an appropriate length, thus creating productivity inefficiency.

Structured and Unstructured Abstracts. Some scientific meetings and journals require a structured abstract, while others call for an unstructured abstract. The **structured abstract** is a research study summary organized by four sections, usually the introduction/background, methods, results, and discussion/conclusions. When called for, these must be included according to the specific headers requested. An **unstructured abstract** is a research summary that does not require specific sections. The headers are not explicitly written, but in general, the flow of the four sections generally follows in an unstructured abstract for empirically conducted research, and it can be written to include the same four sections minus the headers. You may try writing the first draft with headers, and then remove the headers for the final version if you're struggling.

Unique Features and Strategies for Writing a Mixed Methods Abstract. Mixed methods research abstracts have a few unique features (Figure 18.2). The *introduction* (background) provides a rationale for conducting a mixed methods study that is the need for both the qualitative and the quantitative data collection (See Chapter 1). Creswell and Creswell (2018, p. 108) emphasize the "narrative hook" they define as "words that serve to draw, engage, or to hook the reader into a study." With a mixed methods study, the narrative hook ideally would raise a problem or phenomenon alluding to the need for a mixed methods approach. In addition, the study should have a good mixed methods objective where the type of data collected are explicit or at least implied. Chapter 5 reviews effective qualitative and quantitative questions and how they imply specific methods. In the *methods* section, the abstract should include the mixed methods design, both types of data collection and analysis, and the data integration process. The *results* section should depict the mixed findings, possibly as qualitative, quantitative, and mixed, or possibly a series of mixed findings or interpretations of both types of findings (e.g., metainferences). The *discussion* should highlight the study-specific findings of both types of data and the implications for the field. On a positive note, two sentences are approximately 50 words. Depending on the typical abstract length of journals in your field, the total number of sentences can be anticipated. To write a 250-word abstract only requires 10 sentences, or about 14 sentences for a 350-word abstract. On the flip side, there are *only* 10 (or 14) sentences. To write efficiently and avoid overwriting, have in mind the need for succinctness, and keep to the sentence count. From there, it is relatively efficient to wordsmith down to the proper length.

Activity: Writing a Mixed Methods
Research Abstract for a Scientific Meeting or Article

Using Figure 18.2 as a reference, develop your abstract using Workbox 18.3. Use the structured format to record your introduction/background, methods, results, and discussion/conclusion. In particular, be attentive to the word counts/ratios indicated in Figure 18.2. The following seven steps provide guidance for successfully developing an abstract for an empirical mixed methods study.

Workbox 18.3: Writing Your Empirical
Mixed Methods Research Abstract

Word Count	Ratio	Section
10–20		Title:
50	1/5	Introduction/Background
50	1/5	Methods
100	2/5	Results
50	1/5	Discussion/Conclusion

Activity: Checking the Key Elements of a Mixed Methods Abstract

To be certain you have crafted a strong abstract, use the checklist in Workbox 18.4 to review your abstract.

Workbox 18.4: Using a Checklist to Assess for Key Elements
in Your Empirical Mixed Methods Research Abstract

❑ Do you follow the specifications of the scientific program or journal?

❑ Introduction: Do you identify a problem that suggests the need and value for the use of MMR?

❑ Introduction: Does your aim speak/allude to collecting both qualitative and quantitative data?

❑ Methods: Do you include information about the type of mixed methods design?

❑ Methods: Do you include information about both qualitative and quantitative data collection?

❑ Methods: Do you speak to how the qualitative and quantitative data collection are linked?

❑ Results: Do you provide results from both the qualitative and quantitative components of the study?

❑ Results: Do you provide any interpretations/metainferences based on the findings of both the qualitative and quantitative strands?

❑ Discussion: Do you illustrate what using both types of data contributed to your new understanding of the phenomenon you have investigated?

❑ Discussion: Do you allude to the implications for the field as a whole?

❑ If you have already written the article, can all of these elements be found, and do they match what you have written in the text of the article?

Using the Hourglass Model of Mixed Methods to Write the Main Text

Having successfully completed the abstract, now you can focus on writing your article. As before, the hourglass model can guide your mixed methods writing structure (Figure 18.3).

Introduction. Mixed methods studies are unique in needing to consider the different quantitative and qualitative studies, especially with regard to the rationale for conducting the research in light of both qualitative and quantitative findings from the literature. This background should provide the rationale for a mixed methods study

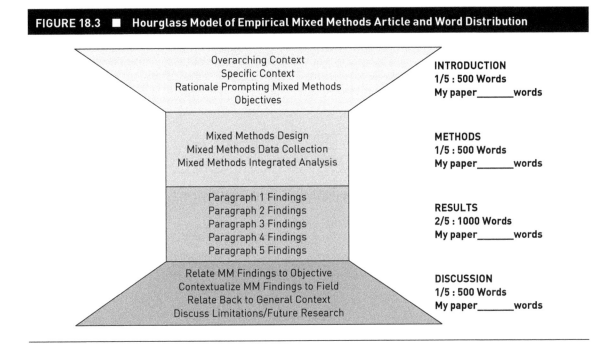

FIGURE 18.3 ■ Hourglass Model of Empirical Mixed Methods Article and Word Distribution

Overarching Context
Specific Context
Rationale Prompting Mixed Methods
Objectives

INTRODUCTION
1/5 : 500 Words
My paper_____words

Mixed Methods Design
Mixed Methods Data Collection
Mixed Methods Integrated Analysis

METHODS
1/5 : 500 Words
My paper_____words

Paragraph 1 Findings
Paragraph 2 Findings
Paragraph 3 Findings
Paragraph 4 Findings
Paragraph 5 Findings

RESULTS
2/5 : 1000 Words
My paper_____words

Relate MM Findings to Objective
Contextualize MM Findings to Field
Relate Back to General Context
Discuss Limitations/Future Research

DISCUSSION
1/5 : 500 Words
My paper_____words

and lead to mixed methods study aims or questions. The expected length of the introduction section for an empirical mixed methods study will be no more than about one-fifth each of the total word count, for example, 500 words (about 2 long or 3 short paragraphs) for a 2,500-word limit journal or about 1,400 words maximum (about 4–5 paragraphs) for a 3,500-word article.

Methods. It is challenging to keep the methods section short in a mixed methods study due to the need to describe the procedures used for the qualitative and quantitative strands. After writing the mixed methods design, there may be overlap in the methodological procedures when describing the setting, participants, sampling, and data collection procedures. When there is overlap in one or more of these dimensions, it is preferable to write about both in the same subsection to avoid repetition. For example, in the MPathic-VR study, the setting, participants, sampling, and data collection procedures could be described for the qualitative and the quantitative data together (Kron et al., 2017). In contrast, in Harper's study on the role of the principal in creating a culture of academic optimism, the setting, participants, sampling, and data collection procedures were different for the quantitative and the qualitative strands (Harper, 2018). The *expected length of the methods* section for an empirical mixed methods study will be about one-fifth of the total word count, for example, 500 words (about 2 paragraphs) for a 2,500-word limit journal or about 700 words maximum (about 3 paragraphs) for a 3,500-word article.

Results. The results section depicts the study findings. Usually, these can be organized by the study tables and figures. The first paragraph is generally demographics of participants. Subsequent sections will be driven by the mixed methods findings. In sequential studies, the order the data are collected make the most sense for presentation of the qualitative and quantitative findings since the first strand creates findings (e.g., survey findings as in Harper's study) that are used to build toward collecting data for the second strand (e.g., qualitative interviews in Harper's study). When possible, presenting mixed findings together proves a very efficient and effective approach. Presentation of findings in a joint display is conducive to explaining mixed findings together. Use of the linking activity in Chapter 14 will facilitate identification of common constructs from the linkages identified between the qualitative and quantitative strands that can lead to an integrated presentation. The expected length of the results section for an empirical mixed methods study will be about two-fifths of the total word count, for example, 1,000 words (about 5 paragraphs) for a 2,500-word limit journal, or about 1,400 words maximum (about 6–7 paragraphs) for a 3,500-word article.

Discussion. An overarching consideration of the discussion is the illustration of how using a mixed methods approach added value. Generally, the section begins with consideration of the mixed methods findings vis-à-vis the mixed methods study aims or questions serves. Mixed methods studies are unique in needing to consider both the quantitative and qualitative findings and are typically based on the literature providing the rationale for the study. Scientific writing typically has a limitations section, and readers will expect this to be included somewhere near the end of the discussion. Use the research integrity considerations raised in Chapter 16 to guide the writing of this section. The expected length of the discussion sections for an empirical mixed methods study will be no more than about one-fifth each of the total word count, for example, 500 words (about 2 long or 3 short paragraphs) for a 2,500-word limit journal or about 1,400 words maximum (about 4–5 paragraphs) for a 3,500-word article.

The structure represented by the hourglass model can be found more or less in many mixed methods articles. Bearing in mind the tasks for each section, the word count limits will serve as a guide as you now turn your attention to writing.

UNIQUE FEATURES AND STRATEGIES FOR WRITING A MIXED METHODS ARTICLE OR CHAPTER

Efficiently Writing Your Mixed Methods Research Article or Chapter

The best way to write an article is to finish it! While this may sound trivial, the academic road is littered with debris of incomplete articles/chapters that all started with the best intentions. Of course, there are many different strategies authors use to successfully finish articles/chapters. The following recommendations can guide your mixed methods writing.

Preparing for Writing

To get started, remember to identify your top three destinations first, if writing an article for submission (see Chapter 17). List these choices on the front page of the manuscript including the word count limits. You may even choose to include a table of manuscripts and choices for submission. Assemble any documents with information about the study, dissertation or thesis proposal, grant submission, figures, tables, previously drafted text, oral presentation slides, posters, or especially previous abstracts. Even if you are writing a dissertation or thesis, planning ahead about where you will submit each chapter for publication can really help move things along.

Drafting an Outline From Writing Templates

To draft an outline of your article, start with your working title from Workbox 18.3. You may have already gone through multiple versions, but anticipate you will make further revisions, as the study title and article direction become clearer. If you have an existing abstract from above Workbox 18.3 or from another source, use it as your first outline. Determine the approximate word counts for each section using Figure 18.2 and based on your first choice of journal for your submission. While working on a dissertation or thesis, it may seem that the word count doesn't matter, but you will be best served to have the chapters as close to submission ready after your successful defense. The less editing required, the more likely for the submission to be completed in a timely matter. There are two primary organizational patterns of empirical mixed methods articles, quantitatively organized and qualitatively organized.

Qualitatively Organized and Quantitatively Organized Writing Structures

Qualitatively organized writing in a mixed methods paper is an approach to recording and presenting study results to convey that the qualitative procedures occurred before the quantitative procedures, for example, with an exploratory sequential design or a convergent design. This approach conveys that the qualitative data collection occurred before the quantitative data collection in a sequential study. In a convergent design, it conveys that the presentation of the study has been structured with the qualitative strand providing the organizing structure. See Workbox 18.5 for a qualitatively organized template. Use the open space in the template for jottings about your planning, and then use a word processor to develop your outline using the elements found in the workbox.

Qualitatively organized should not be confused with the language of qualitatively driven mixed methods research and evaluation (Hesse-Biber, Rodriguez, & Frost, 2015). Qualitatively driven mixed methods inquiry is an approach that privileges the qualitative paradigm through philosophical and theoretical orientation (e.g., constructivism, critical theory, feminist perspectives, and whereby a qualitative approach predominates in the framing, conduct, analysis, and interpretation). Qualitatively driven studies will typically be qualitatively organized, but not all qualitative organized studies will necessarily be qualitatively driven.

Workbox 18.5: Writing With a Template for a Qualitatively Organized Empirical Mixed Methods Article

INTRODUCTION

- Relevant general context (Biggest Picture) (1–2 paragraphs)
- Specific problem
- Rationale for why a mixed methods approach is needed
- Research questions (framed with *qualitative* followed by the *quantitative*)

METHODS

Design: Exploratory or convergent (qualitatively organized) mixed methods research design

Qualitative Phase

- Data collection
- Setting
- Participants
- Instruments
- Data collection

Quantitative phase

- Data collection*
- Setting*
- Participants*
- Instruments
- Data collection

Mixed Methods Integration

RESULTS

Weaving Approach

- 1st integrated mixed methods finding, e.g., QUAL then QUAN
- 2nd integrated mixed methods finding, e.g., QUAL then QUAN
- 3rd integrated mixed methods finding, e.g., QUAL then QUAN
- 4th integrated mixed methods finding, e.g., QUAL then QUAN

OR

Contiguous Approach

- Qualitative findings, e.g., Para 1, Para 2, Para 3
- Quantitative findings, e.g., Para 1, Para 2, Para 3
- Mixed methods findings (optional), e.g., Para 1, Para 2, Para 3

DISCUSSION

- Based on this research we now know. . .
- Implication #1 and relevant literature
- Implication #2 and relevant literature
- Implication #3 and relevant literature
- Limitations
- Final conclusions +/– Future research

*Only use if distinct from the description already written.

Quantitatively organized writing in a mixed methods paper is an approach to recording and presenting study results to convey that the quantitative procedures occurred before the qualitative procedures, for example, in an explanatory sequential design or a convergent design. This approach conveys that the quantitative data collection occurred before the qualitative data in an explanatory sequential study. In a convergent design, it conveys that the presentation of the study has been structured or organized with the quantitative strand providing the organizing structure. See Workbox 18.6 for a quantitatively organized template. Use the open space in the template for jottings about your planning, and then use a word processor to develop your outline using the elements found in the workbox.

Quantitatively organized should not be confused with the language of quantitatively driven MMR and evaluation (Hesse-Biber et al., 2015). Quantitatively driven mixed methods inquiry is an approach that privileges the quantitative paradigm through philosophical and theoretical orientation, for example, postpositivism, and whereby a quantitative approach predominates in the framing, conduct, analysis, and interpretation. While quantitatively driven studies will most likely be quantitatively organized, not all quantitatively organized studies will be quantitatively driven.

Workbox 18.6: Writing With a Template for a Quantitatively Organized Empirical Mixed Methods Article

INTRODUCTION

- Relevant general context (biggest picture) (1–2 paragraphs)
- Specific problem
- Rationale for why a mixed methods approach is needed
- Research questions (framed with *quantitative* followed by the *qualitative*)

METHODS

Design: Explanatory or convergent (quantitatively organized) mixed methods research design

Quantitative **Phase**

- Data collection
- Setting
- Participants
- Instruments
- Data collection

Qualitative Phase

- Data collection*
- Setting*
- Participants*
- Instruments
- Data collection

Mixed Methods Integration

RESULTS

Weaving Approach

- 1st integrated mixed methods finding, e.g., QUAN then QUAL
- 2nd integrated mixed methods finding, e.g., QUAN then QUAL
- 3rd integrated mixed methods finding, e.g., QUAN then QUAL
- 4th integrated mixed methods finding, e.g., QUAN then QUAL

OR

Contiguous Approach

- *Quantitative* findings, e.g., 1 to 3 paragraphs
- *Qualitative* findings, e.g., 1 to 3 paragraphs
- Mixed methods findings (optional) 1 to 3 paragraphs

*Only use if distinct from the description already written.

Activity: Using a Writing Template for Your Mixed Methods Project

For your project, choose a template for organization from Workboxes 18.5 and 18.6. The qualitatively organized template (Workbox 18.5) fits both the exploratory sequential mixed methods design and the qualitatively organized convergent mixed methods design (see Chapter 7). The quantitatively organized template fits for both explanatory sequential and quantitatively organized convergent MMR designs (Workbox 18.6). If you are working on a mixed methods dissertation or thesis, you will also find a comprehensive template to guide the writing of the chapters for your dissertation or thesis in Workbox 18.7.

Recommended Order of Writing Article Sections

Table 18.1 provides a recommendation for the authoring of an article. Emerging scholars are often surprised to find how much front-end work can be done to prepare for writing. Perhaps more surprising seems to be that the ordering of sections in a published article, namely, introduction, methods, results, and discussion, are not necessarily the most efficient order for writing the article. Logically, it seems the writing should begin with the first sentence and end with the last. After many years of living with this format, I received advice from a sage researcher, who advised writing the methods first, then creating the study figures and tables. The results section follows as the figures and tables need to be summarized. The introduction and methods can be written in parallel since much of the cited literature will be the same. Writing by starting with the methods is by far my preferred and recommended approach to writing empirical studies because I find it much easier to record information as the data collection is occurring and the information is fresh, and second, because it helps speed up the writing of the results.

1. **Choose the Appropriate Mixed Methods Template**

The qualitative then quantitative formats (Workbox 18.5) or quantitative then qualitative (Workbox 18.6) provide two general templates for organizing your mixed methods article. Choose the template closest to your own design.

2. **Write the Methods Section**

The rationale for writing the methods before other sections comes down to several reasons. (1) The methods are the first part of the project that are completed. (2) Of all the sections for the article, the structure of the methods most

---

TABLE 18.1 ■ Recommended Steps for Efficiently Writing a Mixed Methods Article or Chapter

1. Choose the appropriate mixed methods template for your design (Workbox 18.5 or 18.6).

2. Write the methods section using the structure from your abstract (Workbox 18.4) outline (Figures 18.5 or 18.6) or an alternative structure.

3. Finalize the study tables and figures.

4. Write the results section by summarizing and explaining the key findings in the tables and figures.

5. Write the introduction and results sections using a parallel approach.

6. Thoroughly edit, revise for consistency, read out loud, and edit again.

7. Check for consistency with the abstract.

8. Send to colleagues or committee members for feedback.

9. Incorporate final edits, submit, and celebrate!

resembles a "recipe" and is most easily written. (3) The flow of the methods usually preface the order of the results section as well. So, if qualitative *methods* are presented first, for consistency, qualitative *results* will come first. If the quantitative methods are presented first, then the results will generally fall in the same order.

I advise writing the methods as soon as you start collecting data for the project. If data collection is long over, then start writing as soon as possible. The details of the data collection process are surprisingly easy to forget. Writing about the methods in detail early can facilitate development of methodological articles/chapters.

3. Finalize the Study Tables, Figures, and Graphs

In most empirical publications, the authors organize the results section based on the study tables, figures, and graphs. Many journals limit the combined number of these visual displays to only five in total. In preparation for writing the results, efficiency requires advanced finalizing of the tables, figures, and graphs. They should be examined for content, organization, and order for best telling the story of the study findings. Using visuals designed for mixed data presentations as a joint display (Chapter 14), or advanced formats (Chapter 15), facilitates achieving efficiency for presenting the mixed methods findings. Use these whenever you can to advance the level of sophistication, and to illustrate use of the most cutting-edge procedures.

4. Craft the Results Section

Writing with consistency throughout a mixed methods article helps avoid confusion. Hence, organizing the results in the same order as presented in the methods generally serves as the best choice. The *weaving* approach integrates both qualitative findings and quantitative findings for each of a series of constructs. The figure illustrates both quantitatively organized and qualitatively organized approaches. The *contiguous* approach presents the quantitative and qualitative sections in adjacent positioning, but content-wise the findings are presented separately. That is, even though the qualitative and quantitative findings sections in the text are contiguous, or adjacent to each other, no interpretation of the meaning of the two types of findings taken together/combined is given until the discussion section (Fetters, Curry & Creswell, 2013).

5. Write the Introduction and Discussion in Parallel

The introduction and the discussion are generally the most difficult components of an article or book chapter to write. The challenge comes from the need to have a good grasp of the literature to indicate the rationale in the introduction, and to reflect about what new knowledge the study produced for the discussion. For any given study, the results will not be known until the study is conducted and the data are analyzed. Since the most important study findings will not be known until the data collection, analysis, and interpretation are completed, authors do not know what to emphasize in the introduction and discussion until interpreting the findings. Hence, efficient writers will wait until the methods, tables, figures, graphs, and results have been organized for the mixed findings. As illustrated in Figure 18.4, there are roughly three structural principles to follow as indicated by the letters (a) to (c). This means that the key elements of the introduction should directly parallel relevant text in the discussion section. As illustrated by the 18.4a arrows, there should be text addressing the article objectives/questions in the beginning of the discussion. As illustrated by 18.4.b arrows, there should be text addressing the rationale and specific context in the discussion. Finally, as illustrated by the 18.4.c arrows, there should be text addressing the overarching context in the discussion section by highlighting limitations and the broader implications of the findings for future research or action.

Primary Study Findings and the Mixed Methods Study Objective (Figure 18.4, "a" arrows). For some studies, the results may not influence the writing of the study objective, while for others it will. Regardless, when the study findings are complete, the researcher should reflect on the extent and how the mixed study findings illuminate the stated study objective. In addition, the rationale prompting the study should be revisited. Particularly, in what way did the mixed methods findings illuminate the mixed methods rationale for the study?

Field Context and Field-Specific Implications (Figure 18.4 "b" arrows). An excellent guide for writing the discussion section is to answer the question, "What do we know because of this research that we did not know before the research?" The researcher needs to answer the question about the implications of the study findings for the field. Thus, while the previous section focused on the degree to which the findings answered the study purpose, the researcher must now think more broadly (as the base of the hourglass broadens) about the meaning of the results beyond the specific findings. This requires recognizing the study findings, as well as the extant literature about this topic. Knowing the findings dramatically helps to focus the literature review and keep it to the approximate word count allocation.

Overarching Context, Limitations, and Broader Implications (Figure 18.4 "c" arrows). In the closing sections of the discussion, both the study limitations and broader implications of the study should be articulated. This content

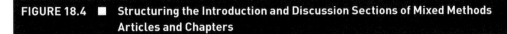

FIGURE 18.4 ■ Structuring the Introduction and Discussion Sections of Mixed Methods Articles and Chapters

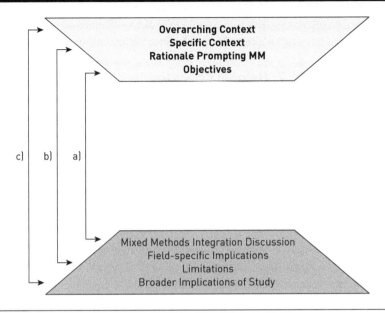

similarly relates to the broad-ranging statements to make in the introduction. Typically, limitations signify areas of future research that can be laid out in the discussion of broader implications. In short, throughout the introduction and the discussion, knowing the actual study findings makes it possible to focus the literature on the key study findings.

6. Thoroughly edit, revise for consistency, read out loud, and edit again. Be certain to fully reread and edit the study. Be sure the structure of the paper overall reflects the mixed methods design you have used. Be conscious that you have used consistent language throughout. That is, have you used the same language to identify the same concept throughout? One approach for ensuring consistency is to create a glossary, and list the words you plan on using. Finally, even in the age of word processing, I still find new mistakes when I read the paper out loud. As a final step, read a written copy as the formatting changes, and your eyes will find mistakes you didn't see before. Virtually guaranteed!

7. Check for consistency with the abstract. While the abstract has helped guide the writing of the manuscript, often key phrases or elements change when writing the actual article. Be sure any text in the abstract has related text in the full article. Especially make sure the key findings haven't changed! Or if they have, update the points in the abstract that you revealed through the writing process.

8. Send to colleagues or committee members for feedback. If you are working on a team, be sure to send a near-final draft to all coauthors. You may want to share with a colleague in your department who can give you an unblinded, pre-peer review to alleviate any really obvious errors. When circulating to coauthors, a fair and good practice is to include a deadline for any edits. If you are working on a dissertation or thesis, have an upfront discussion about when you can send around chapters. Some committee members may like to review drafts as completed, while others may prefer a batch. When you get feedback, remember, most but not all advice is good advice. You may receive conflicting recommendations from different parties. To resolve this issue, consider consulting with your advisor/mentor/senior colleague for assistance to resolve the inevitable conflict of opinions. This review should especially focus on the clarity of the mixed methods writing. Does the text efficiently represent the procedures, and have the integration procedures used been included?

9. Incorporate final edits, submit, and celebrate! Having received all the final edits on your mixed methods article, incorporate the changes. Double check that your word count is not in excess. No matter how important you think your topic must be to you personally, most everyone thinks this. Editors will be loath to make exception. Make sure you recheck that you have prepared the article according to the journal/book/dissertation or thesis guidelines. Then submit 😄! (Just be sure you know where to go next if rejected—see Chapter 17).

Activity: Checking the Key Elements in Your Empirical Mixed Methods Research or Evaluation Article

To ensure you have followed the general expectations for a mixed methods article, fill in and check the word count in Figure 18.2 for each section of your abstract and for your article. In addition, review the elements depicted in Workbox 18.7, as a checklist to assess for elements typically found in a mixed methods article.

Workbox 18.7: Using a Checklist to Assess for Key Elements in Your Empirical Mixed Methods Research Article

☐ Do you follow the specifications of the journal?

☐ Introduction: Do you identify a problem that suggests the need and value for the use of mixed methods research?

☐ Introduction: Do you identify your philosophical stance and the rationale?

☐ Introduction: Do you include your mixed methods rationale?

☐ Introduction: Does your aim speak/allude to collecting both qualitative and quantitative data?

☐ Methods: Do you include information about the type of mixed methods design?

☐ Methods: Do you include information about both qualitative and quantitative data collection?

☐ Methods: Do you speak to how the qualitative and quantitative data collection are related?

☐ Results: Do you provide results from both the qualitative and quantitative components of the study?

☐ Results: Do you use one or more joint displays to present the mixed findings?

☐ Results: Do you provide any interpretations/metainferences based on the findings of both the qualitative and quantitative strands?

☐ Discussion: Do you illustrate what using both types of data contributed to your new understanding of the phenomenon you have investigated?

☐ Discussion: Do you speak to the implications for the field as a whole?

☐ If you have already written the article, can all of these elements be found, and do they match with the way you have written in the text consistently throughout?

CREATING AN OUTLINE FOR YOUR DISSERTATION OR THESIS

Workbox 18.8 provides a template for creating an outline for your mixed methods dissertation or thesis. As illustrated, the template includes five chapters: introduction, literature, methods, results, and discussion. Consider using Workbook Chapter 5 to inform your introduction chapter and Workbook Chapter 3 to inform your literature chapter. For the methods chapter, this template organization most closely fits a quantitatively organized convergent design, as the sample as written implies the subjects would be the same. You may find Workboxes 18.6 and 18.7 helpful for specific chapters. Always bear in mind that the templates function to guide your writing, but not restrict it. You must be the ultimate judge of what structure best fits the needs in your situation. Regarding teamwork on a dissertation, you may find yourself as the mixed methods resource if your advisors have monomethod training in just qualitative research or just quantitative research. If this is the case, it may be advantageous to develop study groups with other graduate students. If there are mixed methods workshops, perhaps you could have an advisor attend with you.

Workbox 18.8: Writing With a Template for Creating an Outline for Your Dissertation or Thesis

(Note: Follow templates and guidance at your university for required sections.)

Introduction Chapter

- Research problem

- Context

- Purpose statement

  o Research questions

Literature Chapter

Methods Chapter

- Identify study design and reference procedural diagram.

- Sample

- Quantitative data collection

  o Measures with description and reliability and validity evidence from past uses

- Qualitative data collection

  o Semistructured interviews with sample interview questions

- Quantitative analysis

  o Chi-square and *t*-tests

  o Significance at alpha .05

  o Using SPSS

- Qualitative analysis

  o Constant comparative method

  o Using QSR N6.0 (now called NVivo)

- Mixed methods integration

  o E.g., related themes to personal characteristics

  o E.g., joint displays

Results Chapter

- Descriptive statistics

- Chi-square and *t*-test results

- Qualitative themes

Discussion Chapter

- Summarize results.

- Discuss limitations.

- Mixed methods integrated analysis

  o Joint display

  o Report integrated results.

  o Discuss and situate major findings in other literature.

- Discuss implications.

  o "The unique contribution of this study is . . ."

Acknowledgment: Reproduced and adapted with permission of Dr. Timothy Guetterman, who adapted previous versions of the writing template for a dissertation or thesis.

Application Activities

1. **Identify an empirical study in your field.** Conduct a literature search to identify an empirical mixed methods study from your field, preferably, one using the same design as yours. Evaluate the article's abstract and full text for the elements identified in Workboxes 18.5 and 18.6. How could the article have been improved? Time permitting, present the article to your class or peers and identify the elements present and the quality of the reporting.

2. **Peer Feedback**. If available, pair up with a peer mentor, and one of you spend about 5 minutes talking about your title, abstract, and article. Take turns talking about your worksheets and giving feedback. If you are working independently, share your protocol with a colleague or mentor.

3. **Peer Feedback Guidance**. As you listen to your partner, you should focus on learning and honing your skills of critiquing. Your goal is to help your partner refine their title, abstract, and article. Help them focus on the mixed methods components of the article and abstract. Focus on what section or area that your partner needs feedback the most.

4. **Group Debrief**. If you are in a classroom or large group setting, take volunteers to present their study titles, abstracts, or papers. Reflect on how these same issues may play out in your own project.

5. **Peer Review**. Distribute blinded abstracts and articles anonymously (blind the article) among your class or peer members, and set a time limit of 30–60 minutes with each person acting as a peer reviewer. Each person should provide written feedback. You can incorporate the feedback, as appropriate.

Concluding Thoughts

Use this checklist to assess your progress in achieving the chapter 18 objectives:

- ☐ I identified my writing strengths and a writing approach.

- ☐ I learned four elements of a mixed methods title that can be incorporated into my writing.

- ☐ I mastered the hourglass model of writing for composing a mixed methods research article.

- ☐ I developed a quantitatively or qualitatively organized outline for writing my mixed methods article.

- ☐ I learned the elements essential in a mixed methods abstract.

- ☐ I understood the essential mixed methods elements to integrate into an article.

- ☐ I organized an outline for my mixed methods dissertation or thesis.

- ☐ I reviewed my Chapter 18 publication planning with a peer or colleague to organize my writing approach.

Workbox 18.2 Suggested Answers

- Views among middle and senior managers in major oil corporations about proactive environmental strategies and competitively valuable corporate strategies: an exploratory sequential mixed methods investigation.

- The views of middle school principals and teachers on the role of the principal in creating a culture of academic optimism: an explanatory sequential mixed methods investigation.

- Use of a virtual human computer simulation for teaching communication skills to 2nd-year medical students: evaluation of a multisite randomized controlled trial using a convergent mixed methods evaluation.

Key Resources

1. **FURTHER READING ON WRITING MIXED METHODS ARTICLES/CHAPTERS**

   - Bazeley, P. (2015). Writing up multimethod and mixed methods research for diverse audiences. In S. Hesse-Biber & R. B. Johnson (Eds.), *The Oxford* *handbook of multimethod and mixed methods research inquiry* (pp. 296–313). New York, NY: Oxford University Press.

   - Bronstein, L. R., & Kovacs, P. J. (2013). Writing a mixed methods report in social work research.

Research on Social Work Practice, 23(3), 354–360.

- Creswell, J. W., & Plano Clark, V. L. (2018). *Designing and conducting mixed methods research* (3rd ed.). Thousand Oaks, CA: Sage.

- Fetters, M. D., & Freshwater, D. (2015). Publishing a methodological mixed methods research article. *Journal of Mixed Methods Research, 9*(3), 203–213. doi:10.1177/1558689815594687

- Guetterman, T. C., & Salmoura, A. (2016). Enhancing text validation through rigorous mixed methods components. In A. J. Moeller, J. W. Creswell, & N. Saville (Eds.), *Second language assessment and mixed methods research (studies in language testing)* (pp. 153–176). Cambridge, UK: Cambridge University Press.

- Leech, N. L. (2012). Writing mixed research reports. *American Behavioral Scientist, 56*(6), 866–881.

- Leech, N. L., & Onwuegbuzie, A. J. (2010). Guidelines for conducting and reporting mixed research in the field of counseling and beyond. *Journal of Counseling & Development, 88*(1), 61–69.

- O'Cathain, A. (2009). Reporting mixed methods projects. *Mixed methods research for nursing and the health sciences.* In S. Andrew & E. J. Halcomb (Eds.), *Mixed methods research for nursing and health sciences* (pp. 135–158). Oxford, UK: Wiley-Blackwell Publishing.

2. **FURTHER READING ON DEVELOPING AND WRITING A MIXED METHODS PROPOSAL, DISSERTATION, OR THESIS.**

- Creswell, J. W., & Plano Clark, V. L. (2018). *Designing and conducting mixed methods research* (3rd ed.). Thousand Oaks, CA: Sage.

- DeCuir-Gunby, J. T., & Schutz, P. A. (2016). *Developing a mixed methods proposal: A practical guide for beginning researchers.* Thousand Oaks, CA: Sage.

APPENDICES

To illustrate the relevance of the Workbook with applied examples, the Workbook features three studies, one from business in Appendix 1 by Sharma and Vredenburg (1998), one from education in Appendix 2 by Harper (2016), and one from the health sciences in Appendix 3 by Kron et al. (2017).

APPENDIX 1. MIXED METHODS RESEARCH IN BUSINESS EXAMPLE

Sanjay Sharma, with a background in commerce, and Harrie Vredenburg, with a background in management, identified that arguments linking corporate environmental responsiveness to organizational capacity and performance were theoretical (Sharma & Vredenburg, 1998). To explore linkages between environmental strategies and the development of capabilities, and understand the nature of any emergent capabilities and competitive outcomes, the authors implemented a two-phase qualitative study. In Phase I, they conducted 19 in-depth interviews with senior and middle management executives to create case studies of seven firms in the Canadian oil and gas industry. In Phase II, they longitudinally interviewed 27 executives between two to five times over 1.5 years. Based on qualitative findings with supplementation from the literature about corporate social performance, environmental strategies, organizational learning, and resource-based views of firms, they identified two environmentally proactive and seven reactive corporations. They further developed hypotheses about linkages between corporate environmental responsiveness to organizational capacity and performance. In a third phase designed to test the hypothesized linkages from the first phase, they distributed a mail-based 95-item, 7-point continuous scale survey to 110 corporations, of whom 99 (response rate 90%) replied, to measure environmental strategies of the Canadian oil and gas industry. Based on their mixed methods approach, they demonstrated that strategies of proactive responsiveness to uncertainties of the interface between business and ecological issues were associated with unique organizational capabilities that had implications for firm competitiveness (Sharma & Vredenburg, 1998).

APPENDIX 2. MIXED METHODS RESEARCH IN EDUCATION EXAMPLE

William A. Harper (2016), with a background in educational leadership, sought to understand how principals can improve student achievement by improving school culture. Noting research demonstrating a positive relationship between academic optimism and student achievement, he assessed this relationship in 26 of Alabama's 218 middle schools by examining high and low categories of student achievement among schools stratified by high, medium, and low socioeconomic status. Using correlation, regression, and recursive partitioning analyses, he found that academic optimism was not a predictor of reading or math achievement but that academic emphasis, a dimension of academic optimism, was a significant predictor of academic achievement. To explain the findings, he then explored qualitatively how three dimensions of academic optimism (i.e., faculty trust, collective efficacy, and academic emphasis) were related to student achievement. Based on interviews with 11 principals of high-achieving middle schools chosen by maximum variation sampling based on school size, socioeconomic status, and geography, he identified five reciprocally interacting strategies—data-based decision making, collaborative team work, principal support of teachers, consistent communication, and routine celebrations of academic excellence—that contributed to a culture of academic optimism. Based on the mixed methods approach, he was able to refine quantitatively academic emphasis as the principle dimension of academic optimism that contributed to academic achievement and then explain further the findings by honing in on five practical strategies principals can use to nurture a culture that promotes academic achievement.

APPENDIX 3. MIXED METHODS RESEARCH IN THE HEALTH SCIENCES EXAMPLE

Noting the profound importance of excellent communication skills for improving health care outcomes according to a variety of measures, Frederick W. Kron (2017), an academic family physician and Hollywood screen writer, formed a multidisciplinary team to address the compelling need to teach empathy to medical learners. Based on pilot work demonstrating the feasibility of teaching empathy using a virtual human system, the team designed a trial that randomized students from three medical schools to either an intervention arm (n = 210), with exposure to virtual human training, or a control arm (n = 211), with exposure to a state-of-the-art computer-based learning module, and then tested student ability to use preferred communication skills in an evaluation of their clinical performance. They found that the students who were in the arm of the trial that exposed them to the virtual human training performed better than students who were in the arm of the trial with a computer-based standard, state-of-the-art communications module. To understand students' experiences with the two types of interventions, all students composed qualitative reflective essays and answered structured survey items about their experiences. These illustrated that a critical difference between the virtual human training and standardized computer-based module training was the interactivity of the virtual human training. Based on their mixed methods trial, the authors were able to demonstrate objectively that the virtual reality intervention worked through a mixed methods evaluation, and for this reason, students who took the virtual human training performed better (Kron et al., 2017).

GLOSSARY

Abstract (structured). A research study summary organized by four sections, usually the introduction/background, methods, results, and discussion/conclusions.

Abstract (unstructured). A research summary written freely that does not require specific sections.

Analysis. The procedures used to make sense of the collected qualitative, quantitative, or mixed methods data.

Ascertaining the need. The collection of qualitative or mixed methods data prior to conducting the main component of a mixed methods research or evaluation study to document the need of the investigation.

Background. The premise for conducting a mixed methods project.

Bias. Deviation in the interpreted value from the actual value.

Brain stretch. An activity designed to trigger thinking beyond the usual data collection procedures and stimulate your grey matter to consider alternatives.

Building. The intention or activity of conducting the data collection and analysis using one form of data to inform the data collection approach of the other type of data collection and analysis.

Candidate journals. The publishing venues for dissemination of MMR and evaluation papers or articles.

Comparing. The collection and analysis of both qualitative and quantitative data about a phenomenon of interest, and then examining how the two types of data relate to each other.

Connecting. The use of one type of data collection to inform selection of participants for the other type of data collection.

Construct. An idea, attribute, mental abstraction, working hypothesis, or theory.

Constructing a case. The collection of qualitative and quantitative data to develop a robust understanding about a specific example under investigation.

Convenience sampling. Selecting for research enrollment study participants most readily available and easy to access.

Convergent mixed methods research design. An approach when collected qualitative and quantitative data where qualitative and quantitative data are collected and analyzed roughly at the same time.

Core mixed methods designs. Three fundamental designs using an integrated approach to qualitative and quantitative data collection and analysis and comprising convergent, explanatory sequential, or exploratory sequential.

Corroborating. Using one type of data to verify the findings of the other form of data.

Data collection inventory. Assembling a comprehensive list of the data collection elements from the qualitative and quantitative data.

Data sources table. A matrix used to identify qualitative and quantitative sources of information for a mixed methods project.

Descriptive mixed methods data analysis. Three approaches used to identify linkages and compare related qualitative and quantitative data that are comprised of spiraling, finding a common thread, and back-and-forth exchanges.

Developing and validating a model. The creation of a theoretical or conceptual framework with one form of data collection and analysis, and then testing its validity with the other form of data collection and analysis.

Diffracting. The search for different cuts or slices of data with qualitative and quantitative data collection.

Directional dimension. The framing of mixed data analysis characterized as unidirectional where the quantitative data or qualitative data frame the analysis, or as bidirectional where both strands frame the analysis.

Domain. An overarching area, sphere of activity, or thought.

Enhancing. The use of information from both the qualitative and quantitative findings to increase interpretability and meaningfulness.

Equivalently driven mixed methods analysis. Investigations equally prioritizing both the qualitative and quantitative strands through the course of the study.

Expanding. The extension of breadth and range of inquiry by using different methods in a mixed methods project.

Expected outcomes. The products anticipated to result from each aim of a mixed methods project.

Explaining. The describing or explicating of initial quantitative findings with subsequent qualitative data collection and analysis.

Explanatory sequential mixed methods research design. An approach first collecting and analyzing quantitative data, followed by collecting and analyzing qualitative data that help explain the initial quantitative findings.

Exploratory sequential mixed methods research design. An approach of first collecting and analyzing qualitative data to explore a phenomenon, followed by collecting and analyzing quantitative data to examine associations or generalizations about the qualitatively generated findings.

Exploring. The intent of using initial qualitative data collection and analysis to discover relevant information prior to conducting a quantitative follow-up study, confirming, or generalizing the initial qualitative findings.

Gap in the literature. A hole/omission in the existing written works that justifies a specific project.

General research objective. A statement of the primary purpose pursued in the investigation that is based on the gap identified.

Generalizability. The extent quantitative findings from the study population can be extrapolated to a broader population; sometimes called *external validity*.

Generalizing. The extension of findings and conclusions drawn from an initial qualitative phase, through the use of a subsequent quantitative phase conducted with a representative population of individuals where findings are assessed by using inferential statistics.

Generating and testing hypotheses. The development of postulations based on one type of data that can then be tested with the other type of data.

Generic questions approach to quality. There are certain features of any design that can be considered with regards to quality criteria.

Geographic information system mapping. The process of solving a spatial question by using digital technologies that store, manage, analyze, and represent spatial information.

Hourglass model of writing. A conceptual structure guiding the writing of findings from research projects.

Human subjects compliance. The state or process of being in accord with regulations designed to protect human subjects engaged in research.

Human subjects review. The process by which a research study is reviewed for compliance with regulations and ethical principles for the ethical conduct of research involving human subjects.

Imitation game. An inherently mixed methods approach from sociology that allows researchers to explore cultural aspects of a phenomenon.

Impact factor. A standardized scoring system designed to describe the influence of the journal.

Implementation matrix. A table or figure that provides a concise overview of a mixed methods research plan with aims, procedures, outcomes, and other optional headings.

Independent data analysis. The process of inferring the meaning of the mixed findings by first examining, exploring, and making interpretations separately within each of the qualitative and quantitative strands, before comparing the two types of findings for an overall interpretation.

Individual components approach to quality. The assertion that attending to rigor and quality of the individual qualitative and quantitative strands will ensure quality in the mixed methods.

Inferences. Conclusions drawn from the findings of the individuals in the sample to the target population.

Information-rich cases. Cases that can illuminate the qualitative question being pursued by virtue of their nature and substance.

Initiating. The intention of searching for paradox and contradiction.

Institutional ethics review board. The organization formally empowered and entrusted to assess the extent that a mixed methods project is compliant with ethical and regulatory requirements for the ethical conduct of research.

Integration intent during mixed methods data collection and analysis. The purposes of linking qualitative and quantitative data as they are gathered and/or examining the findings together for examination during mixed methods studies.

Intent of integration. The purpose of linking qualitative and quantitative approaches and dimensions together to create a new whole, or a more holistic, understanding than achieved by either approach alone.

Interactive data analysis. The process of inferring the meaning of the mixed findings by examining, exploring, and making interpretations iteratively as data collection and analysis occurs based on an emerging understanding of the findings of both types of data.

Intermethod data collection. The gathering of qualitative and quantitative information using *different* procedures.

Intramethod analysis. The process of inferring the meaning of the findings by first examining, exploring, and making interpretations within the strand using the analytics procedures of the respective qualitative and quantitative tradition.

Joint display. A table or figure that represents with structural features in a side-by-side or other type of juxtaposed representation the qualitative and quantitative data collection procedures or findings.

Joint display analysis. The process of identifying linkages between the qualitative and quantitative constructs by developing multiple iterations of a table of qualitative and quantitative findings, and then organizing the structure to optimize understanding of the meaning of the mixed findings.

Joint display linkage activity. The process of organizing the qualitative and quantitative data findings into a table and identifying linkages of related constructs between the two types of data.

Joint display of mixed methods data collection. A table or matrix depicting how both qualitative and quantitative data collection procedures have been matched to ensure collected data address (or will address) related study constructs.

Joint display planning. The process of creating a table or matrix to juxtapose and match the constructs to be addressed through both the qualitative and quantitative data collection processes to ensure that two types of data will be linkable.

Linkages. The bonds held in common through constructs between qualitative and quantitative data.

Linking. An active process of looking for and finding commonality between qualitative and quantitative data in mixed methods projects.

Literature review types. The narrative review, scoping review, meta-analysis, meta-synthesis, mixed methods research synthesis, and meta-integration constitute options for examining published literature.

Matching. Collecting intentionally both qualitative and quantitative data about the *same* domains, constructs, or ideas.

Measurement reliability. Reflects the extent to which the results of a measurement represent the quality of a construct.

Measurement validity. Addresses the extent to which a data collection instrument measures what is intended to assess.

Metainferences. An interpretation about the meaning of qualitative and quantitative results when considered together.

Mixed methods approach to quality. Addressing unique features of mixed methods research and evaluation that require attention for ensuring the integrity.

Mixed methods data analysis. The process of examining both types of findings to identify linkages across the two types of findings that comprise constructs with commonality, and making new interpretations for a more enhanced or holistic understanding.

Mixed methods general multistage (multiphase) designs. A category of scaffolded mixed methods study plans that are conducted as an integrated and sustained program of research.

Mixed methods methodological designs. A category of scaffolded mixed methods study plans that are integrated with a different methodology (e.g., experimental/interventional study, case study, evaluation; survey development; or interactive, user-centered design).

Mixed methods quality (generic questions approach). A view about study rigor presuming that any mixed methods design can be considered with general criteria of excellence.

Mixed methods quality (individual components approach). A view of study rigor maintaining that attention to rigor and excellence of the individual qualitative and quantitative strands will ensure overall quality in a mixed methods study.

Mixed methods research. The integration of qualitative and quantitative approaches in a sustained program of inquiry with due consideration of the philosophical, methodological, and applications in practice.

Mixed methods research integrity. The attributes of rigor and quality with regard to conceptualization, implementation, and interpretation considering the qualitative strand, quantitative strand, the mixed methods, as well as the integration in mixed methodology dimensions.

Mixed methods research protocol. A document containing the key components necessary for conducting a mixed methods research study.

Mixed methods research questions. The concern(s) addressed in an investigation that integrates qualitative and quantitative approaches.

Mixed methods sampling. The strategy used to identify participants for the qualitative and quantitative approaches.

Mixed methods theoretical designs. A category of scaffolded mixed methods study plans that are integrated with an overarching theory (e.g., transformative mixed methods, community-based participatory research, or complexity theory).

Monitoring. Using qualitative or mixed methods data collection and analysis to watch for events during a mixed methods study or evaluation.

Monomethod research. Employing only qualitative procedures or only quantitative procedures in a line of investigation.

Multilevel hierarchical relationship. A relationship where different units or social levels from the hierarchy in an organization are included in the mixed methods project.

Optimizing. Using qualitative or mixed methods data collection and analysis early in a mixed methods research or evaluation study to ensure that study instruments or interventions have been developed effectively.

Overarching context. The circumstances that inform a topic, the most general level of the background.

Peer mentor. A colleague with a similar academic background who will consult with you and provide feedback about your mixed methods project.

Personal background. The entirety of one's cumulative individual, academic, and occupational knowledge and experience.

Personal context. The personal background, theoretical models, and philosophical assumptions researchers bring to their mixed methods projects.

Personal story. The teaching, work, or clinical experience(s) that triggered an interest in a mixed methods topic.

Philosophical assumptions. The beliefs and values about the nature of reality, how one gains knowledge, and the lens through which one sees the world.

Point of integration. The contact of qualitative and quantitative procedures or data interface in a mixed methods study.

Preliminary topic. The initial concern proposed for a mixed methods project.

Probability sampling. A random selection approach to help ensure that the sample chosen can be representative of the target population.

Project aims. The specific achievements aspired for in a mixed methods project.

Project inventory for publication. A written activity to organize study strengths, limitations, order of publications pursuit, and the rationale for the ordering of submission.

Project goal. The overarching purpose of a mixed methods research or evaluation project.

Project procedures. The qualitative and quantitative data collection approaches proposed or used in a mixed methods project.

Publication (candidate journals). The candidate venues for dissemination of mixed methods research and evaluation papers or articles.

Publication categorization of fit. An assessment of the appropriateness of a paper for different journals that can be fit: stretch, good, or safety.

Publication project inventory. A written activity to organize study strengths, limitations, order of publications to pursue, and the rationale for the ordering of submission.

Purposeful sampling. The selection of participants with an explicit intent, rationale, or criteria in a qualitative study.

Qualitative advanced analysis. Advanced analysis using specific methodological approaches, using theory throughout, and/or creating new theories or models.

Qualitative comparative analysis. A theory-driven approach designed to look for solutions to problems by examining the contributions of various conditions and understanding how they lead to a given outcome.

Qualitative primary analysis. The process of iteratively collecting and examining collected text, observations, visuals, or other media data, and making sense of information descriptively to understand a phenomenon of interest.

Qualitative research. The methodology and methods used in the design, data collection, analysis, and presentation of open-ended, textual or visual data.

Qualitatively driven mixed methods projects. Investigations prioritizing the qualitative strand over the qualitative strand and featuring specific qualitative methodology or theory in the data collection and analysis process with less sophisticated quantitative analytics.

Qualitatively organized writing. In a mixed methods paper, the presentation in the methods of the qualitative strand procedures before the quantitative procedures (e.g., with an exploratory sequential design or a convergent design).

Qualitizing data. The transformation of quantitative data into a qualitative form.

Quality (the mixed methods approach). A view of study rigor deeming there are unique features to mixed methods research and evaluation that uniquely require attention.

Quantitative advanced analysis. The use of statistics to answer or model measurement, causality, and relationship-driven research questions.

Quantitative primary analysis. The calculation of descriptive statistics on numerically expressed data such as means, medians, and tabulations.

Quantitative research. The methodology and methods used in the design, data collection, analysis, and presentation of closed-ended or numerical data.

Quantitatively driven mixed methods studies. Investigations prioritizing the quantitative strand over the qualitative strand and featuring advanced inferential statistical analysis and modeling with less sophisticated qualitative analytics.

Quantitatively organized writing. In a mixed methods paper, the presentation in the methods of the quantitative strand procedures before the qualitative procedures (e.g., with an explanatory sequential design or convergent design).

Quantitizing data. The transformation of qualitative data into a quantitative form.

Reflexivity. When a researcher engages in honest, explicit, self-aware analysis of one's own role in the research process.

Relational dimension. The way mixed data are considered relative to each other in the analysis process, either independently with separate analysis of the qualitative and quantitative data, or interactively with the qualitative and quantitative findings iteratively influencing the interpretation of both.

Repertory grid (RepGrid). A written structure used as a cognitive mapping tool to elucidate what people think about a certain topic in a repertory grid analysis study.

Repertory grid analysis. A cognitive mapping approach to interpreting a RepGrid.

Repertory grid dyadic approach. The interview component of a repertory grid study that contrasts only two elements, that is, instances or examples of a topic.

Repertory grid elements. Examples or instances of the topic (i.e., people, objects, or events).

Repertory grid linkages. The way an element is described relative to each construct.

Repertory grid triadic approach. The interview component of a repertory grid study that compares three elements and explains how two are similar and the third is different.

Replicability. The extent that findings from one study are found to be similar to findings of another study where testing is conducted under similar circumstances by others.

Reproducibility. The extent that another researcher who analyzes data from a specific study would have the same findings and reach the same conclusions.

Research topic. The subject of an investigation.

Revised title. A rephrased name for the mixed methods study.

Sample. The individuals drawn from the sampling frame chosen with the intent of representing the individuals of the entire population.

Sampling frame. The individuals from the target population who are available for sampling.

Sampling relationship. How the participants of qualitative and quantitative data collection are related to each other (i.e., identical, nested, enlarged, separate, or hierarchical multilevel).

Sampling timing. The temporal relationship between when the qualitative and the quantitative data are collected, usually synchronous or asynchronous.

Scaffolded mixed methods research designs. The research strategies or plans that collect and analyze both qualitative and quantitative data, are built with a core design or combination of core designs, and are integrated with another application, methodology, and/or theoretical framework.

Scope of previous research. The extent at which previous investigations have addressed a topic of interest.

Search terms. Specific words used to search and identify literature about a topic.

Social network analysis. The process of researchers constructing pictures and diagrams of social relations to reveal patterns not seen by observation, and examining structural properties and the implications for social action.

Spectrum of mixed methods research design structure. A description of the continuum of investigation approaches ranging from emergent as data collection and analysis proceed, or through advanced planning of the data collection procedures.

Study population. Individuals for whom the researcher is taking an interest in a research investigation.

Target journals. Destinations under consideration for submission of mixed methods research and evaluation articles.

Target population. The entire group of individuals as the source from which a smaller number of individuals, the sample, can be drawn.

Theoretical models. The assumptions about or conceptual representations of the nature of topic or phenomenon.

Theory. A system of statements or principles used to explain a phenomenon of interest.

Transferability. The extent the findings can apply to others from the study population or similar background.

Transferring. Conveys the intent to consider the relevance of the findings from the study participants to a larger population, phenomenon of interest, context, or theory.

Transferring. The consideration of the relevance of the findings from a small number of study participants in a qualitative study to another context, larger population, phenomenon of interest, or theory.

Types of data sources. The information bases for mixed methods research projects, including observations, interviews (individual and multiperson interviews, e.g., focus groups), documents, audiovisual, questionnaires, secondary datasets, and biological/medical/engineering/physical sciences data.

Validity threats. The study circumstances or choices that could preclude rigorous, accurate, or robust portrayal of a phenomenon under investigation.

Working title. A provisional name for a mixed methods project.

REFERENCES

Abdelrahim, H., Elnashar, M., Khidir, A., Killawi, A., Hammoud, M., Al-Khal, A. L., & Fetters, M. D. (2017). Patient perspectives on language discordance during healthcare visits: Findings from the extremely high-density multicultural state of Qatar. *Journal of Health Communication, 22*(4), 355–363. doi:10.1080/10810730.2017 .1296507

Alwashmi, M., Hawboldt, J., Davis, E., & Fetters, M. D. (2019). The Iterative Convergent Design for mHealth Usability Testing: Mixed Methods Approach. *JMIR mHealth uHealth. 7*(4):e11656) doi: 10.2196/11656

Angrosino, M. (2007). *Doing ethnographic and observational research.* Thousand Oaks, CA: Sage.

Arabie, P., Carroll, D., & DeSarbo, W. S. (1987). *Three-way scaling: A guide to multidimensional scaling and clustering.* Thousand Oaks, CA: Sage.

Arksey, H., & O'Malley, L. (2002). Scoping studies: Towards a methodological framework. *International Journal of Social Research Methodology, 8*(1), 19–32. doi:10.1080/1364557032000119616

Armenakis, A. A., & Bedeian, A. G. (1999). Organizational change: A review of theory and research in the 1990s. *Journal of Management, 25*(3), 293–315.

Axiology. (n.d.). Retrieved from https://en.oxforddictionaries. com/definition/axiology.

Bandura, A. W. R. (1971). *Social learning theory.* New York, NY: General Learning Press.

Barney, J. B., & Zajac, E. J. (1994). Competitive organizational behavior: Toward an organizationally based theory of competitive advantage. *Strategic Management Journal, 15*(S1), 5–9. doi:10.1002/ smj.4250150902

Bazeley, P. (2012). Integrative analysis strategies for mixed data sources. *American Behavioral Scientist, 56*(6), 814–828. doi:10.1177/0002764211426330

Bazeley, P. (2018). *Integrating analyses in mixed methods research.* Thousand Oaks, CA: Sage.

Bazeley, P., & Kemp, L. (2012). Mosaics, triangles, and DNA: Metaphors for integrated analysis in mixed methods research. *Journal of Mixed Methods Research, 6*(1), 55–72. doi:10.1177/1558689811419514

Beall's List of Predatory Journals and Publishers. (2018). Retrieved from https://beallslist.weebly.com/.

Berger, M. (2017). *Everything you ever wanted to know about predatory publishing but were afraid to ask.* Paper presented at the ACRL 2017, Baltimore, Maryland. Retrieved from https://academic works.cuny.edu/cgi/viewcontent.cgi?referer=https://scholar .google.com/&httpsredir=1&article=1142&context=ny_pubs.

Bernard, H. R. (1995). Choosing research problems, sites, and methods. In *Research methods in anthropology: Qualitative and quantitative approaches* (2nd ed., pp. 102–135). Walnut Creek, CA: AltaMira Press.

Bernard, T., & Flitman, A. (2002). Using repertory grid analysis to gather qualitative data for information systems research. *ACIS 2002 Proceedings*, 98.

Biomarker. (n.d.). *Merriam-Webster dictionary online.* Retrieved from https://www.merriam-webster.com/dictionary/biomarker.

The Biosemantics Group. (2007). JANE, Journal/Author Name Estimator. Retrieved from http://jane.biosemantics.org/index.php.

Boadu, O. S. (2015). A comparative study of behavioural and emotional problems among children living in orphanages in Ghana: A mixed method approach. Dissertation. University of Ghana. Accra, Ghana.

Borg, I., & Groenen, P. J. F. (2005). *Modern multidimensional scaling: Theory and applications (Springer Series in Statistics)* (2nd ed.). New York, NY: Springer.

Bradt, J., Potvin, N., Kesslick, A., Shim, M., Radl, D., Schriver, E., . . . Komarnicky-Kocher, L. T. (2015). The impact of music therapy versus music medicine on psychological outcomes and pain in cancer patients: A mixed methods study. *Support Care Cancer, 23*(5), 1261–1271. doi:10.1007/s00520-014-2478-7

Brinkman, S., & Kvale, S. (2014). *Interviews: Learning the craft of qualitative research interviewing* (3rd ed.). Thousand Oaks, CA: Sage.

Bryman, A. (1988). *Quantity and quality in social research.* London, UK: Unwin Hyman.

Bryman, A. (2006). Integrating quantitative and qualitative research: How is it done? *Qualitative Research, 6*(1), 97–113. doi:10.1177/1468794106058877

Bryman, A. (2007). Barriers to integrating quantitative and qualitative research. *Journal of Mixed Methods Research, 1*(1), 8–22. doi:10.1177/2345678906290531

Bryman, A., Becker, S., & Sempik, J. (2008). Quality criteria for quantitative, qualitative and mixed methods research: A view from social policy. *International Journal of Social Research Methodology, 11*(4), 261–276. doi:10.1080/13645570701401644

Bustamante, C. (2017). TPACK and teachers of Spanish: Development of a theory-based joint display in a mixed methods research case study. *Journal of Mixed Methods Research*, 1–16. doi:10.1177/1558689817712119

Byrne, D., & Uprichard, E. (2013). *Cluster analysis (SAGE benchmarks in social research methods)* (Vol. 4; Volume set ed.). London, UK: Sage.

Callahan, E. J., & Bertakis, K. D. (1991). Development and validation of the Davis observation code. *Family Medicine, 23*(1), 19–24.

Campbell, D. J., Tam-Tham, H., Dhaliwal, K. K., Manns, B. J., Hemmelgarn, B. R., Sanmartin, C., & King-Shier, K. (2017). Use of mixed methods research in research on coronary artery disease, diabetes mellitus, and hypertension: A scoping review. *Circulation: Cardiovascular Quality and Outcomes, 10*(1), 1–11. doi:10.1161/ CIRCOUTCOMES.116.003310

Canadian Institutes of Health Research. (2015). Learning in ethics. Retrieved January 24, 2017, from http://www.cihr-irsc .gc.ca/e/49286.html.

Caputi, P., & Reddy, P. (1999). A comparison of triadic and dyadic methods of personal construct elicitation. *Journal of Constructivist Psychology, 12*(3), 253–264. doi:10.1080/107205399266109

Catallo, C., Jack, S. M., Ciliska, D., & MacMillan, H. L. (2013). Minimizing the risk of intrusion: A grounded theory of intimate partner violence disclosure in emergency departments. *Journal of Advanced Nursing*, 69(6), 1366–1376. doi:10.1111/j.1365-2648.2012.06128.x

Clarivate Analytics—EndNote (n.d.). Manuscript Matcher. Retrieved May 11, 2019, from https://endnote.com/product-details/manuscript-matcher/.

Cochrane, T., & Davey, R. C. (2017). Mixed-methods evaluation of a healthy exercise, eating, and lifestyle program for primary schools. *Journal of School Health*, 87, 823–831. doi:10.1111/josh.12555

Collingridge, D. S. (2013). A primer on quantitized data analysis and permutation testing. *Journal of Mixed Methods Research*, 7(1), 81–97. doi:10.1177/1558689812454457

Collins, H., & Evans, R. (2014). Quantifying the tacit: The imitation game and social fluency. *Sociology*, 48(1), 3–19. doi:10.1177/0038038512455735

Collins, H., Evans, R., Weinel, M., Lyttleton-Smith, J., Bartlett, A., & Hall, M. (2017). The imitation game and the nature of mixed methods. *Journal of Mixed Methods Research*, 11(4), 510–527. doi:10.1177/1558689815619824

Collins, K. M. T. (2015). Validity in multimethod and mixed research. In S. N. Hesse-Biber & B. Johnson (Eds.), *The Oxford handbook of multimethod and mixed methods research inquiry* (pp. 240–256). New York. NY: Oxford University Press.

Collins, K. M. T., Onwuegbuzie, A. J., & Johnson, R. B. (2012). Securing a place at the table: A review and extension of legitimation criteria for the conduct of mixed research. *American Behavioral Scientist*, 56(6), 849–865. doi:10.1177/0002764211433799

Crabtree, B. F., & Miller, W. L. (1999). *Doing qualitative research* (2nd ed., Vol. 3). Newbury Park, CA: Sage.

Crabtree, B. F., Nutting, P. A., Miller, W. L., McDaniel, R. R., Stange, K. C., Jaén, C. R., & Stewart, E. (2011). Primary care practice transformation is hard work: Insights from a 15-year developmental program of research. *Medical Care*, 49, S28. doi:10.1097%2FMLR.0b013e3181cad65c

Creamer, E. G. (2018). *An introduction to fully integrated mixed methods research*. Thousand Oaks, CA: Sage.

Creswell, J. W. (2013). *Qualitative inquiry and research design: Choosing among five approaches* (3rd ed.). Thousand Oaks, CA: Sage.

Creswell, J. W. (2015). *A concise introduction to mixed methods research*. Thousand Oaks, CA: Sage.

Creswell, J. W. (2016). *30 essential skills for the qualitative researcher*. Thousand Oaks, CA: Sage.

Creswell, J. W., & Creswell, J. D. (2018). *Research design: Qualitative, quantitative, and mixed methods approaches* (5 ed., p. 108). Thousand Oaks, CA: Sage.

Creswell, J. W., Fetters, M. D., & Ivankova, N. V. (2004). Designing a mixed methods study in primary care. *Annals of Family Medicine*, 2, 7–12. doi:10.1370/afm.104

Creswell, J. W., Fetters, M. D., Plano Clark, V. L., & Morales, A. (2009). Mixed methods intervention trials. In S. Andrew & E. Halcomb (Eds.), *Mixed methods research for nursing and the health sciences* (pp. 161–180). Oxford, UK: Blackwell Publishing.

Creswell, J. W, Klassen, A. C., Plano Clark, V. L., & Smith, K. C. for the Office of Behavioral and Social Sciences Research. (2011). *Best practices for mixed methods research in the health sciences*. August. National Institutes of Health. Retrieved May 10, 2019, from https://obssr.od.nih.gov/wp-content/uploads/2016/02/Best_Practices_for_Mixed_Methods_Research.pdf.

Creswell, J. W., & Plano Clark, V. L. (2011). *Designing and conducting mixed methods research*. Thousand Oaks, CA: Sage.

Creswell, J. W., & Plano Clark, V. L. (2018). *Designing and conducting mixed methods research* (3rd ed.). Thousand Oaks, CA: Sage.

Creswell, J. W., & Poth, C. N. (2018). *Qualitative inquiry and research design: Choosing among five approaches* (4th ed.). Thousand Oaks, CA: Sage.

Cronin, A., Alexander, V., Fielding, J., Moran-Ellis, J., & Thomas, H. (2008). The analytic integration of qualitative data sources. In P. Alasuutari, L. Bickman, & J. Brannen (Eds.), *The SAGE handbook of social research methods* (pp. 572–584). Thousand Oaks, CA: Sage.

Crooks, V. A., Schuurman, N., Cinnamon, J., Castleden, H., & Johnston, R. (2011). Refining a location analysis model using a mixed methods approach: Community readiness as a key factor in siting rural palliative care services. *Journal of Mixed Methods Research*, 5(1), 77–95. doi:10.1177/1558689810385693

Curry, L. A., & Nunez-Smith, M. (2015). *Mixed methods in health sciences research: A practical primer*. Thousand Oaks, CA: Sage.

DeJonckheere, M., Lindquist-Grantz, R., Toraman, S., Haddad, K., & Vaughn, L. M. (2018). Intersection of mixed methods and community-based participatory research: A methodological review. *Journal of Mixed Methods Research*. https://doi.org/10.1177/1558689818778469

Denzin, N. K. (2010). Moments, mixed methods, and paradigm dialogs. *Qualitative Inquiry*, 16(6), 419–427. doi:10.1177/1077800410364608

DeVellis, R. F. (2012). *Scale development: Theory and applications* (3rd ed.; Vol. 26). Thousand Oaks, CA: Sage.

Directory of Open Access Journals (DOAJ). (n.d.). Retrieved May 11, 2019, from https://doaj.org.

Domagk, S., Schwartz, R. N., & Plass, J. L. (2010). Interactivity in multimedia learning: An integrated model. *Computers in Human Behavior*, 26(5), 1024–1033. doi:10.1016/j.chb.2010.03.003

Dragon, T., Arroyo, I., Woolf, B. P., Burleson, W., el Kaliouby, R., & Eydgahi, H. (2008). Viewing student affect and learning through classroom observation and physical sensors. In B. P. Woolf, E. Aïmeur, R. Nkambou, & S. Lajoie (Eds.), *Intelligent tutoring systems: 9th international conference, ITS 2008, Montreal, Canada, June 23–27, 2008 proceedings* (pp. 29–39). Berlin, Germany: Springer Berlin Heidelberg.

Driscoll, D. L., Appiah-Yeboah, A., Salib, P., & Rupert, D. J. (2007). Merging qualitative and quantitative data in mixed methods research: How to and why not. *Ecological and Environmental Anthropology*, 3(1), 19–28.

Elwood, S., & Cope, M. (2009). Introduction: Qualitative GIS. Forging mixed methods through representations, analytical innovations, and conceptual engagements. In *Qualitative GIS: A mixed methods approach* (pp. 1–12). Thousand Oaks, CA: Sage.

Elwyn, G., Frosch, D., Thomson, R., Joseph-Williams, N., Lloyd, A., Kinnersley, P., . . . Rollnick, S. (2012). Shared decision making: A model for clinical practice. *Journal of General Internal Medicine*, 27(10), 1361–1367. doi:10.1007/s11606-012-2077-6

Elwyn, T. S., Fetters, M. D., Sasaki, H., & Tsuda, T. (2002). Responsibility and cancer disclosure in Japan. *Social Science and Medicine*, 54(2), 281–293. doi:10.1016/S0277-9536(01)00028-4

Epistemology. (n.d.). Retrieved from https://en.oxforddictionaries.com/definition/epistemology.

Ewigman, B. G. (1996). Fire in the belly: Doing what it takes to produce excellent research. *Family Medicine*, 28(4), 289–290.

Fàbregues, S., Paré, M.-H., & Meneses, J. (2018). Operationalizing and conceptualizing quality in mixed methods research: A multiple case study of the disciplines of education, nursing, psychology, and sociology. *Journal of Mixed Methods Research*, 1–22. doi:10.1177/1558689817751774

Federal Trade Commission. (2016). FTC charges academic journal publisher OMICS group deceived researchers. Retrieved from https://www.ftc.gov/news-events/press-releases/2016/08/ftc-charges-academic-journal-publisher-omics-group-deceived.

Fetters, M. D. (2018). Six equations to help conceptualize the field of mixed methods. *Journal of Mixed Methods Research*, *12*(3), 262–267. doi:10.1177/1558689818779433

Fetters, M. D., Curry, L. A., & Creswell, J. W. (2013). Achieving integration in mixed methods designs-principles and practices. *Health Services Research*, *48*, 2134–2156. doi:10.1111/1475-6773.12117

Fetters, M.D. and Detroit Science Center. (2008–2011). Medical Marvels Interactive Translational Research Experience. National Library of Medicine/NIH,R03 LM010052-02.

Fetters, M. D., Elwyn, T. S., Sasaki, H., & Tsuda, T. (2000). 2:"がん告知"—質的研究の例 (Qualitative research Part II: An example of qualitative research on cancer disclosure). *Jpn J Prim Care*, *23*(1), 56–65.

Fetters, M. D., & Freshwater, D. (2015a). The 1 + 1 = 3 integration challenge. *Journal of Mixed Methods Research*, *9*(2), 115–117. doi:10.1177/1558689815581222

Fetters, M. D., & Freshwater, D. (2015b). Publishing a methodological mixed methods research article. *Journal of Mixed Methods Research*, *9*(3), 203–213. doi:10.1177/1558689815594687

Fetters, M. D., & Guetterman, T. C. (forthcoming, 2020). Development of a joint display as mixed analysis. In T. Onwuegbuzie & R. B. Johnson (Eds.), *Reviewer's guide for mixed methods research analysis*. Routledge.

Fetters, M. D., Guetterman, T. C., Scerbo, M. W., & Kron, F. W. (2017). A two-phase mixed methods project illustrating development of a virtual human intervention to teach advanced communication skills and a subsequent blinded mixed methods trail to test the intervention for effectiveness. *International Journals of Multidisciplinary Research Academy*, *10*(1), 748–759.

Fetters, M. D., Ivankova, N. V., Ruffin, M. T., Creswell, J. W., & Power, D. (2004). Developing a website in primary care. *Family Medicine*, *36*(9), 651–659.

Fetters, M.D. and Kron, F.W. (2012–15). Modeling Professional Attitudes and Teaching Humanistic Communication in Virtual Reality (MPathic-VRII). National Center for Advancing Translational Science/NIH 9R44TR000360-04.

Fetters, M.D. and Khidir, A. (2009–12). Providing Culturally Appropriate Health Care Services in Qatar: Development of a Multilingual "Patient Cultural Assessment of Quality" Instrument. Qatar Foundation, NPRP08-530-3-116.

Fetters, M. D., & Molina-Azorin, J. F. (2017a). The journal of mixed methods research starts a new decade: Principles for bringing in the new and divesting of the old language of the field. *Journal of Mixed Methods Research*, *11*, 3–10. doi:10.1177/1558689816682092

Fetters, M. D., & Molina-Azorin, J. F. (2017b). The journal of mixed methods research starts a new decade: The first 10 years in review. *Journal of Mixed Methods Research*, *11*(2), 143–155. doi:10.1177/1558689817696365

Fetters, M. D., & Molina-Azorin, J. F. (2017c). The journal of mixed methods research starts a new decade: The mixed methods research integration trilogy and its dimensions. *Journal of Mixed Methods Research*, *11*(3), 291–307. doi:10.1177/1558689817714066

Fetters, M. D., & Molina-Azorin, J. F. (2019). A call for expanding philosophical perspectives to create a more "worldly" field of mixed methods: The example of yinyang philosophy. *Journal of Mixed Methods Research*, *13*(1), 15–18. https://doi.org/10.1177/1558689818816886

Fetters, M. D., & Rubinstein, E. B. (forthcoming). The 3 Cs of content, context, and concepts: A practical approach to recording unstructured field observations. *Annals of Family Medicine*.

Finlay, L. (2002). "Outing" the researcher: The provenance, process, and practice of reflexivity. *Qualitative Health Research*, *12*(4), 531–545. doi:10.1177/104973202129120052

Frantzen, K. K., & Fetters, M. D. (2015). Meta-integration for synthesizing data in a systematic mixed studies review: Insights from research on autism spectrum disorder. *Quality & Quantity*, *50*(5), 2251–2277. doi: 10.1007/s11135-015-0261-6.

Frantzen, K. K., Lauritsen, M. B., Jørgensen, M., Tanggaard, L., Fetters, M. D., Aikens, J. E., & Bjerrum, M. (2015). Parental self-perception in the autism spectrum disorder literature: A systematic mixed studies review. *Review Journal of Autism and Developmental Disorders*, *3*(1), 18–36.

Franz, A., Worrell, M., & Vögele, C. (2013). Integrating mixed method data in psychological research: Combining Q methodology and questionnaires in a study investigating cultural and psychological influences on adolescent sexual behavior. *Journal of Mixed Methods Research*, *7*(4), 370–389.

Garcia-Castillo, D., & Fetters, M. D. (2007). Quality in medical translations: A review. *Journal of Health Care for the Poor and Underserved (JHCPU)*, *18*(1), 74–84.

Gartner. (n.d.). Gartner IT Glossary: Big Data. Retrieved April 24, 2019, from http://www.gartner.com/it-glossary/big-data/.

Glanz, K., & Bishop, D. B. (2010). The role of behavioral science theory in development and implementation of public health interventions. *Annual Review of Public Health*, *31*, 399–418. doi:10.1146/annurev.publhealth.012809.103604

Gomez-Mejia, L. R., & Balkin, D. B. (2017). Determinants of faculty pay: An agency theory perspective. *Academy of Management Journal*, *35*(5), 921–955. doi:10.5465/256535

Greene, J. C. (2007). *Mixed methods in social inquiry*. San Francisco, CA: Jossey-Bass.

Greene, J. C., & Hall, J. N. (2010). Dialectics and pragmatism: Being of consequence. *Handbook of mixed methods in social and behavioral research* (pp. 119–144). doi:10.4135/9781506335193

Greene, J. C., Caracelli, V. J., & Graham, W. F. (1989). Toward a conceptual framework for mixed-method evaluation designs. *Educational Evaluation and Policy Analysis*, *11*(3), 255–274. doi:10.3102/01623737011003255

Guetterman, T. C., Creswell, J. W., & Kuckartz, U. (2015). Using joint displays and MAXQDA software to represent the results of mixed methods research. In M. McCrudden, G. Schraw, & C. Buckendahl (Eds.), *Use of visual displays in research and testing: Coding, interpreting, and reporting data* (pp. 145–175). Charlotte, NC: Information Age Publishing.

Guetterman, T. C., & Fetters, M. D. (2018). Two methodological approaches to the integration of mixed methods and case study designs: A systemic review. *American Behavioral Scientist*, *62*(7), 900–918. https://doi.org/10.1177/0002764218772641

Guetterman, T. C., Fetters, M. D., & Creswell, J. W. (2015). Integrating quantitative and qualitative results in health science mixed methods research through joint displays. *Annals of Family Medicine*, *13*(6), 554–561. doi:10.1370/afm.1865

Guetterman, T. C., Fetters, M. D., Legocki, L. J., Mawocha, S., Barsan, W. G., Lewis, R. J., . . . Meurer, W. J. (2015). Reflections on the adaptive designs accelerating promising trials into treatments (ADAPT-IT) process—Findings from a qualitative study. *Clinical Research and Regulatory Affairs, 32*(4), 119–128. doi:10.3109/10601 333.2015.1079217

Guetterman, T. C., Kron, F. W., Campbell, T. C., Scerbo, M. W., Zelenski, A. B., Cleary, J. F., & Fetters, M. D. (2017). Initial construct validity evidence of a virtual human application for competency assessment in breaking bad news to a cancer patient. *Advances in Medical Education and Practice, 8*, 505. doi:10.2147/ AMEP.S138380

Haase, M., Becker, I., Nill, A., Shultz, C. J., & Gentry, J. W. (2016). Male breadwinner ideology and the inclination to establish market relationships: Model development using data from Germany and a mixed-methods research strategy. *Journal of Macromarketing, 36*(2), 149–167. doi:10.1177/0276146715576202

Hammoud, M. M., Elnashar, M., Abdelrahim, H., Khidir, A., Elliott, H. A. K., Killawi, A., . . . Fetters, M. D. (2012). Challenges and opportunities of US and Arab collaborations in health services research: A case study from Qatar. *Global Journal of Health Science, 4*, 148–159. doi:10.5539/gjhs.v4n6p148

Harper, W. A. (2016). *Exploring the role of the principal in creating a culture of academic optimism: A sequential QUAN to QUAL mixed methods study* (Dissertation). Birmingham: University of Alabama.

Hart, S. L. (1995). A natural-resource-based view of the firm. *Academy of Management Review, 20*(4), 986–1014. doi:10.2307/258963

Hesse-Biber, S., & Kelly, C. (2010). Post-modernist approaches to mixed methods research. In *Mixed methods research: Merging theory and practice* (pp. 154–730). New York, NY: Guilford Press.

Hesse-Biber, S., Rodriguez, D., & Frost, N. A. (2015). A qualitatively driven approach to multimethod and mixed methods research. In S. N. Hesse-Biber & B. Johnson (Eds.), *The Oxford handbook of multimethod and mixed methods research inquiry* (pp. 3–20). New York, NY: Oxford University Press.

Heyvaert, M., Hammes, K., & Onghena, P. (2017). *Using mixed methods research synthesis for literature reviews.* Thousand Oaks, CA: Sage.

Higgins, J., & Green, S. (2011). *Cochrane handbook for systematic reviews of interventions.* 5.1.0. Retrieved from www.cochrane-handbook.org.

Holtrop, J. S., Potworowski, G., Green, L. A., & Fetters, M. D. (2016). Analysis of novel care management programs in primary care. *Journal of Mixed Methods Research*, 1–28. doi:10.1177/1558689816668689

Hong, Q. N., & Pluye, P. (2018). A conceptual framework for critical appraisal in systematic mixed studies reviews. *Journal of Mixed Methods Research*, 1–15. doi:10.1177/1558689818770058

Hoy, W. K., Tarter, C. J., & Hoy, A. W. (2006). Academic optimism of schools: A force for student achievement. *American Educational Research Journal, 43*(3), 425–446. doi:10.3102/00028312043003425

Hurmerinta-Peltomäki, L., & Nummela, N. (2006). Mixed methods in international business research: A value-added perspective. *Management International Review, 46*(4), 439–459. doi:10.1007/ s11575-006-0100-z

Hwang, H. (2014). The influence of the ecological contexts of teacher education on South Korean teacher educators' professional development. *Teaching and Teacher Education, 43*, 1–14. doi:10.1016/j.tate.2014.05.003

Imenda, S. (2014). Is there a conceptual difference between theoretical and conceptual frameworks? *Journal of Social Sciences, 38*(2), 185–195. doi:10.1080/09718923.2014.11893249

Israel, B. A., Eng, E., Schulz, A. J., & Parker, E. (Eds.). (2012). *Methods for community-based participatory research for health* (2nd ed.). San Francisco, CA: Jossey-Bass.

Israel, B. A., Schulz, A. J., Estrada-Martinez, L., Zenk, S. N., Viruell-Fuentes, E., Villarruel, A. M., & Stokes, C. (2006). Engaging urban residents in assessing neighborhood environments and their implications for health. *Journal of Urban Health, 83*(3), 523–539. doi:10.1007/s11524-006-9053-6

Ivankova, N. V. (2015). *Mixed methods applications in action research: From methods to community action.* Thousand Oaks, CA: Sage.

Ivankova, N. V., Creswell, J. W., & Stick, S. (2006). Using mixed-methods sequential explanatory design: From theory to practice. *Field Methods, 18*(1), 3–20. doi:10.1177/1525822X05282260

Ivankova, N. V., & Stick, S. L. (2007). Students' persistence in a distributed doctoral program in educational leadership in higher education: A mixed methods study. *Research in Higher Education, 48*(1), 93. doi:10.1007/s11162-006-9025-4

Janesick, V. A. (1994). The choreography of qualitative research design: Minuets, improvisations, and crystallization. In N. K. Denzin & Y. S. Lincoln (Eds.), *Handbook of qualitative research* (2nd ed., pp. 379–399). Thousand Oaks. CA: Sage.

Jenson, L. A., & Allen, M. N. (1994). A synthesis of qualitative research on wellness-illness. *Qualitative Health Research, 4*, 349–369. doi:10.1177/104973239400400402

Johnson, B., & Turner, L. A. (2003). Data collection strategies in mixed methods research. In A. Tashakkori & C. Teddlie (Eds.), *Handbook of mixed methods in social and behavioral research* (pp. 297–319). Thousand Oaks, CA: Sage.

Johnson, J. C. (1998). Research design and research strategies. In H. R. Bernard (Ed.), *Handbook of methods in cultural anthropology.* Lanham, MD: AltaMira Press.

Johnson, R. B. (2012). *Dialectical pluralism and mixed research.* Thousand Oaks, CA: Sage.

Johnson, R. B. (2015). Dialectical pluralism: A metaparadigm whose time has come. *Journal of Mixed Methods Research, 11*(2), 156–173. doi:10.1177/1558689815607692

Johnson, R. B., & Christensen, L. (2017). *Educational research: Quantitative, qualitative, and mixed approaches* (6th ed.). Thousand Oaks, CA: Sage.

Johnson, R. B., Onwuegbuzie, A. J., & Turner, L. A. (2007). Toward a definition of mixed methods research. *Journal of Mixed Methods Research, 1*(2), 112–133. doi:10.1177/1558689806298224

Johnson, R. E., Grove, A. L., & Clarke, A. (2017). Pillar integration process: A joint display technique to integrate data in mixed methods research. *Journal of Mixed Methods Research. 13*(3), 301–320. https://doi.org/10.1177/1558689817743108

Jones, G. R. (2012). *Organizational theory, design, and change* (7th ed.). London, UK: Pearson.

Jones, K. (2017). Using a theory of practice to clarify epistemological challenges in mixed methods research: An example of theorizing, modeling, and mapping changing West African seed systems. *Journal of Mixed Methods Research, 11*(3), 355–373. doi:10.1177/1558689815614960

Kahwati, L. & Kane, H. (2020). *Qualitative comparative analysis in mixed methods research and evaluation.* Thousand Oaks, CA: Sage.

Kelle, U. (2015). Mixed methods and the problems of theory building and theory testing in the social sciences. In S. N. Hesse-Biber & R. B. Johnson (Eds.), *The Oxford handbook of multimethod and mixed methods research inquiry* (pp. 594–605). New York, NY: Oxford University Press.

Kelly, G. A. (1955). *The psychology of personal constructs.* New York, NY: W. W. Norton & Co.

Killawi, A., Khidir, A., Elnashar, M., Abdelrahim, H., Hammoud, M., Elliott, H., . . . Fetters, M. D. (2014). Procedures of recruiting, obtaining informed consent, and compensating research participants in Qatar: Findings from a qualitative investigation. *BMC Medical Ethics*, *15*(1), 9–22. doi:10.1186/1472-6939-15-9

Kong, S. Y., Mohd Yaacob, N., & Mohd Ariffin, A. R. (2016). Constructing a mixed methods research design: Exploration of an architectural intervention. *Journal of Mixed Methods Research*, 1–18. doi:10.1177/1558689816651807

Koopmans, M. (2017). Mixed methods in search of a problem: Perspectives from complexity theory. *Journal of Mixed Methods Research*, *11*, 16–18. doi:10.1177/1558689816676662

Kron, F. W., Fetters, M. D., Scerbo, M. W., White, C. B., Lypson, M. L., Padilla, M. A., . . . Becker, D. M. (2017). Using a computer simulation for teaching communication skills: A blinded multisite mixed methods randomized controlled trial. *Patient Education and Counseling*, *100*, 748–759. doi:10.1016/j.pec.2016.10.024

Kron, F. W., Gjerde, C. L., Sen, A., & Fetters, M. D. (2010). Medical student attitudes toward video games and related new media technologies in medical education. *BMC Medical Education*, *10*(50), 1–11. doi:10.1186/1472-6920-10-50

Krueger, R. A., & Casey, M. A. (1994). *Focus groups: A practical guide for applied research* (2nd ed.). Thousand Oaks, CA: Sage.

Legocki, L. J., Meurer, W. J., Frederiksen, S., Lewis, R. J., Durkalski, V. L., Berry, D. A., . . . Fetters, M. D. (2015). Clinical trialist perspectives on the ethics of adaptive clinical trials: A mixed-methods analysis. *BMC Medical Ethics*, *16*(1), 27. doi:10.1186/s12910-015-0022-z

Lincoln, Y. S., & Guba, E. G. (1985). *Naturalistic inquiry*. Newbury Park, CA: Sage.

Lincoln, Y. S., & Guba, E. G. (2000). The only generalization is: There is no generalization. In R. Gomm, M. Hammersley, & P. Foster (Eds.), *Case study method: Key issues, key texts* (pp. 27–44). Thousand Oaks, CA: Sage.

Lucero, J., Wallerstein, N., Duran, B., Alegria, M., Greene-Moton, E., Israel, B., . . . & Pearson, C. (2016). Development of a mixed methods investigation of process and outcomes of community-based participatory research. *Journal of Mixed Methods Research*, *12*, 55–74. doi:10.1177/1558689816633309

Lynch-Sauer, J., Vandenbosch, T. M., Kron, F., Gjerde, C. L., Arato, N., Sen, A., & Fetters, M. D. (2011). Nursing students' attitudes toward video games and related new media technologies. *Journal of Nursing Education*, *50*, 513–523. doi:10.3928/01484834-20110531-04

Mangan, J., Lalwani, C., & Gardner, B. (2004). Combining quantitative and qualitative methodologies in logistics research. *International Journal of Physical Distribution & Logistics Management*, *34*(7), 565–578. doi:10.1108/09600030410552258

Martinez, A., Dimitriadis, Y., Rubia, B., Gómez, E., & de la Fuente, P. (2003). Combining qualitative evaluation and social network analysis for the study of classroom social interactions. *Computers & Education*, *41*(4), 353–368. doi:10.1016/j.compedu.2003.06.001

Maxwell, J., & Mittapalli, K. (2010). *Realism as a stance for mixed methods research* (2nd ed.). Thousand Oaks, CA: Sage.

McKim, C. A. (2017). The value of mixed methods research: A mixed methods study. *Journal of Mixed Methods Research*, *11*(2), 202–222.

McNeill, P. M. (1993). *The ethics and politics of human experimentation*. Cambridge, UK: CUP Archive.

Mertens, D. M. (2007). Transformative paradigm: Mixed methods and social justice. *Journal of Mixed Methods Research*, *1*(3), 212–225. doi:10.1177/1558689807302811.

Mertens, D. M. (2009). *Transformative research and evaluation*. New York, NY: Guilford Press.

Mertens, D. M. (2010). Transformative mixed methods research. *Qualitative inquiry*, *16*, 469–474. doi:10.1177/1077800410364612

Mertens, D. M., Bazeley, P., Bowleg, L., Fielding, N., Maxwell, J., Molina-Azorin, J. F., & Niglas, K. (2016). Expanding thinking through a kaleidoscopic look into the future implications of the mixed methods international research association's task force report on the future of mixed methods. *Journal of Mixed Methods Research*, *10*(3), 221–227. doi: 10.1177/1558689816649719

Methodology. (n.d.). Retrieved from https://en.oxforddictionaries.com/definition/methodology.

Meurer, W. J., Lewis, R. J., Tagle, D., Fetters, M., Legocki, L., Berry, S., . . . Barsan, W. G. (2012). An overview of the Adaptive Designs Accelerating Promising Trials Into Treatments (ADAPT-IT) project. *Annals of Emergency Medicine*, *60*, 451–457. doi:10.1016/j.annemergmed.2012.01.020

Miles, M. B., Huberman, A. M., & Saldaña, J. (2014). *Qualitative data analysis* (3rd ed.). Thousand Oaks, CA: Sage.

Miller, W., & Crabtree, B. (1990). Start with the stories. *Family Medicine Research Updates*, *9*(2), 2–3.

Miller, W. L., Yanoshik, M. K., Crabtree, B. F., & Reymond, W. K. (1994). Patients, family physicians, and pain: Visions from interview narratives. *Family Medicine*, *26*(3), 179–184.

MIT Technology Review. (2013). The big data conundrum: How to define it? Retrieved from https://www.technologyreview.com/s/519851/the-big-data-conundrum-how-to-define-it/.

Moffatt, S., White, M., Mackintosh, J., & Howel, D. (2006). Using quantitative and qualitative data in health services research—what happens when mixed methods findings conflict? *BMC Health Services Research*, *6*(28), 1–10. doi:10.1186/1472-6963-6-28

Moran-Ellis, J., Alexander, V. D., Cronin, A., Dickinson, M., Fielding, J., Sleney, J., & Thomas, H. (2006). Triangulation and integration: Processes, claims and implications. *Qualitative Research*, *6*(1), 45–59. doi:10.1177/1468794106058870

Morgan, D. L. (1997). *The focus group guidebook* (Vol. 1). Thousand Oaks. CA: Sage.

Morgan, D. L. (2007). Paradigms lost and pragmatism regained: Methodological implications of combining qualitative and quantitative methods. *Journal of Mixed Methods Research*, *1*(1), 48–76. doi:10.1177/2345678906292462

Morgan, D. L. (2016). *Essentials of dyadic interviewing*. New York, NY: Routledge.

Morgan, D. L. (2018). Living within blurry boundaries: The value of distinguishing between qualitative and quantitative research. *Journal of Mixed Methods Research*, *12*(3), 268–279. doi:10.1177/1558689816686433

Morgan, D. L., Ataie, J., Carder, P., & Hoffman, K. (2013). Introducing dyadic interviews as a method for collecting qualitative data. *Qualitative Health Research*, *23*(9), 1276–1284.

Morrison, L. G., Hargood, C., Lin, S. X., Dennison, L., Joseph, J., Hughes, S., . . . Michie, S. (2014). Understanding usage of a hybrid website and smartphone app for weight management: A mixed-methods study. *Journal of Medical Internet Research*, *16*, e201. doi:10.2196/jmir.3579

Moseholm, E., & Fetters, M. D. (2017). Conceptual models to guide integration during analysis in convergent mixed methods studies. *Methodological Innovations*, *10*(2), 1–11. doi:10.1177/2059799117703118

Moseholm, E., Rydahl-Hansen, S., Lindhardt, B. O., & Fetters, M. D. (2017). Health-related quality of life in patients with serious non-specific symptoms undergoing evaluation for possible cancer and their experience during the process: A mixed methods study. *Quality of Life Research*, *26*(4), 993–1006. doi:10.1007/s11136-016-1423-2

Nastasi, B. K., & Hitchcock, J. H. (2016). *Mixed methods research and culture-specific interventions: Program design and evaluation.* Thousand Oaks, CA: Sage.

National Center for Education Statistics. (2018). Early Childhood Longitudinal Program. Retrieved from https://nces.ed.gov/ecls/.

National Health Service. (2017). Health research authority. Research ethics service. Retrieved January 24, 2017, from http://www.hra.nhs.uk/about-the-hra/our-committees/res/.

National Institutes of Health. (2012). Human subjects protection and inclusion of women, minorities, and children. Retrieved January 24, 2017, from https://archives.nih.gov/asites/grants/05-29-2015/grants/peer/guidelines_general/Human_Subjects_Protection_and_Inclusion.pdf.

National Institutes of Health. (2016). Resources. Retrieved January 24, 2017, from https://humansubjects.nih.gov/resources.

National Institutes of Health. (2017). *Statement on article publication resulting from NIH funded research.* Notice Number: NOT-OD-18-011. Retrieved May 11, 2019, from https://grants.nih.gov/grants/guide/notice-files/NOT-OD-18-011.html.

National Institutes of Health. (2017–2021) Mission and goals. Retrieved from https://obssr.od.nih.gov/wp-content/uploads/2016/12/OBSSR-SP-2017-2021.pdf.

NIH Office of Behavioral and Social Sciences. (n.d.). About OBSSR. Retrieved May 11, 2019, from https://obssr.od.nih.gov/about/.

NIH Office of Behavioral and Social Sciences. (2018). *Best practices for mixed methods research in the health sciences* (2nd ed). Bethesda: National Institutes of Health. Retrieved May 10, 2019, from https://obssr.od.nih.gov/wp-content/uploads/2018/01/Best-Practices-for-Mixed-Methods-Research-in-the-Health-Sciences-2018-01-25.pdf.

Nilsen, P. (2015). Making sense of implementation theories, models and frameworks. *Implementation Science, 10*(1), 53. doi:10.1186/s13012-015-0242-0

O'Cathain, A. (2009). Reporting mixed methods projects. *Mixed methods research for nursing and the health sciences* (pp. 135–158). Oxford, UK: Blackwell Publishing.

O'Cathain, A. (2010). Assessing the quality of mixed methods research toward a comprehensive framework. In A. Tashakkori & C. Teddlie (Eds.), *SAGE handbook of mixed methods in social & behavioral research* (2nd ed., pp. 531–558). Thousand Oaks. CA: Sage.

O'Cathain, A. (2018). *A practical guide to using qualitative research with randomized controlled trials.* Oxford, UK, Oxford University Press.

O'Cathain, A., Murphy, E., & Nicholl, J. (2010). Three techniques for integrating data in mixed methods studies. *BMJ, 341*, c4587. doi:10.1136/bmj.c4587

O'Cathain, A., Thomas, K., Drabble, S., Rudolph, A., & Hewison, J. (2013). What can qualitative research do for randomised controlled trials? A systematic mapping review. *BMJ open, 3*, e002889. doi:10.1136/bmjopen-2013-002889

Office of Behavioral & Social Sciences Research. Social and Behavioral Theories. (n.d.). Retrieved from http://www.esourceresearch.org/eSourceBook/SocialandBehavioralTheories/1LearningObjectives/tabid/724/Default.aspx.

Ontology. (n.d.). Retrieved from https://en.oxforddictionaries.com/definition/ontology

Onwuegbuzie, A. J., & Johnson, R. B. (2006). The validity issue in mixed research. *Research in the Schools, 13*(1), 48–63.

O'Reilly, M., & Kiyimba, N. (2015). *Advanced qualitative research: A guide to using theory.* Thousand Oaks, CA: Sage.

Oren, G. A. (2017). Predatory publishing: Top 10 things you need to know. Retrieved from http://wkauthorservices.editage.com/resources/author-resource-review/2017/dec-2017.html

Patton, M. Q. (2015). *Qualitative research and evaluation methods* (4th ed.). Thousand Oaks, CA: Sage.

Plano Clark, V. L., Garrett, A. L., & Leslie-Pelecky, D. L. (2010). Applying three strategies for integrating quantitative and qualitative databases in a mixed methods study of a nontraditional graduate education program. *Field Methods, 22*(2), 154–174. doi:10.1177/1525822X09357174

Plano Clark, V. L., & Ivankova, N. V. (2016a). *Mixed methods research: A guide to the field.* Thousand Oaks, CA: Sage.

Plano Clark, V. L., & Ivankova, N. V. (2016b). Why use mixed methods research? Identifying rationales for mixing methods. In *Mixed methods research: A guide to the field.* Thousand Oaks, CA: Sage.

Pluye, P., Grad, R. M., Levine, A., & Nicolau, B. (2009). Understanding divergence of quantitative and qualitative data (or results) in mixed methods studies. *International Journal of Multiple Research Approaches, 3*, 58–72. doi:10.5172/mra.455.3.1.58

Pluye, P., & Hong, Q. N. (2014). Combining the power of stories and the power of numbers: Mixed methods research and mixed studies reviews. *Annual Review of Public Health, 35*(1), 29–45. doi:10.1146/annurev-publhealth-032013-182440

Poth, C. N., (2018a). Innovation in mixed methods research—a practical guide to integrative thinking with complexity. Thousand Oaks, CA: Sage.

Poth, C. N. (2018b). The curious case of complexity: Implications for mixed methods research practices. *International Journal of Multiple Research Approaches.*

Prochaska, J. O. (2008). Decision making in the transtheoretical model of behavior change. *Medical Decision Making, 28*(6), 845–849. doi:10.1177/0272989X08327068

Prosessor, J. (2011). Visual methodology: Toward a more seeing research. In N. K. Denzin & Y. S. Lincoln (Eds.), *The SAGE handbook of qualitative research* (4th ed., pp. 479–496). Thousand Oaks, CA: Sage.

Ragin, C. C., Shulman, D., Weinberg, A., & Gran, B. (2003). Complexity, generality, and qualitative comparative analysis. *Field Methods, 15*(4), 323–340. doi:10.1177/1525822X03257689

Rhetoric. (n.d.). Retrieved from https://en.oxforddictionaries.com/definition/rhetoric.

Richardson, L. (1994). Writing: A method of inquiry. In N. K. Denzin & Y. S. Lincoln (Eds.), *Handbook of qualitative research* (pp. 516–529). Thousand Oaks, CA: Sage.

Rogers, B., & Ryals, L. (2007). Using the repertory grid to access the underlying realities in key account relationships. *International Journal of Market Research, 49*(5), 595–612. doi:10.1177/147078530704900506

Rosenstock, I. M. (1974). Historical origins of the health belief model. *Health Education Monographs, 2*(4), 328–335. doi:10.1177/109019817400200403.

Rothman, David J. (1991). *Strangers at the bedside: A history of how law and bioethics transformed medical decision making.* New York, NY: Basic Books.

Roux, B. L. L., & Rouanet, H. (2009). *Multiple correspondence analysis.* Thousand Oaks, CA: Sage.

Salkind, N. J. (2017). *Statistics for people who (think they) hate statistics* (6th ed.). Thousand Oaks, CA: Sage.

Sandelowski, M., Docherty, S., & Emden, C. (1997). Focus on qualitative methods qualitative metasynthesis: Issues and techniques. *Research in Nursing and Health, 20*, 365–372.

Schoonenboom, J. (2017). A performative paradigm for mixed methods research. *Journal of Mixed Methods Research. 13*(3), 284–300. https://doi.org/10.1177/1558689817722889

Schulz, A. J., Israel, B. A., Coombe, C. M., Gaines, C., Reyes, A. G., Rowe, Z., . . . Weir, S. (2011). A community-based participatory planning process and multilevel intervention design: Toward eliminating cardiovascular health inequities. *Health Promotion Practice, 12*(6), 900–911.

Scimago. (2007). Scimago Journal & Country Rank (SJR). Retrieved from http://www.webcitation.org/76BVoeWUs.

Scott, J. (2017). *Social network analysis* (4th ed.). Thousand Oaks, CA: Sage.

Scott, J., Tallia, A., Crosson, J. C., Orzano, A. J., Stroebel, C., DiCicco-Bloom, B., . . . Crabtree, B. (2005). Social network analysis as an analytic tool for interaction patterns in primary care practices. *Annals of Family Medicine, 3*(5), 443–448. doi:10.1370/afm.344

Shannon-Baker, P. (2016). Making paradigms meaningful in mixed methods research. *Journal of Mixed Methods Research, 10*(4), 319–334. doi:10.1177/1558689815575861

Sharma, S., & Vredenburg, H. (1998). Proactive corporate environmental strategy and the development of competitively valuable organizational capabilities. *Strategic Management Journal*, 729–753. doi:10.1002/(SICI)1097-0266(199808)19:8<729::AID-SMJ967>3.0.CO;2-4

Shell, D. F., Brooks, D. W., Trainin, G., Wilson, K. M., Kauffman, D. F., & Herr, L. M. (2010). *The unified learning model: How motivational, cognitive, and neurobiological sciences inform best teaching practices*. Dordrecht, The Netherlands: Springer.

Shultz, C. G., Chu, M. S., Yajima, A., Skye, E. P., Sano, K., Inoue, M., . . . & Fetters, M. D. (2015). The cultural context of teaching and learning sexual health care examinations in Japan: A mixed methods case study assessing the use of standardized patient instructors among Japanese family physician trainees of the Shizuoka Family Medicine Program. *Asia Pacific Family Medicine, 14*, 8. doi:10.1186/s12930-015-0025-4

Simões, C., Dibb, S., & Fisk, R. P. (2005). Managing corporate identity: An internal perspective. *Journal of the Academy of Marketing Science, 33*, 153–168. doi:10.1177/0092070304268920

Sorden, S. D. (2012). The cognitive theory of multimedia learning. *Handbook of educational theories* (pp. 1–31). Charlotte, NC: Information Age Publishing.

Stange, K. C., Crabtree, B. F., & Miller, W. L. (2006). Publishing multimethod research. *Annals of Family Medicine, 4*(4), 292–294. doi:10.1370/afm.615

Swain, A. K. (2016). Mining big data to support decision making in healthcare. *Journal of Information Technology Case and Application Research, 18*(3), 141–154.

Tashakkori, A., & Teddlie, C. (1998). *Mixed methodology: Combining qualitative and quantitative approaches*. Thousand Oaks, CA: Sage.

Teddlie, C., & Tashakkori, A. (2006). A general typology of research designs featuring mixed methods. *Research in the Schools, 13*(1), 12–28.

Teddlie, C., & Tashakkori, A. (2009a). Considerations before collecting your data. In *Foundations of mixed methods research:*

Integrating quantitative and qualitative approaches in the social and behavioral sciences (pp. 197–216). Thousand Oaks, CA: Sage.

Teddlie, C., & Tashakkori, A. (2009b). *Foundations of mixed methods research: Integrating quantitative and qualitative approaches in the social and behavioral sciences*. Thousand Oaks, CA: Sage.

Think. Check. Submit. (2018). Retrieved from http://thinkcheck submit.org/check/.

Tsushima, R. (2012). *The mismatch between educational policy and classroom practice: EFL teachers' perspectives on washback in Japan*. McGill University, Retrieved from ProQuest Digital Dissertations. (MR84313).

Tsushima, R. (2015). Methodological diversity in language assessment research: The role of mixed methods in classroom-based language assessment studies. *International Journal of Qualitative Methods, 14*, 104–121. doi:10.1177/160940691501400202

U.S. Department of Health & Human Services. (2009). Code of federal regulations. Title 45 Public Welfare. Part 46: Protection of Human Subjects. Department of Health and Human Services. Retrieved from https://http://www.hhs.gov/ohrp/regulations-and-policy/regulations/45-cfr-46/index.html - 46.101(b)

University of Michigan. (2018). *I. f. S. R. health and retirement study: A study of longitudinal study of health, retirement, and aging*. Retrieved from http://hrsonline.isr.umich.edu/.

Uprichard, E., & Dawney, L. (2016). Data diffraction challenging data integration in mixed methods research. *Journal of Mixed Methods Research, 13*(1), 19–32. doi:10.1177/1558689816674650

Vence, T. (2017). On blacklists and whitelists. Retrieved from https://www.the-scientist.com/?articles.view/articleNo/49903/title/On-Blacklists-and-Whitelists/.

Venkatesh, V., Brown, S. A., & Bala, H. (2013). Bridging the qualitative-quantitative divide: Guidelines for conducting mixed methods research in information systems. *MIS Quarterly, 37*, 21–54.

von Bartheld, C. S., Houmanfar, R., & Candido, A. (2015). Prediction of junior faculty success in biomedical research: Comparison of metrics and effects of mentoring programs. *PeerJ, 3*, e1262. doi:10.7717/peerj.1262

Vygotsky, L. S. (1978). *Mind in society: The development of higher psychological processes*. Cambridge, MA: Harvard University Press.

Wakai, T., Simasek, M., Nakagawa, U., Saijo, M., & Fetters, M. D. (2018). Screenings during well-child visits in primary care: A mixed methods intervention quality improvement study. *Journal of the American Board of Family Medicine, 31*(4), 558–569. doi:10.3122/jabfm.2018.04.170222

Walsh, M., & Wigens, L. (2003). *Foundations in nursing and health care: Introduction to research*. Cheltenham, UK: Nelson Thornes.

Wang, R. R. (2012). *Yinyang: The way of heaven and earth in Chinese thought and culture* (Vol. 11). New York, NY: Cambridge University Press.

Ward, J. S., & Barker, A. (2013), Undefined by data: A survey of big data definitions. Retrieved April 24, 2019, from https://arxiv.org/pdf/1309.5821.pdf.

Weiss, H. B., Kreider, H., Mayer, E., Hencke, R., & Vaughan, M. A. (2005). Working it out: The chronicle of a mixed methods analysis. In T. S. Weisner (Ed.), *Discovering successful pathways in children's development: Mixed methods in the study of childhood and family life* (pp. 47–64). Chicago, IL: University of Chicago Press.

Windsor, L. C. (2013). Using concept mapping in community-based participatory research: A mixed methods approach. *Journal of Mixed Methods Research, 7*(3), 274–293.

Wisdom, J. P., & Fetters, M. D. (2015). Funding for mixed methods research: Sources and strategies. In S. Hesse-Biber & R. B. Johnson (Eds.), *The Oxford handbook of multimethod and mixed methods research inquiry* (pp. 314–332). New York, NY: Oxford University Press.

World Health Organization. (n.d.). Recommended format for a research protocol. Retrieved May 10, 2019, from http://www.who .int/rpc/research_ethics/format_rp/en/

Worthley, M. R., Gloeckner, G. W., & Kennedy, P. A. (2016). A mixed-methods explanatory study of the failure rate for freshman STEM calculus students. *PRIMUS, 26*(2), 125–142. doi:10.1080/10511970.2 015.1067265

Wu, J. (2017-22). Improving Contraceptive Care for Women with Chronic Conditions: A Novel: Web-Based Decision Aid in Primary Care. National Institute of Child Development and Human Health. 1 K23 HD084744-01A1.

Wu, J. P., Damschroder, L. J., Fetters, M. D., Zikmund-Fisher, B. J., Crabtree, B. F., Hudson, S. V., . . . Taichman, L. S. (2018). A web-based decision tool to improve contraceptive counseling for women with chronic medical conditions: Protocol for a mixed methods implementation study. *JMIR Research Protocols, 7*(4), e107. doi:10.2196/resprot.9249

Yang, S., Keller, F. B., & Zheng, L. (2017). *Social network analysis: Methods and examples*. Thousand Oaks, CA: Sage.

Yardley, L., Williams, S., Bradbury, K., Garip, G., Renouf, S., Ware, L., . . . Little, P. (2012). Integrating user perspectives into the development of a web-based weight management intervention. *Clinical Obesity, 2*, 132–141. doi:10.1111/cob.12001

Yin, R. K. (2014). *Case study research: Design and methods* (5th ed.). Thousand Oaks, CA: Sage.

Yuki, G. (1989). Managerial leadership: A review of theory and research. *Journal of Management, 15*(2), 251–289.

INDEX

Milton Keynes UK
Ingram Content Group UK Ltd.
UKHW020241070923
428182UK00003B/14